C0-AZW-440

BIBLIOTHÈQUE DU PAVILLON DES FEMMES
WOMEN'S PAVILION LIBRARY, F4-24

Inherited Bleeding Disorders in Women

BIBLIOTHÈQUE DU PAVILLON DES FEMMES
WOMEN'S PAVILION LIBRARY, F4-24

Inherited Bleeding Disorders in Women

Christine A Lee
Oxford Haemophilia and Thrombosis Centre
Churchill Hospital
Old Road
Headington
Oxford
UK

Rezan A Kadir
Royal Free Hospital
Pond Street
London
UK

Peter A Kouides
Mary M Gooley Hemophilia Centre
Rochester General Hospital
Rochester
New York
USA

⟨W⟩ WILEY-BLACKWELL

A John Wiley & Sons, Ltd., Publication

This edition first published 2009, © 2009 by Blackwell Publishing Ltd

Blackwell Publishing was acquired by John Wiley & Sons in February 2007. Blackwell's publishing program has been merged with Wiley's global Scientific, Technical and Medical business to form Wiley-Blackwell.

Registered office: John Wiley & Sons Ltd, The Atrium, Southern Gate, Chichester, West Sussex, PO19 8SQ, UK

Editorial offices: 9600 Garsington Road, Oxford, OX4 2DQ, UK
The Atrium, Southern Gate, Chichester, West Sussex, PO19 8SQ, UK
111 River Street, Hoboken, NJ 07030-5774, USA

For details of our global editorial offices, for customer services and for information about how to apply for permission to reuse the copyright material in this book please see our website at www.wiley.com/wiley-blackwell

The right of the author to be identified as the author of this work has been asserted in accordance with the Copyright, Designs and Patents Act 1988.

All rights reserved. No part of this publication may be reproduced, stored in a retrieval system, or transmitted, in any form or by any means, electronic, mechanical, photocopying, recording or otherwise, except as permitted by the UK Copyright, Designs and Patents Act 1988, without the prior permission of the publisher.

Wiley also publishes its books in a variety of electronic formats. Some content that appears in print may not be available in electronic books.

Designations used by companies to distinguish their products are often claimed as trademarks. All brand names and product names used in this book are trade names, service marks, trademarks or registered trademarks of their respective owners. The publisher is not associated with any product or vendor mentioned in this book. This publication is designed to provide accurate and authoritative information in regard to the subject matter covered. It is sold on the understanding that the publisher is not engaged in rendering professional services. If professional advice or other expert assistance is required, the services of a competent professional should be sought.

The contents of this work are intended to further general scientific research, understanding, and discussion only and are not intended and should not be relied upon as recommending or promoting a specific method, diagnosis, or treatment by physicians for any particular patient. The publisher and the author make no representations or warranties with respect to the accuracy or completeness of the contents of this work and specifically disclaim all warranties, including without limitation any implied warranties of fitness for a particular purpose. In view of ongoing research, equipment modifications, changes in governmental regulations, and the constant flow of information relating to the use of medicines, equipment, and devices, the reader is urged to review and evaluate the information provided in the package insert or instructions for each medicine, equipment, or device for, among other things, any changes in the instructions or indication of usage and for added warnings and precautions. Readers should consult with a specialist where appropriate. The fact that an organization or Website is referred to in this work as a citation and/or a potential source of further information does not mean that the author or the publisher endorses the information the organization or Website may provide or recommendations it may make. Further, readers should be aware that Internet Websites listed in this work may have changed or disappeared between when this work was written and when it is read. No warranty may be created or extended by any promotional statements for this work. Neither the publisher nor the author shall be liable for any damages arising herefrom.

Library of Congress Cataloging-in-Publication Data

Lee, Christine A.
    Inherited bleeding disorders in women / Christine A. Lee, Rezan A. Kadir, Peter A. Kouides.
        p. ; cm.
    Includes bibliographical references.
    ISBN 978-1-4051-6915-8
    1. Blood coagulation disorders. 2. Women–Diseases. 3. Blood coagulation disorders in pregnancy.
I. Kadir, Rezan A. II. Kouides, Peter A. III. Title.
    [DNLM: 1. Blood Coagulation Disorders, Inherited. 2. Women's Health. WH 322 L477i 2009]
    RC647.C55L44 2009
    616.1'57–dc22

                                                                                                    2008035471

A catalogue record for this book is available from the British Library.

Set in 9/11.5 Sabon by Graphicraft Limited, Hong Kong
Printed in Singapore by Fabulous Printers Pte Ltd

1   2009

Contents

Contributors

Claudia Chi
Department of Obstetrics and Gynaecology
Royal Free Hospital
Pond Street
London, UK

H Marijke van den Berg
Meander Medisch Centrum
Amersfoort, The Netherlands

Måns Edlund
Department of Obstetrics and Gynaecology
Karolinska University Hospital Solna
Stockholm, Sweden

Adrian England
Department of Anaesthetics
Royal Free Hospital
Pond Street
London, UK

Rezan A Kadir
Department of Obstetrics and Gynaecology
Royal Free Hospital
Pond Street
London, UK

Peter Kouides
Mary M Gooley Hemophilia Center
Rochester General Hospital
Portland Avenue
Rochester, New York, USA

Christine Lee
Oxford Haemophilia and Thrombosis Centre
Churchill Hospital
Old Road
Headington
Oxford, UK

Jane Matheson
Haemophilia Society
Hatton Gardens
London, UK

Ann-Marie Nazzaro
National Hemophilia Foundation US
West 32nd Street
New York, New York, USA

Flora Peyvandi
Fondazione Luigi Villa
Via Pace
Milan, Italy

Claire Philipp
Division of Hematology
University of Medicine and Dentistry of New Jersey
Robert Wood Johnson Medical School
New Brunswick, New Jersey, USA

Edward Tuddenham
Haemophilia Centre and Thrombosis Unit
Royal Free Hospital
Pond Street
London, UK

Rochelle Winikoff
Division of Hematology
CHU Sainte-Justine
Côte Ste-Catherine Road
Montreal, Quebec, Canada

Preface

In 1926 Erik von Willebrand described a large kindred from the Aland Islands, an archipelago in the Baltic sea, many of whom had a bleeding disorder. The index case was a little girl called Hjordis, who presented with severe epistaxis and died at the onset of her fourth menstrual period. Her maternal grandmother died from haemorrhage after childbirth in her only pregnancy. von Willebrand wrote that the condition was particularly prevalent in women. This first description of von Willebrand disease underlined the haemostatic challenges of menstruation and childbirth for those women with an inherited bleeding disorder.

Until recently, the predominant issue for men with haemophilia has been safe and effective treatment, and most effort has been directed to the resolution of transfusion-transmitted disease. Furthermore, since haemophilia is a sex-linked disorder there has been a failure to recognise that women have inherited bleeding disorders. Thus, the substantial morbidity caused in women with inherited bleeding disorders has only recently been addressed in a comprehensive way. It is important that collaboration in the care and research of bleeding disorders in women continue as many challenges remain. The main task now is to identify those women who do not realise they may have a treatable condition. The patient advocacy organisations are crucial to this endeavour. There also remains the challenge of developing more effective, tolerable and widely available therapies in controlling menorrhagia and post-partum haemorrhage.

This book is written by haematologists, obstetrician–gynaecologists, an anaesthetist and those involved in patient advocacy. It covers the gynaecological and obstetric issues for carriers of haemophilia, women with von Willebrand's disease, rare bleeding disorders and inherited platelet disorders. We hope that this book is a modest step towards safe motherhood and provision of quality of care for women with bleeding disorders world-wide and that all those providing care for these women, as well as the women themselves, will find it useful.

Acknowledgement

Cover image 'Menorrhagia Healing' © Barbara Bruch 1991

Christine A Lee
Rezan A Kadir
Peter A Kouides
December 2008

1

Approach to the patient with an inherited bleeding disorder

Peter A Kouides and Claire Philipp

Introduction

At the time of injury to the endothelium, the integrity of the high-pressure circulatory system is maintained through the hemostatic mechanism. In general terms, a "plug" of platelets is covered over by a "net" of fibrin, resulting in the formation of a clot (Fig. 1.1). The resultant clot normally leads to cessation of bleeding. Bleeding occurs when there is a precipitant such as direct traumatic injury to the endothelium or in the case of menstruation hormonal-induced shedding of the endothelium, so "injuring" the endothelium.

The understanding of hemostasis can be simplified into two steps: first (step 1) the formation of the platelet "plug" at the initial site of injury and second (step 2) the formation of a "net" of fibrin covering the platelet plug. An evolving cell-based model of hemostasis augments the historical description of coagulation focused on enzymatic activation of a sequence of coagulant proteins as a "cascade." The cell-based model includes the crucial role of tissue factor (TF)-bearing cells at the site of bleeding [1, 2]. The two main components within the blood exposed to the injured endothelium in step 1 are von Willebrand factor (VWF) and platelets. At the time of vessel injury, there is exposure of free-flowing blood through the injured endothelium to two subendothelial constituents, collagen and TF, involved respectively in platelet plug formation and fibrin generation.

Formation of the platelet "plug"

The flowing blood is subjected to a high shear stress rate upon exposure of subendothelial collagen following injury to the endothelium. The high shear stress leads to "unfolding" of VWF with subsequent exposure of the A1 and A3 domains [3]. The A1 domain primarily recognizes and binds to the glycoprotein Ib_α/IX receptor on the platelet surface whereas the A3 domain primarily recognizes and binds to subendothelial type I and type III collagen [3]. In essence, VWF localizes the platelets to the site of bleeding by binding to collagen and also to platelets that are traveling though the injured opening of the endothelium. The VWF protein is capable of binding to both platelets and collagen because it is a large, multimeric molecule. The binding of platelets to collagen by VWF leads to the subsequent aggregation and formation of a platelet plug.

Formation of fibrin

Adequate clot formation is necessary to fully stop bleeding; thus, a patient with a clotting factor deficiency, such as hemophilia, bleeds even though the platelet count and function and VWF are normal. At the time of injury factor VIIa (FVIIa) within the flowing blood at the injured site is exposed to subendothelial TF. This imitates thrombin generation resulting in fibrin formation. This leads to the formation of the VIIa–TF complex on the surface of platelets which are acting as a "scaffold," and then converts FX to activated FXa (termed the "extrinsic pathway" as depicted in Fig. 1.2). In turn, FXa is localized to the

Inherited Bleeding Disorders in Women, 1st edition. By CA Lee, RA Kadir and PA Kouides. Published 2009 by Blackwell Publishing, ISBN: 978-1-4051-6915-8.

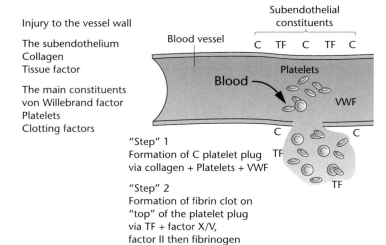

Injury to the vessel wall

The subendothelium
Collagen
Tissue factor

The main constituents
von Willebrand factor
Platelets
Clotting factors

"Step" 1
Formation of C platelet plug
via collagen + Platelets + VWF

"Step" 2
Formation of fibrin clot on
"top" of the platelet plug
via TF + factor X/V,
factor II then fibrinogen

Fig. 1.1 Steps in hemostasis. C, collagen; TF, tissue factor; VWF, von Willebrand factor.

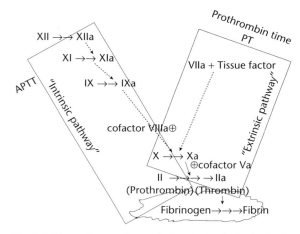

Fig. 1.2 The pathways of coagulation: the intrinsic (*in vitro*) pathway as measured by the activated partial thromboplastin time (APTT) and the extrinsic (*in vivo*) pathway as measured by the prothrombin time.

platelet surface by the cofactor, factor V (FV). This enzyme complex of FX + FV can then convert circulating coagulation factor II (prothrombin) to IIa (thrombin). Thrombin is the main enzyme of the coagulation cascade, and cleaves circulating fibrinogen to fibrin, which polymerizes to form a "net" of fibrin around the platelet plug. Patients with a deficiency of FVIII (hemophilia A) or FIX (hemophilia B) bleed even though these patients should have an adequate amount of FVII as well as FII, FV, FX, and fibrinogen.

This is because such patients do not have amplification of the coagulation cascade by FIX with cofactor VIII. The FIX/FVIII complex activates X to Xa, and is termed the propagation phase of coagulation.

Bleeding: inherited platelet disorders and von Willebrand disease

A quantitative defect of platelets (thrombocytopenia) as in the case of immune thrombocytopenic purpura (ITP) or acute leukemia, or a qualitative defect (i.e., dysfunction) of platelets ("thrombocytopathy") as in the case of uremia or aspirin use can lead to bleeding. Another cause of bleeding related to step 1 of hemostasis would be a quantitative or qualitative deficiency of VWF termed von Willebrand disease (VWD). von Willebrand disease is an inherited bleeding disorder. A mild to moderate (~15–50% VWF level) deficiency with normal multimer structure of VWF is termed type 1; a qualitative deficiency with dysfunctional VWF is type 2 [4]. In type 2, the qualitative defect can be classified further as a loss of high and intermediate weight multimers (type 2A); a loss of high molecular weight multimers (type 2B) usually with associated thrombocytopenia; or normal VWF multimers (type 2M). Type 2N VWD involves a mutation leading to decreased binding of FVIII with resultant FVIII deficiency and this is often misdiagnosed as hemophilia A. Finally, a severe quantitative deficiency of VWF with undetectable VWF protein is termed type 3.

The severe forms of VWD usually have a detectable genetic mutation whereas a third to a half of cases of type 1 VWD have a normal genotype implying extragenetic factors in the pathogenesis of VWD in these cases [5, 6]. Many of these cases (usually with VWF levels ~30–50%) with a normal genotype are related to ABO blood group O [7]. In turn, 15% of ABO blood group O patients have VWF levels <50% [8]. Consequently, given the ~40% prevalence of blood group O in the general population, ~5% of the general population will have "subnormal" VWF levels.

Bleeding: inherited coagulation factor deficiencies

Bleeding may result from a deficiency of any of the clotting factors of the coagulation cascade from factor I (fibrinogen) to factor XI. Inherited clotting factor deficiencies are due to a mutation in the gene coding for the respective coagulation protein resulting in a lower than normal level adequate for hemostasis.

Clinical presentation of the bleeding patient

Inherited platelet disorders and VWD are associated with "mucocutaneous" bleeding. Typical bleeding frequently involves nosebleeds (epistaxis), bleeding related to surgical invasive procedures including dental work, easy bruising and menorrhagia. In contrast, patients with an inherited coagulation factor deficiency such as hemophilia will have primarily deep tissue (ecchymoses) and muscle/joint bleeding. A previously undiagnosed mild disorder such as mild hemophilia A with a low factor VIII level can be "unmasked" in the setting of surgery.

Table 1.1 The prevalence of various bleeding symptoms in the general population, adapted from Sadler [9] with permission

Symptom	Healthy controls (%)
Epistaxis	5–39
Gum bleeding	7–51
Bruising	12–24
Bleeding from trivial wounds	0.2–2
Dental extraction related bleeding	1–13
Post-tonsillectomy bleeding	2–11
Post-partum bleeding	6–23
Menorrhagia	23–44

The challenge for the clinician when encountering the bleeding patient is to determine whether the bleeding symptom is due to an underlying disorder of hemostasis. Many bleeding symptoms may be quite prevalent in the general "healthy" population with a prevalence of bleeding symptoms reported ranging from 0.2% (bleeding from trivial wounds) to 51% (gingival bleeding) [9] as summarized in Table 1.1. However, only a relatively small proportion of these patients will have a true underlying disorder of hemostasis. Consequently, the discriminatory power of the various bleeding symptoms in predicting an underlying disorder of hemostasis varies from poor to excellent as depicted in Table 1.2, based on the authors collective clinical experience and published studies of bleeding risk [9–12].

These symptoms have been refined and incorporated into a scoring system (termed the bleeding score assessment) by the International Society of Hemostasis and Thrombosis network [13] and then modified by the European Union VWD project [14] (Appendix i). The main principles underlying this bleeding assessment

Table 1.2 The relative discriminatory value of bleeding symptoms

Good	Fair	Poor
Family members with established bleeding disorder	Bruising	Family members with bleeding symptoms
Profuse bleeding of small wounds	Epistaxis	Gum bleeds
Profuse surgical-related bleeding esp. T&A, dental	Menorrhagia	Hematuria
Muscle/joint-related bleeding	Post-partum hemorrhage	Bright blood per rectum

T&A, tonsillectomy and adenoidectomy.

are that the likelihood of a laboratory diagnosis of VWD is increased if (a) the bleeding symptom is of such severity that medical attention was sought and/or an intervention made, or (b) multiple bleeding symptoms are present. Ten bleeding symptoms were graded from 0 to 3 and, in general, a score of 2 was given if the respective bleeding symptom required medical attention whereas a score of 3 indicated the symptom necessitated a medical intervention. If the resultant total score was >3 in males or >5 in females, the sensitivity, specificity, and positive and negative predictive values for type 1 VWD were respectively 45%, 100%, 100% and 99.5 %. Subsequently, in a further modification of the bleeding score assessment tool, a −1 score was introduced to account for situations associated with a high bleeding risk, such as tooth extraction, where bleeding did not occur even though prophylaxis was not given. On further analysis, an inverse relationship was noted between the score and the VWF levels [14].

Studies are ongoing to determine the utility of the bleeding score in the diagnostic evaluation of other hemostatic disorders, such as platelet function defects, and in the pediatric population [15].

Recent studies demonstrate that nearly 50% of "idiopathic" menorrhagia patients will have a laboratory abnormality of hemostasis, including most frequently VWD or a platelet function defect [16, 17]. If we assume that knowledge of such an abnormality will have clinical benefit, then it becomes a public health issue [18] to test for disorders of hemostasis in all menorrhagia patients. Thus, modifications of the EU bleeding score (range −3 to 45) [13, 14] or other assessment tools [19] for screening women may be a cost-effective measure. In 42 women with documented VWD in London, the mean bleeding score was 9.7 compared with a mean score of 0 in 10 control subjects, a resultant sensitivity of 83% for a bleeding score >5 [20].

A recently developed screening tool appears promising in identifying which women with menorrhagia warrant referral for comprehensive hemostatic testing [19]. Based on analysis of a 12-page bleeding and menstrual symptom questionnaire in 146 menorrhagia patients undergoing hemostasis testing [21], there was a relatively high sensitivity of 81% (95% CI 74–89%) and positive predictive value 71% (95% CI 63–71%) if one of the following four criteria were met: (a) duration of menses >7 days and either "flooding" or impairment of daily activities with most periods; (b) a history of treatment of anemia; (c) family history of a diagnosed bleeding disorder; (d) history of excessive bleeding with tooth extraction, delivery or miscarriage or surgery. Furthermore, the addition of a pictorial blood assessment chart score (see Appendix ii) >100 increased the sensitivity of the screening tool to 93% (95% CI 89–98%) [19].

Since VWD and platelet function defects are the most common bleeding disorders in females [21, 22], the bleeding symptoms associated with these disorders of hemostasis will be discussed in further detail.

Epistaxis
This occurs predominantly in childhood and decreases in frequency and severity as the patient enters adulthood [23]. Epistaxis is "significant" if excessive bleeding necessitates medical attention, particularly packing and/or cautery. The typical duration is >10 minutes and the typical frequency is at least yearly, particularly in childhood, adolescence and young adulthood.

Dental work-related bleeding
Excessive bleeding at the time of wisdom tooth extraction or other invasive dental procedures is associated with bleeding disorders. A history of intervention by the dentist for continued/recurrent bleeding after dental extraction is probably significant [13].

Skin-related bleeding
This includes easy bruising and bleeding from trivial cuts.

Bruising Bruising is a very subjective bleeding symptom and a significant proportion of women in a general primary care practice report easy bruising. In one study 24% of reproductive age control women compared with 78% of women with VWD reported easy bruising [24]. Significant features of bruising appear to be: (a) atraumatic bruising, (b) bruising occurring at least weekly, and (c) bruises greater than 5 cm.

Bleeding from cuts Prolonged bleeding >5 minutes from trivial cuts [13] such as a paper cut or shaving appears to be significant.

Menorrhagia
Menorrhagia is the most common symptom in females with VWD. Approximately 80% of patients with

VWD report that they regard their periods as heavy [24–26]. Women with a deficient amount of VWF protein are unable to form adequate platelet plugs and formation of the platelet plug is critical in resolving menstrual blood loss. Consequently, the pre-test probability of "true" menorrhagia (>80 mL blood loss per menstrual cycle objectively documented by spectrophotometric analysis of collected pads and tampons) would appear to be quite high in a female with VWD. This is unlike the general population of females reporting a history of menorrhagia, where the positive predictive value of excessive menstrual loss may be anywhere from 25% to 75% [27]. In the (general) female population, a complaint of menorrhagia requiring a trial of oral contraceptive does not reliably predict excessive menstruation by objective measurement [28]. Table 1.3 outlines features that probably have a positive predictive value for menorrhagia in patients with VWD reporting heavy menses.

Menstrual blood flow can be measured objectively by the spectrophotometric method, which involves collection of all menstrual pads and dissolving them in an alkaline solution to convert the heme into hematin. Surrogate estimates of menstrual blood flow have been developed using the pictorial blood assessment chart [29], as described further in Appendix ii. Iron deficiency anemia may correlate with true menorrhagia and is present in at least two-thirds of women with menorrhagia [30]. Serum ferritin status, clots, and the pad changing rate have been demonstrated to be predictive of objectively defined menstrual loss in 76% of women [28].

Postpartum hemorrhage

A >500 mL loss of blood occurs in the first 24 hours following delivery in about 4% of the general population whereas blood loss after 24 hours greater than the normal "lochial" loss occurs in 1.3% of the general population [31]. Hemostasis testing should be performed in patients if there is a family history of bleeding or a history of postpartum hemorrhage (PPH) so severe that it necessitates blood transfusion. In a survey of type 1 VWD patients, one-quarter required red blood cell transfusions [24].

Approach to a female who has a "positive" bleeding history

The bleeding history is important in the diagnosis of a bleeding disorder. Laboratory assessment is required to confirm the diagnosis. A synthesis of the history, physical examination and laboratory assessment is presented in Fig. 1.3.

History

The history should include (a) the patient's past and present history of bleeding symptoms, and (b) a family history of bleeding.

A past personal history of bleeding is suggestive of an inherited bleeding disorder. The history should include easy bruising, prolonged bleeding with trivial cuts, extensive oral cavity bleeding, epistaxis, bleeding at the time of dental work or any surgical procedure, PPH, and menorrhagia (as depicted in Table 1.4).

A positive family history suggests an inherited bleeding disorder. Even though VWD is inherited, there can be variable penetrance as well as spontaneous mutations, and the patient may not have a family history

---

Table 1.3 The salient details of menses in women with bleeding disorders.

Audit of prior medical interventions
? history of hormonal therapy, dilation and curettage, endometrial ablation, levonorgestrel intrauterine device, hysterectomy

Details of menses
? use of (super) absorbent pads
? use of two pads or tampons at a time or both
? changing pad or tampon q 0.5–2.0 hours
? frequently stain clothes or bed sheets
? clots the size of a quarter (pence)
? time lost from work/school
? iron requirement

Quality of life assessment: on a scale of 0 to 10, to what degree, if any, does menses interfere with general activity
Ability to go to work or school
Family activities
Ability to enjoy life
Sleep
Mood
Overall quality of life

Pain assessment
? mid-cycle pain
? degree of pain during menses

Combined approach to the bleeding patient

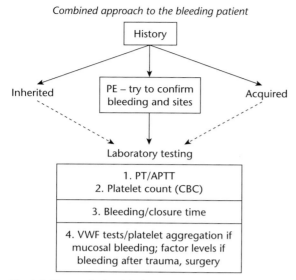

Fig. 1.3 The synthesis of the history and laboratory examination in a patient with a suspected bleeding disorder. PE, physical examination; PT, prothrombin time; APTT, activated partial thromboplastin time.

of excessive bleeding. If the family history for bleeding is limited to males, females may be carriers of the hemophilia gene. Female carriers of the hemophilia gene can be symptomatic and themselves manifest mild symptoms [11] (see Chapter 3).

Physical examination

If the patient reports bruising, this can be confused with a drug-induced rash, rash from another cause, or skin discoloration [32]. A distinction has been made between bleeding from a platelet/VWF deficiency and bleeding from a coagulation factor deficiency. The former patients will have "mucocutaneous bleeding"; therefore, careful examination of the nose and gums are important. The latter patients will have a tendency to bleed in the joints and deep tissue, requiring careful examination for joint swelling or even contracture formation.

It is possible that a patient, particularly with VWD, may unmask an underlying anatomical/pathological lesion in the uterus and the pelvic examination may be abnormal [24, 25, 33, 34].

Table 1.4 Suggested list of symptoms for history taking of the bleeding patient

Bleeding symptoms	Ever experienced symptom?		If yes, provider intervention required ever?	
	Yes	No	Yes	No
More than one nosebleed per year lasting 10 minutes or longer	☐	☐	☐	☐
Oral mucosal bleeding lasting 10 minutes or longer	☐	☐	☐	☐
Bleeding during or after dental procedures of concern to healthcare provider	☐	☐	☐	☐
Bleeding from minor cuts lasting 5 minutes or longer	☐	☐	☐	☐
Bruises larger than a quarter size occurring at least once a month without trauma	☐	☐	☐	☐
Bleeding after surgery of concern to healthcare provider	☐	☐	☐	☐
Menstrual bleeding that required protection change at least every 2 hours on heaviest day	☐	☐	☐	☐
Bleeding with pregnancy/post-partum of concern to healthcare provider	☐	☐	☐	☐
Joint bleeding	☐	☐	☐	☐
Muscle bleeding	☐	☐	☐	☐
Central nervous system bleeding	☐	☐	☐	☐
Gastrointestinal bleeding	☐	☐	☐	☐

Laboratory assessment

Accurate hemostasis testing is important because the specificity of bleeding symptoms may be poor, and many "normal" patients without an identifiable disorder of hemostasis will report bleeding symptoms [9, 24].

Initial screening tests in the female with a "positive" bleeding history would include the following.

1 Full blood count (FBC): iron deficiency can first be detected by a decreased mean cell volume (MCV). The FBC includes a platelet count.

2 Prothrombin time (PT), activated partial thromboplastin time (APTT): these are standard, readily available tests of hemostasis carried out in the evaluation of the bleeding patient. However, in general, these tests carry a very low positive and negative predictive value for an underlying bleeding disorder [35].

Clinicians generally use the FBC and PT/APTT in the evaluation of a patient who presents with a bleeding history with the erroneous assumption that normal PT/APTT values rule out an underlying bleeding disorder. Whereas the sensitivity of a prolonged APTT for VWD is less than 40% [36], for the severe recessive clotting factor deficiency, factors I, II, V, VII, X, XI, the PT and APTT are an adequate screen [37].

A prolonged APTT necessitates a mixing study with pooled normal plasma to distinguish further between a deficiency state such as hemophilia or an inhibitor. An inhibitor, such as a lupus anticoagulant or acquired hemophilia A, a potentially life-threatening bleeding diathesis, would not demonstrate a corrected APTT on mixing with normal plasma.

3 VWF testing (VWF antigen, VWF ristocetin cofactor and factor VIII levels). The ~13% (95% CI 11.1–15.6%) prevalence [22, 38–41] of VWD in females with menorrhagia warrants VWF and FVIII levels as part of the initial hemostasis evaluation. The FVIII level can be reduced in VWD as VWF protects FVIII from proteolytic cleavage [42]. Factor VIII deficiency with normal VWF levels may also be associated with menorrhagia (i.e., female carriers of hemophilia A, von Willebrand Normandy) [11, 25].

VWF analysis ideally should be done on site with immediate on-site processing. Frequent misdiagnosis of VWF deficiency occurs when specimens are transported to another site far from where the blood was drawn with subsequent activation/degradation of the sample [43]. In the USA, this is a growing concern among hematologists because VWF levels are drawn through managed care contracted laboratories where the plasma sample may be sent thousands of miles away and be exposed to extreme temperatures [43]. Cold storage of whole blood can lead to artifactually low VWF levels [44]. Such patients may then be given an erroneous laboratory diagnosis of VWD that ultimately is disproved on referral to the hematologist/laboratory scientist capable of on-site processing and complex analysis of the plasma sample. Ideally, primary care physicians should refer the patient directly to a hemostasis laboratory.

Furthermore the clinician must be aware that VWF and FVIII levels can fluctuate during the menstrual cycle. The use of exogenous hormones such as the oral contraceptive (OC) may change these levels [45]. The laboratory diagnosis of VWD is discussed further in Chapter 4.

Testing in relation to the menstrual cycle

There have been reports in a relatively small number of patients that show a decrease in VWF levels during menstruation [46, 47]. The practitioner should note the time in the menstrual cycle of VWF testing and whether the results are at the mean or below the reference range. Repeat testing should be performed in the first 4 days of menstruation.

Testing and oral contraceptive use

It has been suggested that OC use can mask the diagnosis of VWD based on an observation that estrogen can raise VWF levels in patients with VWD [48]. However, there is a lack of evidence demonstrating a definite effect of the current combination OCs (which are of lower dose potency than the estrogen preparations used in the initial case reports associating estrogen with raising the VWF levels). A practical approach would be to test women prior to starting the OC, if possible, but to obtain VWF testing if OCs have already been started.

Adjustment for the ABO blood type

It is well known that patients with blood type O have 25% lower VWF and FVIII levels [8]. Adjusting normal ranges for ABO blood type would require a lower threshold VWF and FVIII level for blood type O patients with bleeding symptoms. However, it has been shown that type O patients with VWF levels between 35% and 50% had similar bleeding symptoms to non-O patients in that range [49]. Whether the laboratory diagnosis of VWD necessitates ABO adjustment remains controversial. Probably a significant proportion of cases that have been diagnosed as mild "VWD" are non-genetic and related to the blood type [50]. Perhaps, in the future, a better descriptive term of patients with subnormal VWF levels and bleeding symptoms would be the classification of von Willebrand deficiency based on the demonstration of a subnormal VWF antigen and/or ristocetin cofactor compared with the non-ABO-adjusted local laboratory range [51]. ABO typing may still be advisable, as the finding of blood type O allows the clinician to emphasize to the patient that their subnormal VWF level is most likely secondary, at least in part, to being blood type O. Recent US guidelines do not advise ABO adjustment [52].

In those patients with a low VWF antigen and/or ristocetin cofactor VWF multimer analysis and ristocetin-induced platelet aggregation should be carried out for further subtyping of VWD [45].

Because of the association of hypothyroidism with acquired VWD, the patient should be screened for hypothyroidism [53, 54]. In hypothyroidism, thyroid replacement can result in resolution of the VWF deficiency [55].

Bleeding time and/or platelet function analyzer-100 closure time

The bleeding time (BT) and the platelet function analyzer-100 closure time (CT) have a relatively poor sensitivity for mild VWF deficiency [56] and platelet function disorders [56–58]. However the platelet function analyzer-100 CT may be useful for monitoring treatment [59].

Platelet aggregation and release studies

If initial hemostasis testing is normal, platelet aggregation and release, preferably off all medication, should be performed [60]. This is warranted on the basis of a relatively high prevalence of platelet function abnormalities in patients with menorrhagia. The abnormalities were far more prevalent in the black population [21]. Such a patient may respond to desmopressin [61] and shortening of the CT can be seen [62].

Additional coagulation studies may be considered if platelet aggregation and release studies are within normal limits. This would include testing for factors II, V, VII, X and XI deficiencies. Approximately 1–4% of women with menorrhagia have been found to have mild single factor coagulation deficiency other than VWD [16, 18, 37]. Additional coagulation studies such as testing for factor XIII deficiency [37] and tests for fibrinolysis such as the euglobulin lysis test [63] and more specific assays for α_2-anti-plasmin or plasminogen activator inhibitor deficiency may be indicated. Increased fibrinolysis, in general, has been reported in menorrhagia patients [64–66], but whether fibrinolysis is localized to the uterus or present systemically has not been fully studied. Patients with bleeding diatheses, including menorrhagia, associated with deficiencies in plasminogen activator inhibitor 1 and α_2-plasmin inhibitor have been reported [67–69].

Finally, when all of the above tests for hemostasis return normal, the clinician should reconsider the history in terms of a bleeding disorder. In particular, it is possible that what the patient reports as bruising is a drug-induced rash or a disorder of the endothelium, such as scurvy or vasculitis, or a connective tissue disorder, such as hereditary hemorrhagic telangiectasia. If all these possibilities are absent, the patient may have a disorder of hemostasis yet undiscovered and on occasion in cases with a very convincing bleeding history, e.g., multiple mucocutaneous bleeding symptoms of severity necessitating medical attention/intervention in the past, consideration for semi-empiric hemostatic therapy can be considered at the time of invasive procedures.

References

1 Hoffman M, Monroe DM, III. A cell-based model of hemostasis. *Thromb Haemost* 2001; **85**: 958–965.
2 Hoffman M, Monroe DM. Coagulation **2006:** a modern view of hemostasis. *Hematol Oncol Clin North Am* 2007; **21**: 1–11.
3 Tsai HM. Shear stress and von Willebrand factor in health and disease. *Semin Thromb Hemost* 2003; **29**: 479–488.
4 Sadler JE, Budde U, Eikenboom JC, *et al.* Update on the pathophysiology and classification of von Willebrand disease: a report of the Subcommittee on von Willebrand Factor. *J Thromb Haemost* 2006; **4**: 2103–2114.

5 James PD, Notley C, Hegadorn C, et al. The mutational spectrum of type 1 von Willebrand disease: results from a Canadian cohort study. Blood 2007; 109: 145–154.

6 Goodeve A, Eikenboom J, Castaman G, et al. Phenotype and genotype of a cohort of families historically diagnosed with type 1 von Willebrand disease in the European study, Molecular and Clinical Markers for the Diagnosis and Management of Type 1 von Willebrand Disease (MCMDM-1VWD). Blood 2007; 109: 112–121.

7 James PD, Paterson AD, Notley C, et al. Genetic linkage and association analysis in type 1 von Willebrand disease: results from the Canadian type 1 VWD study. J Thromb Haemost 2006; 4: 783–792.

8 Gill JC, Endres-Brooks J, Bauer PJ, et al. The effect of ABO blood group on the diagnosis of von Willebrand disease. Blood 1987; 69: 1691–1695.

9 Sadler JE. Von Willebrand disease type 1: a diagnosis in search of a disease. Blood 2003; 101: 2089–2093.

10 Sramek A, Eikenboom JC, Briet E, et al. Usefulness of patient interview in bleeding disorders [see comments]. Arch Intern Med 1995; 155: 1409–1415.

11 Plug I, Mauser-Bunschoten EP, Brocker-Vriends AH, et al. Bleeding in carriers of hemophilia. Blood 2006; 108: 52–56.

12 Eikenboom JC, Rosendaal FR, Briet E. Value of the patient interview: all but consensus among haemostasis experts. Haemostasis 1992; 22: 221–223.

13 Rodeghiero F, Castaman G, Tosetto A, et al. The discriminant power of bleeding history for the diagnosis of type 1 von Willebrand disease: an international, multicenter study. J Thromb Haemost 2005; 3: 2619–2626.

14 Tosetto A, Rodeghiero F, Castaman G, et al. A quantitative analysis of bleeding symptoms in type 1 von Willebrand disease: results from a multicenter European study (MCMDM-1 VWD). J Thromb Haemost 2006; 4.

15 Rodeghiero F, Tosetto A, Castaman G. How to estimate bleeding risk in mild bleeding disorders. J Thromb Haemost 2007; 5 (Suppl 1): 157–166.

16 Miller CH, Heit J, Kouides PA, et al. Laboratory characteristics of women with menorrhagia participating in a multi-site United States Menorrhagia Management Study [Abstract]. J Thromb Haemost 2007.

17 Kouides PA, Kadir RA. Menorrhagia associated with laboratory abnormalities of hemostasis: epidemiological, diagnostic and therapeutic aspects. J Thromb Haemost 2007; 5 (Suppl 1): 175–182.

18 James AH, Ragni MV, Picozzi VJ. Bleeding disorders in premenopausal women: (another) public health crisis for hematology? Hematol Am Soc Hematol Educ Program 2006; 474–485.

19 Philipp CS, Faiz A, Dowling N, et al. Development of a screening tool in women presenting with unexplained menorrhagia. Am J Obstet Gynecol 2007; 198: e1–e8.

20 Chi C, Riddell A, Griffioen A, et al. Bleeding score as screening tool for the identification and assessment of von Willebrand disease in women [Abstract]. Thromb Res 2007; 119 (Suppl 1): S101.

21 Philipp CS, Dilley A, Miller CH, et al. Platelet functional defects in women with unexplained menorrhagia. J Thromb Haemost 2003; 1: 477–484.

22 Shankar M, Lee CA, Sabin CA, et al. von Willebrand disease in women with menorrhagia: a systematic review. Br J Obstet Gynaecol 2004; 111: 734–740.

23 von Willebrand EA. Hereditar pseudohemofili. Finska Lakarsallskapets Handl 1926; 67: 7–112.

24 Kouides PA, Burkhart P, Phatak P, et al. Gynecological and obstetrical morbidity in women with Type I von Willebrand disease: results of a patient survey. Haemophilia 2000; 6: 643–648.

25 Kadir RA, Economides DL, Sabin CA, et al. Assessment of menstrual blood loss and gynaecological problems in patients with inherited bleeding disorders. Haemophilia 1999; 5: 40–48.

26 Ragni MV, Bontempo FA, Cortese Hassett A. von Willebrand disease and bleeding in women. Haemophilia 1999; 5: 313–317.

27 Fraser IS, McCarron G, Markham R. A preliminary study of factors influencing perception of menstrual blood loss volume. Am J Obstet Gynecol 1984; 149: 788–793.

28 Warner PE, Critchley HO, Lumsden MA, et al. Menorrhagia I: measured blood loss, clinical features, and outcome in women with heavy periods: a survey with follow-up data. Am J Obstet Gynecol 2004; 190: 1216–1223.

29 Higham JM, O'Brien PM, Shaw RW. Assessment of menstrual blood loss using a pictorial chart. Br J Obstet Gynaecol 1990; 97: 734–739.

30 Hallberg L, Hogdahl AM, Nilsson L, Rybo G. Menstrual blood loss and iron deficiency. Acta Med Scand 1966; 180: 639–650.

31 James AH, Jamison MG. Bleeding events and other complications during pregnancy and childbirth in women with von Willebrand disease. J Thromb Haemost 2007; 5: 1165–1169.

32 Eisen D, Hakim MD. Minocycline-induced pigmentation. Incidence, prevention and management. [Review]. Drug Safety 1998; 18: 431–440.

33 Kirtava A, Drews C, Lally C, et al. Medical, reproductive and psychosocial experiences of women diagnosed with von Willebrand's disease receiving care in haemophilia treatment centres: a case-control study. Haemophilia 2003; 9: 292–297.

34 James AH. More than menorrhagia: a review of the obstetric and gynaecological manifestations of bleeding disorders. *Haemophilia* 2005; **11**: 295–307.

35 Fricke W, Kouides P, Kessler C, *et al.* A multicenter clinical evaluation of the Clot Signature Analyzer. *J Thromb Haemost* 2004; **2**: 763–768.

36 Montgomery RR, Coller BS. von Willebrand disease. In: Colman RW, Hirsh J, Marder VJ, Salzman EW (eds). *Hemostasis and thrombosis: basic principles and practice.* Philadelphia, PA: JB Lippincott Co, 1994: 134–168.

37 Mannucci PM, Duga S, Peyvandi F. Recessively inherited coagulation disorders. *Blood* 2004; **104**: 1243–1252.

38 Edlund M, Blomback M, von Schoultz B, Andersson O. On the value of menorrhagia as a predictor for coagulation disorders. *Am J Hematol* 1996; **53**: 234–238.

39 Kadir RA, Economides DL, Sabin CA, *et al.* Frequency of inherited bleeding disorders in women with menorrhagia. *Lancet* 1998; **351**: 485–489.

40 Dilley A, Drews C, Miller C, *et al.* von Willebrand disease and other inherited bleeding disorders in women with diagnosed menorrhagia. *Obstet Gynecol* 2001; **97**: 630–636.

41 Woo YL, White B, Corbally R, *et al.* von Willebrand's disease: an important cause of dysfunctional uterine bleeding. *Blood Coagul Fibrinolys* 2002; **13**: 89–93.

42 Federici AB. The factor VIII/von Willebrand factor complex: basic and clinical issues [Review]. *Haematologica* 2003; **88**: EREP02.

43 Lipton RA. Misdiagnosis by milk box. *Haemophilia* 2003; **9**: 235.

44 Bohm M, Taschner S, Kretzschmar E, *et al.* Cold storage of citrated whole blood induces drastic time dependent losses in factor VIII and von Willebrand factor: potential for misdiagnosis of haemophilia and von Willebrand disease. *Blood Coagul Fibrinolys* 2006; **17**: 39–46.

45 Federici AB. Mild forms of von Willebrand disease: diagnosis and management. *Curr Hematol Rep* 2003; **2**: 373–380.

46 Mandalaki T, Louizou C, Dimitriadou C, Symeonidis P. Variations in factor VIII during the menstrual cycle in normal women [Letter]. *N Engl J Med* 1980; **302**: 1093–1094.

47 Blomback M, Eneroth P, Landgren BM, *et al.* On the intraindividual and gender variability of haemostatic components. *Thromb Haemost* 1992; **67**: 70–75.

48 Alperin JB. Estrogens and surgery in women with von Willebrand's disease. *Am J Med* 1982; **73**: 367–371.

49 Nitu-Whalley IC, Lee CA, Griffioen A, *et al.* Type 1 von Willebrand disease – a clinical retrospective study of the diagnosis, the influence of the ABO blood group and the role of the bleeding history. *Br J Haematol* 2000; **108**: 259–264.

50 Bauduer F, Ducout L. Is the assessment of von Willebrand disease prevalence an achievable challenge? The example of the French Basque Country where blood group O and factor XI deficiency are highly prevalent. *J Thromb Haemost* 2004; **2**: 1724–1726.

51 Sadler JE. Slippery criteria for von Willebrand disease type 1. *J Thromb Haemost* 2004; **2**: 1720–1723.

52 Nichols WL, Hultin MB, James AH, *et al.* Von Willebrand Disease Guidelines [Personal communication]. 2007.

53 Coccia MR, Barnes HV. Hypothyroidism and acquired von Willebrand disease. *J Adolesc Health* 1991; **12**: 152–154.

54 Blesing NE, Hambley H, McDonald GA. Acquired von Willebrand's disease and hypothyroidism: report of a case presenting with menorrhagia. *Postgrad Med J* 1990; **66**: 474–476.

55 Michiels JJ, Schroyens W, Berneman Z, Van der Planken M. Acquired von Willebrand syndrome type 1 in hypothyroidism: reversal after treatment with thyroxine. *Clin Appl Thromb Hemost* 2001; **7**: 113–115.

56 Posan E, Nichols WL, McBane RD, *et al.* Comparison of the PFA-100 testing and the bleeding time for detecting platelet hypofunction and von Willebrand disease. *J Thromb Haemost* 2003; **90**: 483–490.

57 Quiroga T, Goycoolea M, Munoz B, *et al.* Template bleeding time and PFA-100 have low sensitivity to screen patients with hereditary mucocutaneous hemorrhages: comparative study in 148 patients. *J Thromb Haemost* 2004; **2**: 892–898.

58 Philipp CS, Miller CH, Faiz A, *et al.* Screening women with menorrhagia for underlying bleeding disorders: the utility of the platelet function analyser and bleeding time. *Haemophilia* 2005; **11**: 497–503.

59 Koscielny J, von Tempelhoff GF, Ziemer S, *et al.* A practical concept for preoperative management of patients with impaired primary hemostasis. *Clin Appl Thromb Hemost* 2004; **10**: 155–166.

60 Bick RL. Platelet function defects: a clinical review [Review]. *Semin Thromb Hemost* 1992; **18**: 167–185.

61 DiMichele DM, Hathaway WE. Use of DDAVP in inherited and acquired platelet dysfunction. *Am J Hematol* 1990; **33**: 39–45.

62 Rose SS, Faiz A, Miller CH, *et al.* Laboratory response to intranasal desmopressin in women with menorrhagia and platelet dysfunction. *Haemophilia* 2008; **14**: 571–578.

63 Smith AA, Jacobson LJ, Miller BI, *et al.* A new euglobulin clot lysis assay for global fibrinolysis. *Thromb Res* 2003; **112**: 329–337.

64 Hahn L, Cederblad G, Rybo G, *et al.* Blood coagulation, fibrinolysis and plasma proteins in women with normal and with excessive menstrual blood loss. *Br J Obstet Gynaecol* 1976; **83**: 974–980.

65 Winkler UH. Menstruation: extravascular fibrinolytic activity and reduced fibrinolytic capacity. *Ann NY Acad Sci* 1992; **667**: 289–290.

66 Edlund M, Blomback M, He L. On the correlation between local fibrinolytic activity in menstrual fluid and total blood loss during menstruation and effects of desmopressin. *Blood Coagul Fibrin* 2003; **14**: 593–598.

67 Repine T, Osswald M. Menorrhagia due to a qualitative deficiency of plasminogen activator inhibitor-1: case report and literature review. *Clin Appl Thromb Hemost* 2004; **10**: 293–296.

68 Fay WP, Parker AC, Condrey LR, Shapiro AD. Human plasminogen activator inhibitor-1 (PAI-1) deficiency: characterization of a large kindred with a null mutation in the PAI-1 gene. *Blood* 1997; **90**: 204–208.

69 Favier R, Aoki N, de Moerloose P. Congenital alpha(2)-plasmin inhibitor deficiencies: a review. *Br J Haematol* 2001; **114**: 4–10.

2 Physiology of menstruation and menorrhagia

Måns Edlund

Menstrual physiology

Introduction

The shedding of the endometrium, menstrual bleeding, is the physiological consequence of ovulation in women when fertilization and implantation does not occur. This is a significant and normally regular event in the human reproductive cycle, and one of the unique physiological properties in the human species. From an evolutionary perspective, it is interesting that menstrual bleeding does, with two exceptions, occur only in humans and non-human primates. The exceptions are the elephant shrew and some species of bats. Thus, menstruation is an evolutionary and recently developed physiological process. In species that have menstrual bleedings, one important characteristic that seems to develop in parallel to menstrual bleeding is a more invasive form of placental invasion during gestation. Other viviparous animals including primates that do not menstruate have a less invasive form of implantation [1].

The issues of menstrual bleeding and aberrations in bleeding patterns have been focused upon for the last few decades. Better methods for investigation of the pathophysiology of menstrual bleeding are being developed, and treatment of menstrual bleeding disorders has improved. Furthermore, in developed countries the average woman today is expected to menstruate more than 400 times before menopause. This can be compared with approximately 40 menstruations during a normal lifespan of women in less developed countries or with the situation during the nineteenth century when women were amenorrheic throughout most of their lives due to late puberty, numerous pregnancies, prolonged lactation, and early menopause [2].

Menstruation therefore is the process by which the endometrium is discarded each month if no pregnancy occurs and the regular menstrual bleeding is the outward manifestation of cyclical ovarian function. During a normal menstrual cycle the endometrium is under cyclical control of the ovarian hormones. The ovaries are in turn under neuroendocrine control of the pituitary gland and the hypothalamus.

The premenarcheal development

In the fetus, the primordial germ cells have migrated to the genital ridge by the sixth week of gestation. Through mitosis the number of cells increases and between the eighth and the twentieth week of gestation they multiply and reach a maximum number of 7 million in total [3]. Primordial follicles now start to form and at birth approximately 2 million oocytes, arrested in the meiotic prophase, have developed.

Throughout a woman's life until menopause, when the reservoir is emptied, primordial follicles start growing and undergo atresia. This is a continuous process that is not affected by other ovarian events, e.g., ovulation, pregnancy, or anovulation due to hormonal treatment. The rate at which the primordial follicles are consumed in this process decreases over the years and is related to the remaining pool of primordial follicles. At puberty only 300 000 follicles

Inherited Bleeding Disorders in Women, 1st edition. By CA Lee, RA Kadir and PA Kouides. Published 2009 by Blackwell Publishing, ISBN: 978-1-4051-6915-8.

remain to last the 400 potential ovulations during a woman's fertile life [4].

Hormonal development

In the fetus, from the tenth week of gestation, gonadotropin-releasing hormone (GnRH) is present in the hypothalamus and luteinizing hormone (LH) and follicle-stimulating hormone (FSH) are present in the pituitary gland. Gonadotropin levels are elevated, and at birth gonadotropin and sex steroid concentrations are high, but the levels decline during the first weeks of life and remain low during the prepubertal years. The hypothalamic–pituitary axis appears to be suppressed by the extremely low levels of gonadal steroids present in childhood.

Early in puberty, there is increased sensitivity of LH to GnRH and basal levels of both FSH and LH increase through puberty. LH levels eventually become greater than FSH levels. Although gonadotropins are always secreted in an episodic or pulsatile fashion, even before puberty, the pulsatile secretion of gonadotropins is more easily documented as puberty progresses and basal levels increase [5].

Menarche

It is not fully understood what triggers the changes that result in menarche. A mechanism best described as a central nervous system program has been hypothesized. In childhood the hypothalamus and pituitary gland seem to be insensitive to the estradiol feedback mechanisms, but they become very sensitive after puberty. It appears that the hypothalamic–pituitary–gonadal axis in girls develops in two distinct stages during puberty. First, sensitivity to the negative or inhibitory effects of the low levels of circulating sex steroids present in childhood decreases early in puberty. Second, late in puberty, there is maturation of the positive or stimulatory feedback response to estrogen, which is responsible for the ovulatory mid-cycle surge of LH. It is only in the last stages of puberty that gonadotropins come into play in the maturation of the follicle. Based on this theory, the neuroendocrine control of puberty is mediated by GnRH-secreting neurons in the medial basal hypothalamus, which together act as an endogenous pulse generator. At puberty, the GnRH pulse generator is reactivated (i.e., disinhibited), leading to increased amplitude and frequency of GnRH pulses. At first these are detected during the sleep period but eventually the episodic release of LH and FSH increase into pulsations that can be detected throughout the 24 hours. In turn, the increased GnRH secretion results in increased gonadotropin and then gonadal steroid secretion. What causes this "disinhibition" of GnRH release is unknown.

Anovulatory cycles are common in the first years after menarche [6]. There is a reported prevalence of 55% anovulation in the first 2 years after menarche that decreases to 20% anovulatory cycles by the fifth year. This also leads to an initial irregularity in the menstrual pattern. During these first years of frequent anovulatory cycles it is also not uncommon to have a prolonged cycle length, prolonged estrogenic exposure and hyperplasia of the endometrium, and a subsequent very heavy bleeding (see "Adolescent menorrhagia").

The ovaries

The time of development from primordial follicle to ovulation is approximately 85 days. In the ovaries there is a continuous and hormone-independent development of primordial follicles whereof a majority undergoes atresia. During a limited time-span in the menstrual cycle, some 12–14 days before ovulation, a group of follicles starts to respond to hormone stimulation and continues to grow to preantral, antral, and preovulatory follicles. In these stages there are vast changes in the surrounding cell layers involving production of hormone receptors, notably the receptors for FSH and LH and the production of estrogen. During a typical cycle 3–11 follicles are developed in each ovary [7].

The ovarian cycle is regulated by internal and external hormones in the circulation. FSH and LH from the anterior pituitary are released in response to the GnRH, which is produced in the arcuate nucleus of the hypothalamus and secreted in a pulsatile fashion into the portal circulation. As the ovarian follicular development moves from a period of gonadotropin independence to a phase of FSH dependence, the corpus luteum of the previous cycle fades and luteal production of progesterone decreases, allowing FSH levels to rise.

In response to the FSH stimulus, the follicles grow and differentiate and secrete increasing amounts of estrogen. Estrogen stimulates growth and differentiation of the functional layer of the endometrium, which prepares for implantation. Estrogens also work with FSH in stimulating follicular development, and rising estrogen levels negatively feed back on the pituitary gland and hypothalamus and decrease the secretion of FSH.

The one follicle destined to ovulate each cycle is called the dominant follicle. It has relatively more FSH receptors and produces a larger concentration of estrogens than the follicles that will undergo atresia. Therefore, it is able to continue to grow despite falling FSH levels.

Sustained high estrogen levels cause a surge in pituitary LH secretion that triggers ovulation, progesterone production, and the shift to the secretory, or luteal, phase.

Luteal function is dependent on the presence of LH. However, the corpus luteum secretes estrogen, progesterone, and inhibin-A, which serve to maintain gonadotropin suppression. Without continued LH secretion, the corpus luteum will regress after 12–14 days. The resulting loss of progesterone secretion results in menstruation (Fig. 2.1).

If pregnancy occurs, the embryo secretes human chorionic gonadotropin (hCG), which mimics the action of LH in sustaining the corpus luteum. The corpus luteum continues to secrete progesterone and supports the secretory endometrium, allowing the pregnancy to continue to develop.

The menstrual cycle

During the first 14 days of the cycle the endometrium grows under the influence of estrogen (proliferatory phase) and during the following 14 days, under the influence of estrogen and progesterone that is secreted from the corpus luteum. The endometrium matures (secretory phase) in preparation to receive a fertilized egg. Without a pregnancy progesterone production in the ovaries ceases and the matured endometrium is expelled as menstrual bleeding. Thus, menstruation is an unusual physiological process that involves the expulsion and regeneration of healthy tissue lining the uterus. In the endometrium, the morphological changes during these processes have been thoroughly studied and described over the years. Modern research is focused on the molecular biology and immunology of the changing endometrium under endocrine regulation [8].

The physiological events in the uterus leading to shedding of the endometrium, subsequent bleeding, and repair have been studied for more than a century. Corner and Allen [9] presented a synthesis on the relation between estradiol, progesterone, and the changes

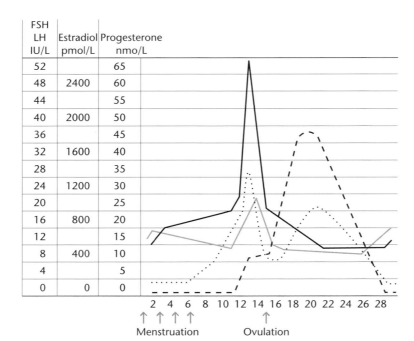

Fig. 2.1 Graph showing the relationship between progesterone and menstruation. Gray, follicle-stimulating hormone; black, luteinizing hormone; dotted, estradiol; dashed, progesterone.

in endometrial structure and function throughout the cycle. In 1940 J. Eldridge Markee [10] presented a classical and extensive work on intraocular endometrial transplants in the rhesus monkey. In these studies he established the relationship between the fall in estrogen (estrone) and progesterone and the contractions in the coiled (also called spiral) arteries of the endometrium. The key event in inducing menstrual bleeding was found to be progesterone withdrawal.

In the 1960s the concept of constriction and subsequent dilation of the coiled arteries as a vital mechanism for menstruation was questioned [11], and since then several different theories on the physiology of menstrual bleeding have evolved. These theories have in common that the onset of menstrual bleeding can be partly a consequence of an inflammatory process. Both menstruation and implantation after fertilization have been shown to share some properties of the inflammatory process [12, 13]: prostaglandins and cytokines are involved [14] and leukocytes are activated [15]. One result of this is expression of a particular class of enzymes, the matrix metalloproteinases (MMPs) in the endometrium.

The onset of menstrual bleeding is presently regarded as a combination of three major events: vasoconstriction, inflammation, and tissue degradation. The link between progesterone withdrawal, the inflammatory response, and tissue destruction is fairly well studied and understood [16–18], whereas the link between progesterone withdrawal and vasoconstriction is less clear [19]. One mechanism may involve the progesterone withdrawal-induced upregulation of prostaglandin production via cyclooxygenase 2 (COX2), the inducible form of prostaglandin synthetase [20]. Another possible vasoconstrictor is the 21 amino acid polypeptide endothelin (ET).

Vasoconstriction
The effects of progesterone on cells in endometrial tissue can theoretically be exerted in two ways. First, there is signaling via the progesterone receptors A and B [21], the classical, slow steroid receptor signaling via genomic activation. Second, the progesterone effect can be mediated through membrane-bound receptors giving a fast non-genomic response. In neuronal tissues, progesterone can signal via gamma-aminobutyric acid (GABA) A chloride channels, thereby evoking an immediate answer [22]. However, to date no reports exist on such a membrane-bound receptor

in endometrial tissue and there are reports on the absence of progesterone receptors in the vascular endothelium of the actual coiled arteries [23–25].

It has been shown that progesterone, at physiological concentrations, potentiates the thrombin-induced cellular response by upregulation of protease activated receptor 1 (PAR-1) in aortic cells [26]. The result is increased vasoconstriction despite an unchanged level of thrombin. When uterine endothelial cells are exposed to progesterone withdrawal, upregulation of the thrombin receptor is found (Fig 2.2) [27]. When progesterone levels decrease after the demise of the corpus luteum the endothelium in the uterine vessels should consequently become more sensitive to thrombin. In accordance with these findings, it has been shown that in endometrial tissue downregulation of the PAR-1 gene was seen as a response to exposure to the progesterone levonorgestrel [28].

Thrombin is a serine protease and one of the most important enzymes in the blood-clotting cascade. In addition to its action in hemostasis, thrombin has been found to act as a cofactor in response to sex steroids [29–31]. Thrombin both upregulates the endothelin-converting enzyme (ECE-1) that processes ET from its precursor peptide pre-proendothelin [32] and stimulates ET release [33].

Previous work has shown that ET may be involved in regulation of menstruation, but compelling evidence of the role of ET is lacking. It has previously been shown that ET has a crucial role in the regulation of vessel contractility [34] in several organ systems including the urogenital tract. ET contracts vascular and myometrial smooth muscle in the uterus [35] and has been shown to be more potent in contracting small branches of the uterine artery than in contracting the main stem [36]. These steps provide a chain of events that link progesterone withdrawal to the contraction of small endometrial vessels, the last observation being one of the first influential findings in the early works on menstrual physiology [9–11].

In addition to this, menstrual bleeding is regulated on several other levels. Two phases of menstruation have been proposed. The early events in the onset of menstruation are vasoconstriction and a process resembling inflammation [14] induced by progesterone withdrawal by direct or indirect action. This is followed by activation of lytic mechanisms that presumably are partly a consequence of hypoxia and subsequent tissue degradation and inflammation.

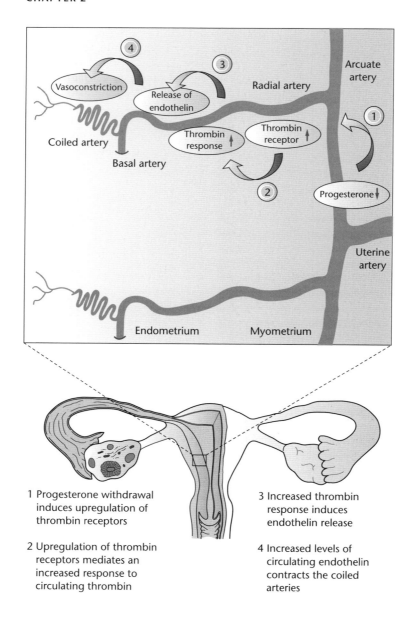

Fig. 2.2 Vascular events in menstrual physiology. Redrawn with permission from Eva Andersson.

1 Progesterone withdrawal induces upregulation of thrombin receptors

2 Upregulation of thrombin receptors mediates an increased response to circulating thrombin

3 Increased thrombin response induces endothelin release

4 Increased levels of circulating endothelin contracts the coiled arteries

Tissue degradation

The breakdown of the endometrial extracellular matrix (ECM) involves enzymes, the MMPs [15, 37, 38]. MMPs consist of a group of 24 protease-like proteins that degrade the ECM and basement membrane [18]. Stromal cells in the upper endometrial zones secrete MMPs after 48 hours after progesterone withdrawal [39, 40].

MMPs are significantly increased in the endometrium at menstruation compared with other stages of the cycle [41], and withdrawal of progesterone under experimental conditions does upregulate the MMPs [40]. A cyclicity has also been found for the physiological inhibitors of MMP, tissue inhibitors of MMP (TIMP) [42, 43]. The link between progesterone withdrawal and MMP upregulation and secretion has been unclear. A candidate for this connection has now however been presented in LEFTY-A [44]. LEFTY-A is a member of the transforming growth factor-β family, identified originally as an endometrial bleeding associated factor (EBAF) [45]. LEFTY-A increases the expression of MMPs during menstruation. Progesterone exerts an inhibition on the LEFTY-A effect on MMPs on two levels [44]: upstream by inhibiting LEFTY-A expression and downstream by suppressing its stimulatory effect on MMPs.

Another link between progesterone withdrawal and MMP upregulation and secretion is thrombin, a substance that has also been studied with regard to its proliferative effect on cultured human vascular endothelial cells [46]. Furthermore, thrombin has been shown to exert specific proliferative effects on endometrial cells [47]. The ability to regulate levels of MMP1, MMP2, and MMP3 [48–50] makes thrombin especially interesting. It has been shown that a progesterone, medroxyprogesterone acetate, strongly inhibits MMP-1 levels in endometrial stromal cells [51]. However, thrombin overcomes this suppression, resulting in MMP-1 levels that are several-fold higher than in controls. Thus it seems as if thrombin signaling, either by increased levels of thrombin or by an upregulation of the thrombin receptor, may have a central role in endometrial ECM breakdown as well as in the chain of events in menstrual physiology leading to vasoconstriction.

Inflammation
Progesterone withdrawal induces endometrial changes that can be regarded as an inflammatory process [12]. There is an influx of leukocytes [52] and release of prostaglandins. Endometrial and peripheral blood leukocytes do not express progesterone receptors, indicating that recruitment of leukocytes into the endometrium is mediated indirectly [53]. COX2 is the inducible form of prostaglandin synthetase; it is present in the human endometrium and is expressed mainly during the menstrual phase [20] when prostaglandin levels have been shown to rise. Several substances related to inflammation correlate with the onset of menstrual bleeding in the endometrium, such as the chemokine interleukin 8 (IL-8), chemotactic for neutrophils and NK cells [54], and the monocyte chemotactic peptide (MCP-1) [55]. A cyclic variation of the proinflammatory cytokine tumor necrosis factor alpha (TNF-α) has been shown in the plasma [56] and in the endometrium [57]. The effects of the inflammatory substances on menstrual bleeding are either direct, such as for prostaglandins that induce vascular permeability changes, or indirect, such as for IL-8 and MCP-1, which attract cells that activate and release MMPs.

In summary, monthly occurring menstrual bleeding is normally a remarkably well-controlled event. Abnormal uterine bleeding in regularity, frequency, or amount happens, on the other hand, to most women at some stage during their reproductive years.

Disturbance in menstrual bleeding is not a disease by itself but a symptom of an underlying disorder. Menorrhagia is a regular but abundant period. Irregular and heavy bleeding is called metrorrhagia and is often caused by hormonal disturbances due to irregularities in ovulation. Other causes of metrorrhagia are infections and benign or malignant tumors. Irregular bleeding in the beginning of a pregnancy, normal or pathological, e.g. ectopic pregnancy, can also be misinterpreted as a metrorrhagia.

Menorrhagia

The most common pathology of menstrual bleeding is menorrhagia, heavy but regular menstrual bleeding. Menorrhagia is the most common reason for examination and treatment in gynecology. It is also a very important issue in general health. Menorrhagia is the most common cause of iron deficiency, anemia, in fertile women worldwide. As menorrhagia is a symptom of an underlying disease, it is crucial that treatment is preceded by an adequate examination to ensure provision of the most appropriate therapy for all women.

Definition

When describing menstrual abnormalities there is a need for simple terminology and definitions that can be accepted and understood worldwide. The terminology used in this chapter is the one used by health professionals in most parts of Europe, the USA and other English-speaking parts of the world (Table 2.1). The use of Latin, Greek, and ill-defined terms such as dysfunctional uterine bleeding (DUB) makes it difficult to compare descriptions between clinicians and the general population. As a result of this, an international group of experts on disorders of menstruation has

Table 2.1 Current terminology describing menstrual abnormalities

Regular bleeding (cyclic bleeding)	Irregular bleeding (acyclic bleeding)
Menorrhagia, excessive regular periods	Metrorrhagia, irregular periods
Oligomenorrhea, infrequent regular periods	Menometrorrhagia, irregular excessive periods
Polymenorrhea, frequent regular periods	Contact (coital) bleeding, bleeding after intercourse
Amenorrhea, no periods at all	Postmenopausal bleeding, bleeding more than 1 year after menopause (last regular period)

initiated an international debate and consultation process in order to find clear, simple terminologies and definitions that have the potential for wide acceptance [58].

Menorrhagia is traditionally defined as heavy regular menstrual bleeding. Since the 1960s there have been several studies on the subject of menorrhagia. Normal menstrual blood loss (MBL) is on average 40 mL per month [59, 60]. Recommendations for an upper limit of normal blood loss have ranged from 60 mL of MBL to 120 mL [61] per month. The most accepted definition is a monthly MBL exceeding 80 mL. This definition was established by studying how much an otherwise healthy woman could bleed every month without becoming iron deficient or anemic [62]. Regularity in bleeding does require ovulation; anovulatory bleedings do quite soon become irregular. There is sometimes an intraindividual variation, up to 3 days, in cycle length, which is not considered as an irregularity. Furthermore, there are also interindividual variations, and the defined normal range is 23 to 35 days. Thus the definition for menorrhagia is a MBL exceeding 80 mL in ovulatory cycles.

Adolescent menorrhagia

As menstrual periods in adolescents are often irregular due to frequent anovulation, the condition "adolescent menorrhagia" is quite often in fact a menometrorrhagia, i.e., heavy and at least to some extent irregular bleeding. The condition is normally not severe and does not require treatment. If irregularity continues for several periods or if the blood loss causes anemia, hormonal treatment is advisable. The most convenient treatment option in these young women is the combined contraceptive pill, provided there are no risk factors for venous thromboembolism. Rarely, teenagers may have an organic pathology such as carcinomas of the cervix or vagina, or ovarian tumors leading to estrogen production and heavy menstrual loss. A persistent and continuously changing bleeding pattern is a reason for a thorough examination. Adolescents with a more or less regular bleeding pattern and heavy menstrual blood loss should always be examined for coagulation deficiency, see "Treatment of menorrhagia" and Chapter 7.

Prevalence

Menorrhagia is one of the most common gynecological symptoms and a common reason for consulting gynecologists or general practitioners [63, 64]. The prevalence of objectively verified menorrhagia is around 10% [65]. The prevalence increases with age until menopause, often with an increasing tendency of menometrorrhagia, heavy and irregular bleeding, towards the end. There is a wide range in the prevalence of subjectively experienced menorrhagia and on average 30% of women do at some occasion experience heavy regular bleeding [66, 67]. As a result of this discrepancy, up to 50% of women complaining of menorrhagia have an objective blood loss of less than 80 mL [68]. Thus one difficulty in the management of menorrhagia is to get a reliable quantification of the MBL.

Quality of life

Surprisingly, impact from menorrhagia on the quality of life (QoL), which is the predominant cause for complaint among suffering women, has not been studied extensively. Even more surprising is the poor quality of QoL follow-up in association with different medical and/or surgical treatments. A validated tool for specific menorrhagia-related QoL is lacking, but the Short Form 36 (SF 36) has shown to be reliable and valid in the general population, in chronically ill people [69, 70], and in women with menorrhagia [71]. A patient-administered questionnaire for menorrhagia based on the type of questions asked when taking a gynecological history has also been developed [72]. Even the most simplified form of satisfaction follow-up can be of value, especially in connection to treatment evaluation outside of clinical trials. One set of questions that could be used was presented by Winkler [73].

1 Do you feel that your social activities have been impaired because of your menstrual bleeding, e.g. less swimming, tennis, theater, leisure plans? (1, impaired; 5, not impaired).

2 Do you feel your work performance to be impaired because of your menstrual bleeding? (1, impaired; 5, not impaired).

3 Do you feel tired or exhausted during your menstruation? (1, tired, exhausted; 5, fit, active).

4 Do you feel less productive during your menstruation? (1, less productive; 5, very productive).

5 Do you feel unclean or unhygienic during your menstruation? (1, unclean, unhygienic; 5, very clean).

6 Do you feel depressed during your menstruation? (1, depressed, low spirits; 5, no depressive feeling).

7 Do you feel that your action radius is limited during your menstruation? (1, action radius limited; 5, no limitations).

8 Do you feel generally impaired by your menstruation? (1, impaired by the heavy bleeding; 5, in no way impaired).

The nature of these questions does give insight into these women's severe limitations in daily living and the impact on quality of life that menorrhagia has (see also Chapter 7).

Measurement of menstrual blood loss

The discrepancy between objectively measured MBL and the subjective estimation of the MBL necessitates verifiable methods to measure the actual MBL. Neither the duration of menses nor the number of sanitary tampons and pads used accurately corresponds to the actual MBL [74, 75]. Furthermore there is an intraindividual variation in MBL [74],

especially in women with menorrhagia. Therefore, an optimal assessment is only obtained with repeated measurements.

Alkaline hematin method
The most accurate method, the alkaline hematin method, described by Hallberg and Nilsson [76] and modified by Newton and co-workers [77], can determine the actual blood loss with precision. It gives a value of the exact amount of hemoglobin lost during one menstrual period.

The patient is rigorously instructed that all blood lost during a menstrual period must be collected. This means for example that a tampon or white cotton should be used during showers and all toilet visits. The collected blood material is packed in plastic bags (a bag for every 24 hours). Menstrual blood is then extracted from the sanitary material with 5% sodium hydroxide. In the sodium hydroxide the sanitary material is homogenized and the hemoglobin content of the menstrual blood is transformed to alkaline hematin. Subsequently the homogenate is measured spectrophotometrically at 540 nm and, with knowledge of the venous hemoglobin concentration of the patient, the corresponding volume of MBL for that period of 24 hours can be calculated.

The method is however laborious and is therefore used exclusively in research. As a result of this there has been a need for alternative objective or semi-objective methods.

Pictorial blood loss assessment chart
The pictorial blood loss assessment chart (PBAC) or the menstrual pictogram was developed by Higham and co-workers [78] in order to simplify measurement of MBL in a way that it could be used not only for research but also for routine clinical use (Appendix ii). It has been developed as a simple scoring system, taking account of the number of sanitary tampons and pads used as well as the degree of soiling. Higham obtained a sensitivity of 86% and a specificity of 81–89% compared with the "gold standard," the alkaline hematin method. Use of this method has become widespread and instructions and charts can be found for downloading from the Internet for home assessment. The method has, however, been criticized. Follow-up studies for validation have been few and with differing results from the initial study. One main issue seems to be at which cut-off score menorrhagia will be

correctly diagnosed [79, 80]. Further discussion is found in Chapters 3, 4, 5, 7 and Appendix ii.

Menstrual fluid volume measurement
As menstrual "blood" consists not only of blood, but also of serous fluid and endometrial debris, it has not been considered reliable to estimate the blood loss by weighing the sanitary tampons and pads. Fraser and co-workers [81] however showed that careful measurement of the total menstrual fluid volume is sufficiently accurate for estimation of MBL for clinical purposes. This method needs however to be further evaluated.

Etiology
Menorrhagia is a symptom. Traditionally, menorrhagia has been considered to signal a local gynecological disorder. However, 80% of women treated for menorrhagia have no anatomically perceptible pathology and in 50% of women undergoing hysterectomy as treatment for menorrhagia, no uterine pathology is found [82].

The complexity of the matter is even increased by the fact that two or several etiologies can coexist and complicate the investigation. For example a woman with impaired coagulation who has most likely suffered from menorrhagia since menarche. If the correct diagnosis is not found (probably because it is not looked for) or if symptomatic treatment with, for example, combined contraceptives has been initiated at an early stage she may go undiagnosed up to an age of over 30 years. If then an additional condition such as a uterine myoma is added this can tip her over the edge, lead to anemia and an impaired QoL. The subsequent investigation will meet the challenge of unmasking the underlying conditions causing menorrhagia (Fig. 2.3).

Uterine causes
Local pelvic pathology (such as leiomyoma, adenomyosis, and endometrial polyps) is estimated to be the main cause of approximately 25–30% of all cases of menorrhagia, leiomyomas being the most common cause [83]. These data are derived from statistics on women who have undergone a hysterectomy for heavy periods. However, most women going through surgery for this reason do not actually have objective menorrhagia. Furthermore, leiomyomas are also very common conditions in women with normal menstrual

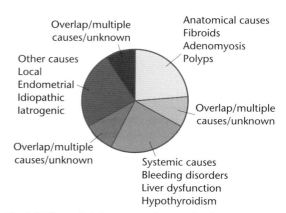

Fig. 2.3 The underlying causes of menorrhagia.

blood loss. The location of the myoma is probably important: intrauterine or submucosal myomas are more likely to affect the amount of blood lost at menstruation. These types of fibroids are associated with an increased endometrial surface that contributes to the increased bleeding. The same reasoning goes for endometrial polyps and adenomyosis.

Systemic causes
Systemic causes have previously been considered to be an uncommon underlying condition in women with the symptoms of menorrhagia. The association between hypothyroidism and menorrhagia has been well known for decades, and approximately 1–2% of women with menorrhagia suffer from hypothyroidism [84]. Apart from that, bleeding disorders, inherited as well as acquired, have earlier been considered to be an obvious but uncommon cause of menorrhagia. However, several articles published in the last 10 years have clearly pointed out that there is a relatively high probability of finding an undiagnosed bleeding disorder when properly examining a patient with menorrhagia [85–89]. This is further discussed in Chapter 7.

Iatrogenic causes
The use of a non-hormonal intrauterine device (IUD) increases average menstrual blood loss by 45% [90] and bleeding problems remain the most frequent single reason for the removal of an IUD. Treatment with anticoagulants increases the risk of menorrhagic bleeding. Medical treatment influencing the function of platelets, notably non-steroidal anti-inflammatory drugs (NSAIDs), including acetylic salicylic acid (ASA),

induce increased MBL in some women. This effect is most often seen in women with defective coagulation such as mild von Willebrand disease (VWD) or mild platelet dysfunction.

Idiopathic or unexplained menorrhagia

No matter how hard we try to find the underlying cause there will still be a significant proportion of women with menorrhagia that cannot be explained. With increasing skill and technology to investigate menorrhagia, the proportion of idiopathic menorrhagia diminishes. Ultrasound, hysteroscopic techniques and increased awareness and availability to perform hematological work-ups have reduced the fraction of unexplained menorrhagia from well above 50% to perhaps 25%.

Local changes in the endometrium associated with menorrhagia

There are also hypotheses on endometrial factors contributing to menorrhagic bleeding. Excessive MBL has, for example, been ascribed to abnormal uterine levels of prostaglandins [91]. The endometrium of women with excessive menstrual bleeding has been found to have higher levels of prostaglandin E2 and prostaglandin F2α than the endometrium of women with normal menses [92]. There is further evidence of deranged hemostasis such as an elevated ratio of prostaglandin E2 to F2 [93] and the ratio of prostacyclin to thromboxane [94]. These substances are present both in the endometrium and in the myometrium, although the exact mechanism by which the excessive blood loss occurs remains speculative.

Plasminogen activators are a group of substances that cause fibrinolysis. An increase in the levels of plasminogen activators has been found in the endometrium of women with heavy menstrual bleeding compared with those with normal menstrual loss [95–97]. Whether these local factors are actually causing the heavy MBL or are a result of the heavy MBL or may be only a coexisting observation without connection is yet to be proven.

The local endometrial environment is, as described, undergoing thorough changes during the whole menstrual cycle, and menstrual bleeding acts as a crescendo in a biological firework. Treatments initially used *ex juvantibus*, e.g., NSAIDs and antifibrinolytic treatment, for unknown menorrhagia were found to have therapeutic effect. Several substances have, after this,

been studied in relation to menorrhagia, notably prostaglandins and markers of fibrinolytic activity.

Previously described physiological events in menstrual regulation where dysregulation could cause menorrhagia mainly involve hormonal dysfunction. Progesterone dysfunction however is predominantly reported to cause irregular bleeding [98, 99]. Dysfunctional uterine bleedings may result from both high and low levels of estrogen and progesterone. Furthermore, there is a possibility that changes in receptor density distribution or function could cause bleeding disturbances. However, studies on endometrial and myometrial histology using immunohistochemistry [100, 101] have not shown any significant differences in the amount or distribution of estrogen or progesterone receptors between women with normal menstruation and women with menorrhagic blood loss.

The steps following progesterone withdrawal resulting in increased vascular contraction have been little focused upon. The hypothesis that upregulation of the thrombin receptor is involved has been studied with regard to menorrhagia. Thrombin signaling may also be a possible link between vascular events and tissue degradation [51], although a previous study showed no variation in thrombin levels in peripheral circulation during spontaneous cycles or during progesterone treatment [102, 103].

A cyclic normal or abnormal variation in the expression of the thrombin receptor would offer an explanation for dysregulation in the endometrial control of bleeding [27]. The link between thrombin and ET, with its presumed role in regulation of uterine bleeding and endometrial repair [104], necessitates further studies on the influence of the variation in thrombin receptor density, distribution, or function on menstrual control. Thrombin signaling could influence endometrial bleeding also by another mechanism. Plasminogen activators (t-PA) are a group of substances that give rise to fibrinolysis. Endothelial cells store t-PA in specific vesicles from which it can be released after exposure to thrombin [105]. Since fibrinolytic activity in tissues and blood is largely determined by the concentration of t-PA [106, 107], it is interesting that increased local fibrinolytic activity has been found in women with menorrhagia [95, 97, 108].

Increased local fibrinolytic activity in menorrhagia

Presence of plasminogen activators in the endometrium was reported in 1966 [108]. In the process of degrading blood clots, t-PA transforms plasminogen to plasmin, which degrades fibrin. Previous studies have shown that there is normally high fibrinolytic activity in the endometrium and in menstrual blood in humans, and a further increase is seen in some conditions associated with menorrhagia [95, 109–111]. To a large extent, increased local endometrial fibrinolytic activity is also seen in idiopathic menorrhagia. This has been shown in the endometrium and in the menstrual fluid [95, 112–114].

There are few earlier studies on the exact relationship between local fibrinolytic activity and the amount of menstrual bleeding [95, 97]. In these studies, measurement of local fibrinolytic activity has been made on endometrial tissue. After the finding of a positive correlation between MBL and fibrinolytic activity, the increase in local fibrinolysis has been considered to be an important factor in idiopathic menorrhagia. The efficacy of antifibrinolytic drugs (e.g., tranexamic acid) on menorrhagia is regarded as supporting this. Whether local fibrinolytic activity causes heavy MBL or whether it is a result of heavy MBL or may even be a coexisting observation without causal nexus is a question that remains to be answered.

In a recent study [115] a highly significant correlation was found between the actual MBL and the fibrinolytic activity in menstrual fluid. This correlation was applicable to women with normal MBL as well as to women with menorrhagia.

Evaluation and investigation

The evaluation of the patient seeking help and treatment for menorrhagia has two main goals. First, we have to establish whether the MBL is excessive or not. If it is found (after taking a thorough history and that may also be a semi-objective measurement of the MBL) not to be an excessive MBL, then the task will be to educate and inform the patient about the normal physiology of menstrual bleeding. It is also important at this stage to separate menorrhagia from other period-related problems such as dysmenorrhea and premenstrual dysphoric disorder. If the subjective problem remains, it is of course possible to try a medical treatment with an unspecific effect, but only after confirming that the effect experienced will be small.

Second, we must establish the cause of heavy MBL. This is a prerequisite for successful treatment whether it will be medical or surgical.

Menstrual history and assessment of MBL

It is important to find out when menorrhagia was first experienced. Menorrhagia since menarche is seldom caused by pelvic pathology but more likely to be attributed to bleeding disorders. It is important to find out about the consequences on daily life. A woman who uses several sanitary pads or a tampon and pad simultaneously, needs to change several times at night, and bleeds through her protection is probably suffering from menorrhagia. If menstruation means regular sick leave or that meetings, social events, or travel plans are cancelled, this is also valuable information in our efforts to quantify the menstrual bleeding. Often this is the closest that we can get to evaluate the amount of blood loss. Some clinicians have worked up a routine with the PBAC as a support in the diagnosis of menorrhagia, but most of the time estimation relies on information: to what extent does the bleeding impair the woman's daily activities. If the bleeding is irregular, is it a metrorrhagia or a menometrorrhagia. These conditions may have a completely different pathophysiology and the underlying causes will not be thoroughly discussed here.

Clinical assessment

All women presenting with menorrhagia should undergo a gynecological examination (Fig. 2.4). An exception can be made for young girls with adolescent menorrhagia who have not become sexually active. A routine evaluation includes an ultrasound examination, preferably vaginally. Ultrasound can sometimes overlook small polyps. The diagnostic accuracy of ultrasound is better during the early follicular phase of the menstrual cycle when the endometrium is thin. Better results are obtained with hydrosonography when the uterine cavity is filled and distended with a saline solution. The saline solution acts as a sonographic contrast and most intrauterine aberrations are detectable. A good result is also obtained if the endometrium can be examined visually, through diagnostic hysteroscopy. With a diagnostic hysteroscopy, a targeted biopsy of the endometrium or a visualized focal pathology can also be obtained. All these examinations can be performed at the outpatient clinic. In all women over the age of 40 and in women with an irregular bleeding pattern, an endometrial sample should be obtained. Endometrial aspiration cytology has now replaced dilation and curettage for this purpose. A cervical PAP smear should also be assessed.

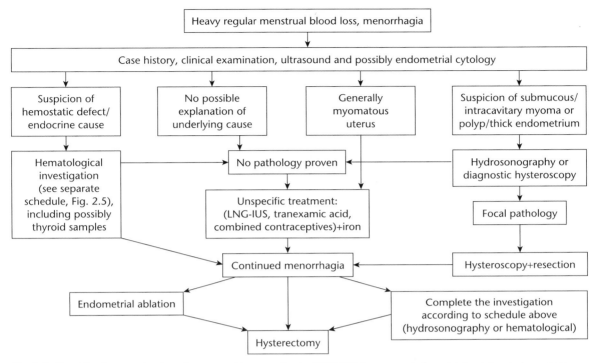

Fig. 2.4 Algorithm for examination of women with menorrhagia. LNG-IUS, levonorgestrel-containing intrauterine system.

Blood samples

Blood samples to evaluate the hemoglobin level and, when indicated, iron studies are useful for early detection and management of iron deficiency. Thyroid function tests should be performed on suspicion of hypothyroidism. If the history, including the family history, indicates a possibility of a defective coagulation system, a coagulation screen designed to reveal the most common mild coagulation deficiencies such as VWD and platelet dysfunction (Fig. 2.5) should also be performed. The circumstances around blood sampling, the pre-analytical conditions, are important [116]. Since there is evidence that some of the coagulation factors change cyclically during the menstrual cycle and reach their nadir during the menstrual phase, it is recommended that blood sampling should be performed at this period of the cycle [117].

When signs of a bleeding disorder are found, the patient should be referred to a hematologist for further evaluation. When the hematological work-up is concluded and an underlying bleeding disorder has not been verified, then gynecological evaluation and treat-ment should continue. Sometimes both a bleeding disorder and a local uterine pathology are found. In these cases, it is of course advisable to conclude the hematological investigation and to commence medical treatment before embarking on any surgical treatment option.

Treatment of menorrhagia

There exists controversy on the subject of menorrhagia treatment: medical management or surgical cure. One must keep in mind that menorrhagia is only a symptom; the underlying cause of heavy menstrual blood loss will determine the treatment.

Surgical treatment of menorrhagia

Hysterectomy Surgical treatment of menorrhagia includes hysterectomy or endometrial ablation. Hysterectomy is one of the most frequently performed major surgical procedures among women of reproductive age. In the USA approximately 500 000 to 600 000 hysterectomies are performed each year

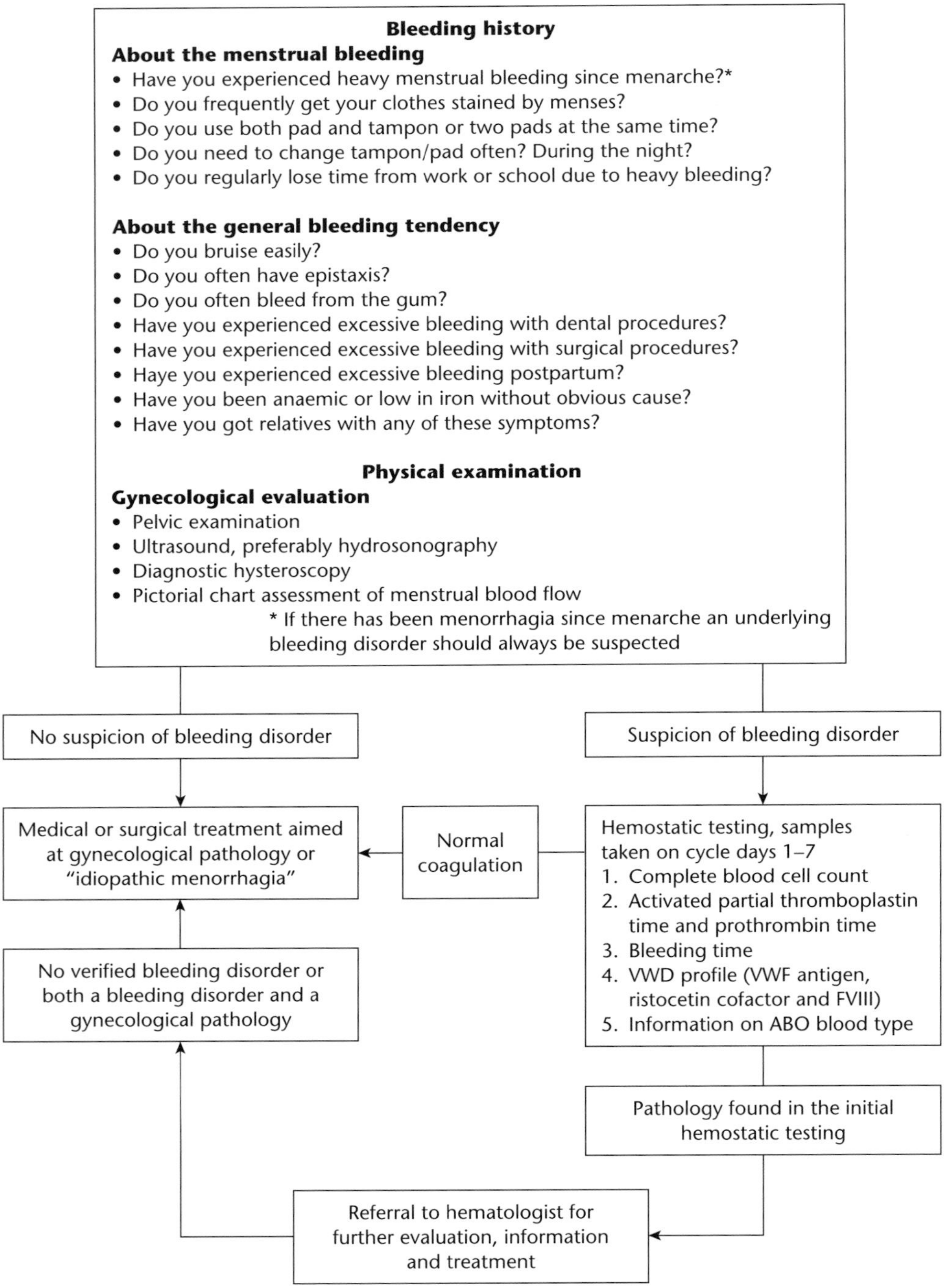

Bleeding history

About the menstrual bleeding
- Have you experienced heavy menstrual bleeding since menarche?*
- Do you frequently get your clothes stained by menses?
- Do you use both pad and tampon or two pads at the same time?
- Do you need to change tampon/pad often? During the night?
- Do you regularly lose time from work or school due to heavy bleeding?

About the general bleeding tendency
- Do you bruise easily?
- Do you often have epistaxis?
- Do you often bleed from the gum?
- Have you experienced excessive bleeding with dental procedures?
- Have you experienced excessive bleeding with surgical procedures?
- Have you experienced excessive bleeding postpartum?
- Have you been anaemic or low in iron without obvious cause?
- Have you got relatives with any of these symptoms?

Physical examination

Gynecological evaluation
- Pelvic examination
- Ultrasound, preferably hydrosonography
- Diagnostic hysteroscopy
- Pictorial chart assessment of menstrual blood flow

* If there has been menorrhagia since menarche an underlying bleeding disorder should always be suspected

---

No suspicion of bleeding disorder

Suspicion of bleeding disorder

Medical or surgical treatment aimed at gynecological pathology or "idiopathic menorrhagia"

Normal coagulation

Hemostatic testing, samples taken on cycle days 1–7
1. Complete blood cell count
2. Activated partial thromboplastin time and prothrombin time
3. Bleeding time
4. VWD profile (VWF antigen, ristocetin cofactor and FVIII)
5. Information on ABO blood type

No verified bleeding disorder or both a bleeding disorder and a gynecological pathology

Pathology found in the initial hemostatic testing

Referral to hematologist for further evaluation, information and treatment

Fig. 2.5 Extended examination on women with menorrhagia where initial examination has indicated the possibility of a pathologically increased bleeding tendency as a sole or contributing cause. VWD, von Willebrand disease; VWF, von Willebrand factor.

[118]. It is reported that in 25–70% [119, 120] of cases, menorrhagia and dysmenorrhea are the indications for this major surgery. More than a quarter of the US female population undergoes hysterectomy before age 60 years [121]. Even if hysterectomy effectively cures the symptoms of menorrhagia, it can leave the patient with an underlying cause untreated. Furthermore, hysterectomy is accompanied by significant morbidity and even mortality [122]. Different methods for endometrial ablation have evolved over the past 20 years, and probably to some extent reduced the use of hysterectomy in the treatment of menorrhagia.

Endometrial destruction Irreversible endometrial ablation is achieved through several methods. The methods include the traditional hysteroscopic transcervical resection (TCRE) and more recently non-hysteroscopic techniques such as thermal balloon hydrothermal ablation (TBA), cryotherapy and microwave ablation. Endometrial ablation is usually used as second-line therapy in patients for whom medical treatment is not successful or not suitable, especially those with a high surgical risk. TRCE and TBA are the most commonly used techniques and are equally and highly efficient [123], but after 4 years the difference from medically treated patients is small [124].

Transcervical myomectomy Hysteroscopic resection of myomas (TCRM) that are accessible from the uterine cavity (i.e., submucosal fibroids) is an efficient method to reduce MBL without performing a full-scale hysterectomy [125]. However, 20–30% of these patients will undergo an additional operation within 3 years. Risk factors for repeated operations are a large uterus, multiple myomas and a disadvantageous location of the myomas [126].

Medical treatment of menorrhagia
Medical treatment of menorrhagia can be divided into hormonal and non-hormonal treatment. The medical treatments are with some exceptions administered orally. Exceptions are the hormone-containing intrauterine system (IUS) and combined contraceptives, either transdermally or vaginally. It is also possible but uncommon, because of poor cycle control, to treat menorrhagia by administering progesterones parenterally, e.g., by injections or implants. However, improved cycle control has been reported when continuous progesterone is combined with intermittent antiprogesterone treatment[127, 128]. This may provide an alternative when contraception is also desired. The four most effective and best accepted medical treatments are listed in Table 2.2.

Hormonal treatment of menorrhagia

Intrauterine progesterone compounds The levonorgestrel-containing intrauterine system (LNG-IUS) Mirena/Levonova is the most effective medical treatment for menorrhagia [129]. Its action is to reduce the endometrial growth by continuous release of levonorgestrel, 20 μg/24 hours. The device lasts for 5 years. It reduces MBL by up to 96% [130–132] and induces amenorrhea in 20% of users. The LNG-IUS is also a highly efficient contraceptive with a pearl index of 0.09–0.18 [133, 134]. The most common reason

Table 2.2 Medical treatment of menorrhagia

Most effective medical treatments for pure menorrhagia		
Therapy	Reduction on MBL (%)	Side-effects
Intrauterine levonorgestrel	90–96	Irregular bleeding
Combined oral contraceptives	43	VTE, breast tenderness, nausea, weight gain
Antifibrinolytics	50–53	Gastrointestinal side-effects (nausea, stomach ache, diarrhea)
NSAIDs	25–47	Gastrointestinal side-effects (peptic ulcer). Increased bleeding due to undiagnosed bleeding disorder

MBL, menstrual blood loss; NSAIDs, non-steroidal anti-inflammatory drugs; VTE, venous thromboembolism.

for discontinuation of treatment is bleeding irregularities, often during the first 3 months of treatment. Discontinuation rate can be reduced with thorough pretreatment counseling.

Combined contraceptives Combined contraceptive hormones, containing both estrogen and a progestagen, reduce MBL by inducing regular shedding of a thinner endometrium and inhibiting ovulation. The average effect of combined oral contraceptives (COCs) on MBL is a reduction of approximately 43% [135]. The most serious side-effect is venous thromboembolism (VTE), the incidence being approximately doubled in otherwise healthy users [136]. The development of combined contraceptives administered dermally or vaginally has further broadened their use.

By induction of "extended cycles," i.e., treatment without discontinuation for 3 months or more, the reduction in MBL has further improved [137]. The effect depends on the cycle design but amenorrhea for up to 12 months can be achieved. One drawback is uncontrolled breakthrough bleeding if the cycle length is too long.

Oral progesterone compounds Cyclical treatment with oral progesterones can have a certain effect on MBL in women with anovulatory bleeding disturbances. Pure menorrhagia however is normally not treated with cyclical oral progesterones. To achieve an effect it is necessary to prolong the treatment period to 22 days per cycle, which can give a reduction of up to 87% on MBL [132]. Owing to side-effects, only one-quarter of the treated patients want to continue treatment after 3 months.

Gonadotropin-releasing hormone agonists GnRH agonists induce anovulation and reduce MBL, often amenorrhea. It is routinely used in the treatment of endometriosis and as pretreatment before some types of uterine surgery, such as TCRM, TCRE, or abdominal myomectomy. However the treatments have side-effects associated with hypoestrogenicity, such as vaginal dryness and hot flushes [138], and treatment is limited to 6 months due to the risk of excessive bone demineralization.

Androgens Danazol is an androgenic substance that reduces MBL by up to 80% [139] by its action on the hypothalamic–pituitary–ovarian axis suppressing ovarian function. It also exerts a direct suppression on the endometrium and induces atrophy. However, the androgenic side-effects are severe, and notably to a large extent irreversible. As permanently changed hair growth and a deepened voice is not acceptable by women, the treatment is hardly used nowadays.

Antiprogesterone The antiprogesterone mifepristone (RU486) as well as other antigestagens are licensed and routinely used for termination of pregnancy in a number of nations worldwide. It has been shown that it is also possible to use it as a contraceptive [140], with the beneficial effect of reduced MBL. Ovulation was suppressed in 60–70% of women and 65–90% were amenorrheic. Six percent of the women experienced hot flushes during the 3-month treatment. Further studies are needed to evaluate the usefulness of mifepristone for these indications.

Non-hormonal treatment of menorrhagia

Antifibrinolytics The use of antifibrinolytic therapy in menorrhagia is based on augmented local fibrinolysis due to an increased concentration of plasminogen activator in the endometrium. Antifibrinolytic compounds displace plasminogen from the surface of fibrin, thereby preventing its activation by fibrin-bound tissue activators [141]. The clinically used fibrinolytic compounds are epsilon-aminocaproic acid (EACA, e.g., Amicar) and tranexamic acid (TA; amino-methyl-cyclohexane-carboxylic acid, AMCHA; e.g., Cyklokapron, Cyklo-F). TA, which is six to eight times more potent than EACA [142], is associated with fewer side-effects and thus a better treatment option.

TA reduces menstrual blood loss dose dependently up to 50–53% [143, 144]. Its use is widespread mainly in the Scandinavian countries. Although it is an efficient treatment, it has until recently been one of the least frequently prescribed therapies in the United Kingdom and it is not used for treatment of menorrhagia in primary care in the USA. In the USA a study has been performed to evaluate the effect and improvement in the QoL with a sustained-release formulation of TA. This earlier reluctance to prescribe antifibrinolytics may be due to possible side-effects of the drugs. As these medications slow the breakdown of clots, there has been concern that antifibrinolytic agents may be associated with an increased risk of

VTE. However, studies in Sweden [145, 146], as well as international studies [147], have shown that the incidence of thrombosis in women treated with TA is comparable with the spontaneous frequency of thrombosis in untreated women. There are some common but less severe side-effects. Gastrointestinal side-effects domin-ate, e.g., nausea, abdominal pain, and diarrhea. This is related to relatively poor gastrointestinal absorption, giving the drug a bioavailability of 35%. Gastrointes-tinal side-effects are the most common reason for discontinuing treatment and a main reason for reducing the dose, resulting in reduced effect. It is also the rationale for developing sustained-release for-mulations. A prodrug of TA with an improved uptake and bioavailability has also been studied but has never been developed for the market, despite promising preliminary results [148].

NSAIDs Individual NSAIDs used for the treatment of heavy menstrual bleeding include mefenamic acid, naproxen, ibuprofen, flurbiprofen, meclofenamic acid, diclofenac, indomethacin, and acetylsalicylic acid. Studies have not been able to show a consistent difference in clinical efficacy between individual prostaglandin inhibitors, although there are individual women who seem to respond well to one agent but less well to another. The range in effect on reduced MBL with NSAIDs is from 25% to 47%, depending on the agent and the dosage used [149, 150]. The main side-effect of NSAIDs is gastrointestinal symptoms and they increase the risk of peptic ulceration. In individuals with reduced platelet function or a hemorrhagic diathesis such as mild VWD and platelet dyusfunction, NSAIDs increase the risk of bleeding because of their antiplatelet effect.

Desmopressin With increased awareness of the high prevalence of bleeding disorders in women with menorrhagia there is a need for new therapeutic tools: effect-ive, harmless medical treatment aiming at correcting the underlying cause of menorrhagia. Desmopressin (DDAVP, 1-desamino-8-D-arginine vasopressin) is a treatment option that has been used for patients with hemophilia A and mild VWD since the early 1980s. Desmopressin is a synthetic analog of the antidiuretic hormone vasopressin. It releases von Willebrand factor (VWF) from the endothelium and increases the level in circulation [151–153]. It also increases plasma concentrations of coagulation FVIII. Furthermore, there is an increase in platelet adhesiveness. The maximal hemostatic effect is achieved with a dosage of 0.3 µg/kg intravenously [152]. Intranasal administration of 300 µg desmopressin by nasal spray (Octostim) gives a slightly lower response and is comparable to 0.2 µg/kg intravenously [152, 154, 155]. The intravenous route (0.3 µg/kg) is used mostly in connection with surgery or large bleedings, whereas the intranasal spray (300 µg) is used for home treatment, for bleedings such as epistaxis or menorrhagia, after minor trauma, or as cover for tooth extractions or minor surgery.

Two articles have reported a positive effect of desmopressin on menorrhagia given to women without a known bleeding disorder [156, 157]. These studies showed that nasal desmopressin might be a possible complement in the treatment of menorrhagia. Further studies are needed to evaluate efficacy, optimal dosage, and safety.

Further discussion on the treatment of menorrhagia in women with different bleeding disorders is found in Chapters 3–7.

References

1 Fraser IS. Regulating menstrual bleeding. A prime function of progesterone. *J Reprod Med* 1999; **44** (2 Suppl): 158–164.

2 Short RV (ed). *Oestrous and menstrual cycles*. Cambridge: Cambridge University Press, 1984.

3 Gondos B, Bhiraleus P, Hobel CJ. Ultrastructural observations on germ cells in human fetal ovaries. *Am J Obstet Gynecol* 1971; **110**: 644–652.

4 Peters H, Byskov AG, Grinsted J. Follicular growth in fetal and prepubertal ovaries of humans and other primates. *Clin Endocrinol Metab* 1978; **7**: 469–485.

5 Penny R, Olambiwonnu NO, Frasier SD. Episodic fluctuations of serum gonadotropins in pre- and postpubertal girls and boys. *J Clin Endocrinol Metab* 1977; **45** (2): 307–311.

6 Apter D, Vihko R. Serum pregnenolone, progesterone, 17-hydroxyprogesterone, testosterone and 5 alpha-dihydrotestosterone during female puberty. *J Clin Endocrinol Metab* 1977; **45** (5): 1039–1048.

7 Pache TD, Wladimiroff JW, de Jong FH, *et al*. Growth patterns of nondominant ovarian follicles during the normal menstrual cycle. *Fertil Steril* 1990; **54**: 638–642.

8 Jabbour HN, Kelly RW, Fraser HM, Critchley HO. Endocrine regulation of menstruation. *Endocrine Rev* 2006; **27** (1): 17–46.

9 Corner GW, Allen WM. Physiology of the corpus luteum. II. Production of a special uterine reaction (progestational proliferation) by extracts of the corpus luteum. *Am J Physiol* 1929; **88**: 326–339.

10 Markee JE. Menstruation in intraocular endometrial transplants in the rhesus monkey. Contribution to *Embryology, Carnegie Institute of Washington* 1940; **28**: 219–308.

11 Hisaw FL, Hisaw FLJ. Action of estrogen and progesterone on the reproductive tract of lower primates. In: Young WC (ed.). *Sex and internal secretions*. Baltimore, MD: Williams and Wilkins, 1961: 556–568.

12 Finn CA. Implantation, menstruation and inflammation. *Biol Rev Camb Philos Soc* 1986; **61**: 313–328.

13 Kelly RW. Pregnancy maintenance and parturition: the role of prostaglandin in manipulating the immune and inflammatory response. *Endocr Rev* 1994; **15**: 684–706.

14 Kelly RW, King AE, Critchley HO. Cytokine control in human endometrium. *Reproduction* 2001; **121** (1): 3–19.

15 Salamonsen LA, Woolley DE. Menstruation: induction by matrix metalloproteinases and inflammatory cells. *J Reprod Immunol* 1999; **44** (1–2): 1–27.

16 Critchley HO, Kelly RW, Brenner RM, Baird DT. The endocrinology of menstruation – a role for the immune system. *Clin Endocrinol* 2001; **55**: 701–710.

17 Kelly RW, King AE, Critchley HO. Inflammatory mediators and endometrial function – focus on the perivascular cell. *J Reprod Immunol* 2002; **57** (1–2): 81–93.

18 Goffin F, Munaut C, Frankenne F, *et al.* Expression pattern of metalloproteinases and tissue inhibitors of matrix-metalloproteinases in cycling human endometrium. *Biol Reprod* 2003; **69**: 976–984.

19 Hickey M, Fraser I. Human uterine vascular structures in normal and diseased states. *Microsc Res Tech* 2003; **60**: 377–389.

20 Jones RL, Kelly RW, Critchley HO. Chemokine and cyclooxygenase-2 expression in human endometrium coincides with leukocyte accumulation. *Human Reprod* 1997; **12**: 1300–1306.

21 Clarke CL, Sutherland RL. Progestin regulation of cellular proliferation. *Endocr Rev* 1990; **11** (2): 266–301.

22 Majewska MD, Harrison NL, Schwartz RD, *et al.* Steroid hormone metabolites are barbiturate-like modulators of the GABA receptor. *Science* 1986; **232**: 1004–1007.

23 Perrot-Applanat M, Deng M, Fernandez H, *et al.* Immunohistochemical localization of estradiol and progesterone receptors in human uterus throughout pregnancy: expression in endometrial blood vessels. *J Clin Endocrinol Metab* 1994; **78** (1): 216–224.

24 Kohnen G, Campbell S, Jeffers MD, Cameron IT. Spatially regulated differentiation of endometrial vascular smooth muscle cells. *Human Reprod* 2000; **15** (2): 284–292.

25 Critchley HO, Brenner RM, Henderson TA, *et al.* Estrogen receptor beta, but not estrogen receptor alpha, is present in the vascular endothelium of the human and nonhuman primate endometrium. *J Clin Endocrinol Metab* 2001; **86**: 1370–1378.

26 Herkert O, Kuhl H, Sandow J, *et al.* Sex steroids used in hormonal treatment increase vascular procoagulant activity by inducing thrombin receptor (PAR-1) expression: role of the glucocorticoid receptor. *Circulation* 2001; **104**: 2826–2831.

27 Edlund M, Andersson E, Fried G. Progesterone withdrawal causes endothelin release from cultured human uterine microvascular endothelial cells. *Human Reprod* 2004; **19**: 1272–1280.

28 Hague S, Oehler MK, MacKenzie IZ, *et al.* Protease activated receptor-1 is down regulated by levonorgestrel in endometrial stromal cells. *Angiogenesis* 2002; **5** (1–2): 93–98.

29 Henrikson KP, Jazin EE, Greenwood JA, Dickerman HW. Prothrombin levels are increased in the estrogen-treated immature rat uterus. *Endocrinology* 1990; **126** (1): 167–175.

30 Henrikson KP. Thrombin as a hormonally regulated growth factor in estrogen-responsive tissue. *Semin Thromb Hemost* 1992; **18** (1): 53–9.

31 Henrikson KP, Hall ES, Lin Y. Cellular localization of tissue factor and prothrombin in the estrogen-treated immature rat uterus. *Biol Reprod* 1994; **50**: 1145–1150.

32 Eto M, Barandier C, Rathgeb L, *et al.* Thrombin suppresses endothelial nitric oxide synthase and upregulates endothelin-converting enzyme-1 expression by distinct pathways: role of Rho/ROCK and mitogen-activated protein kinase. *Circ Res* 2001; **89**: 583–590.

33 Ohlstein EH, Storer BL. Oxyhemoglobin stimulation of endothelin production in cultured endothelial cells. *J Neurosurg* 1992; **77** (2): 274–278.

34 Yanagisawa M, Kurihara H, Kimura S, *et al.* A novel potent vasoconstrictor peptide produced by vascular endothelial cells. *Nature* 1988; **332**: 411–415.

35 Fried G, Samuelson U. Endothelin and neuropeptide Y are vasoconstrictors in human uterine blood vessels. *Am J Obstet Gynecol* 1991; **164**: 1330–1336.

36 Ekström P, Alm P, Åkerlund M. Differences in vasomotor responses between main stem and smaller branches of the human uterine artery. *Acta Obstet Gynecol Scand* 1991; **70**: 429–433.

37 Schatz F, Papp C, Aigner S, *et al.* Biological mechanisms underlying the clinical effects of RU 486: modulation of cultured endometrial stromal cell stromelysin-1 and

prolactin expression. *J Clin Endocrinol Metab* 1997; **82** (1): 188–193.

38 Lockwood CJ, Krikun G, Hausknecht VA, *et al.* Matrix metalloproteinase and matrix metalloproteinase inhibitor expression in endometrial stromal cells during progestin-initiated decidualization and menstruation-related progestin withdrawal. *Endocrinology* 1998; **139**: 4607–4613.

39 Hampton AL, Salamonsen LA. Expression of messenger ribonucleic acid encoding matrix metalloproteinases and their tissue inhibitors is related to menstruation. *J Endocrinol* 1994; **141** (1): R1–3.

40 Rudolph-Owen LA, Slayden OD, Matrisian LM, Brenner RM. Matrix metalloproteinase expression in Macaca mulatta endometrium: evidence for zone-specific regulatory tissue gradients. *Biol Reprod* 1998; **59**: 1349–1359.

41 Zhang J, Salamonsen LA. In vivo evidence for active matrix metalloproteinases in human endometrium supports their role in tissue breakdown at menstruation. *J Clin Endocrinol Metab* 2002; **87**: 2346–2351.

42 Chegini N, Rhoton-Vlasak A, Williams RS. Expression of matrix metalloproteinase-26 and tissue inhibitor of matrix metalloproteinase-3 and -4 in endometrium throughout the normal menstrual cycle and alteration in users of levonorgestrel implants who experience irregular uterine bleeding. *Fertil Steril* 2003; **80**: 564–570.

43 Vincent AJ, Zhang J, Ostor A, *et al.* Decreased tissue inhibitor of metalloproteinase in the endometrium of women using depot medroxyprogesterone acetate: a role for altered endometrial matrix metalloproteinase/tissue inhibitor of metalloproteinase balance in the pathogenesis of abnormal uterine bleeding? *Hum Reprod* 2002; **17**: 1189–1198.

44 Cornet PB, Picquet C, Lemoine P, *et al.* Regulation and function of LEFTY-A/EBAF in the human endometrium. mRNA expression during the menstrual cycle, control by progesterone, and effect on matrix metalloproteinases. *J Biol Chem* 2002; **277**: 42496–42504.

45 Kothapalli R, Buyuksal I, Wu SQ, *et al.* Detection of ebaf, a novel human gene of the transforming growth factor beta superfamily association of gene expression with endometrial bleeding. *J Clin Invest* 1997; **99**: 2342–2350.

46 Zetter BR, Antoniades HN. Stimulation of human vascular endothelial cell growth by a platelet-derived growth factor and thrombin. *J Supramol Struct* 1979; **11**: 361–370.

47 Asselin E, Fortier MA. Influence of thrombin on proliferation and prostaglandin production in cultured bovine endometrial cells. *J Cell Physiol* 1996; **168**: 600–607.

48 Klein-Soyer C, Duhamel-Clerin E, Ravanat C, *et al.* PF4 inhibits thrombin-stimulated MMP-1 and MMP-3 metalloproteinase expression in human vascular endothelial cells. *C R Acad Sci III* 1997; **320**: 857–868.

49 Fernandez-Patron C, Martinez-Cuesta MA, Salas E, *et al.* Differential regulation of platelet aggregation by matrix metalloproteinases-9 and -2. *Thromb Haemost* 1999; **82**: 1730–1735.

50 Haslinger B, Mandl-Weber S, Sitter T. Thrombin suppresses matrix metalloproteinase 2 activity and increases tissue inhibitor of metalloproteinase 1 synthesis in cultured human peritoneal mesothelial cells. *Perit Dial Int* 2000; **20**: 778–783.

51 Rosen T, Schatz F, Kuczynski E, *et al.* Thrombin-enhanced matrix metalloproteinase-1 expression: a mechanism linking placental abruption with premature rupture of the membranes. *J Matern Fetal Neonatal Med* 2002; **11** (1): 11–17.

52 Loke YW, King A. Immunology of human placental implantation: clinical implications of our current understanding. *Mol Med Today* 1997; **3** (4): 153–159.

53 Salamonsen LA, Zhang J, Brasted M. Leukocyte networks and human endometrial remodelling. *J Reprod Immunol* 2002; **57** (1–2): 95–108.

54 Critchley HO, Kelly RW, Kooy J. Perivascular location of a chemokine interleukin-8 in human endometrium: a preliminary report. *Hum Reprod* 1994; **9**: 1406–1409.

55 Critchley HO, Jones RL, Lea RG, *et al.* Role of inflammatory mediators in human endometrium during progesterone withdrawal and early pregnancy. *J Clin Endocrinol Metab* 1999; **84** (1): 240–248.

56 Brännström M, Fridén BE, Jasper M, Norman RJ. Variations in peripheral blood levels of immunoreactive tumor necrosis factor alpha (TNFalpha) throughout the menstrual cycle and secretion of TNFalpha from the human corpus luteum. *Eur J Obstet Gynecol Reprod Biol* 1999; **83** (2): 213–217.

57 Cork BA, Tuckerman EM, Li TC, Laird SM. Expression of interleukin (IL)-11 receptor by the human endometrium in vivo and effects of IL-11, IL-6 and LIF on the production of MMP and cytokines by human endometrial cells in vitro. *Mol Hum Reprod* 2002; **8**: 841–848.

58 Fraser IS, Critchley HO, Munro MG, Broder M. A process designed to lead to international agreement on terminologies and definitions used to describe abnormalities of menstrual bleeding. *Fertil Steril* 2007; **87**: 466–476.

59 Hallberg L, Högdahl AM, Nilsson L, Rybo G. Menstrual blood loss: a population study. *Acta Obstet Gynecol Scand* 1966; **45**: 25–56.

60 Cole SK, Billewicz WZ, Thomson AM. Sources of variation in menstrual blood loss. *J Obstet Gynaecol Br Commonw* 1971; **78**: 933–939.

61 Janssen CA, Scholten PC, Heintz AP. Reconsidering menorrhagia in gynecological practice. Is a 30-year-old definition still valid? *Eur J Obstet Gynecol Reprod Biol* 1998; **78** (1): 69–72.

62 Rybo G. Clinical and experimental studies on menstrual blood loss. *Acta Obstet Gynecol Scand* 1966; **45**: 1–23.

63 Vihko KK, Raitala R, Taina E. Endometrial thermoablation for treatment of menorrhagia: comparison of two methods in outpatient setting. *Acta Obstet Gynecol Scand* 2003; **82**: 269–274.

64 Oehler MK, Rees MC. Menorrhagia: an update. *Acta Obstet Gynecol Scand* 2003; **82**: 405–422.

65 van Eijkeren MA, Christiaens GH, Scholten PC, Sixma JJ. Menorrhagia. Current drug treatment concepts. *Drugs* 1992; **43**: 201–209.

66 Rees MC. Role of menstrual blood loss measurements in management of complaints of excessive menstrual bleeding. *Br J Obstet Gynaecol* 1991; **98**: 327–328.

67 Edlund M, Magnusson C, von Schoultz B. Quality of life: a Swedish survey of 2200 women. In: Smith SK (ed.). *Dysfunctional uterine bleeding*. London: The Royal Society of Medicine Press Limited, 1994: 36–37.

68 Gannon MJ, Day P, Hammadieh N, Johnson N. A new method for measuring menstrual blood loss and its use in screening women before endometrial ablation. *Br J Obstet Gynaecol* 1996; **103**: 1029–1033.

69 Jenkinson C, Wright L, Coulter A. Criterion validity and reliability of the SF-36 in a population sample. *Qual Life Res* 1994; **3** (1): 7–12.

70 Sullivan M, Karlsson J. The Swedish SF-36 Health Survey III. Evaluation of criterion-based validity: results from normative population. *J Clin Epidemiol* 1998; **51**: 1105–1113.

71 Clark TJ, Khan KS, Foon R, et al. Quality of life instruments in studies of menorrhagia: a systematic review. *Eur J Obstet Gynecol Reprod Biol* 2002; **104** (2): 96–104.

72 Ruta DA, Garratt AM, Chadha YC, et al. Assessment of patients with menorrhagia: how valid is a structured clinical history as a measure of health status? *Qual Life Res* 1995; **4** (1): 33–40.

73 Winkler UH. The effect of tranexamic acid on the quality of life of women with heavy menstrual bleeding. *Eur J Obstet Gynecol Reprod Biol* 2001; **99** (2): 238–243.

74 Haynes PJ, Hodgson H, Anderson AB, Turnbull AC. Measurement of menstrual blood loss in patients complaining of menorrhagia. *Br J Obstet Gynaecol* 1977; **84**: 763–768.

75 Chimbira TH, Anderson AB, Turnbull A. Relation between measured menstrual blood loss and patient's subjective assessment of loss, duration of bleeding, number of sanitary towels used, uterine weight and endometrial surface area. *Br J Obstet Gynaecol* 1980; **87**: 603–609.

76 Hallberg L, Nilsson L. Determination of menstrual blood loss. *Scand J Clin Lab Invest* 1964; **16**: 244–248.

77 Newton J, Barnard G, Collins W. A rapid method for measuring menstrual blood loss using automatic extraction. *Contraception* 1977; **16**: 269–282.

78 Higham JM, O'Brien PM, Shaw RW. Assessment of menstrual blood loss using a pictorial chart. *Br J Obstet Gynaecol* 1990; **97**: 734–739.

79 Janssen CA, Scholten PC, Heintz AP. A simple visual assessment technique to discriminate between menorrhagia and normal menstrual blood loss. *Obstet Gynecol* 1995; **85**: 977–982.

80 Reid PC, Coker A, Coltart R. Assessment of menstrual blood loss using a pictorial chart: a validation study. *Br J Obstet Gynaecol* 2000; **107** (3): 320–322.

81 Fraser IS, Warner P, Marantos PA. Estimating menstrual blood loss in women with normal and excessive menstrual fluid volume. *Obstet Gynecol* 2001; **98**: 806–814.

82 Clarke A, Black N, Rowe P, et al. Indications for and outcome of total abdominal hysterectomy for benign disease: a prospective cohort study. *Br J Obstet Gynaecol* 1995; **102** (8): 611–620.

83 Fraser IS, Arachchi GJ. Aetiology and investigation of menorrhagia. In: Sheth S, Sutton C (eds). *Menorrhagia*. Oxford: Isis Medical Media, 1999: 1–9.

84 Wilansky DL, Greisman B. Early hypothyroidism in patients with menorrhagia. *Am J Obstet Gynecol* 1989; **160**: 673–677.

85 Dilley A, Drews C, Miller C, et al. von Willebrand disease and other inherited bleeding disorders in women with diagnosed menorrhagia. *Obstet Gynecol* 2001; **97**: 630–636.

86 Edlund M, Blombäck M, von Schoultz B, Andersson O. On the value of menorrhagia as a predictor for coagulation disorders. *Am J Hematol* 1996; **53**: 234–238.

87 Kadir RA, Economides DL, Sabin CA, et al. Frequency of inherited bleeding disorders in women with menorrhagia. *Lancet* 1998; **351**: 485–489.

88 Kouides P, Phatak P, Sham RL, et al. The prevalence of subnormal von Willebrand Factor levels in menorrhagia patients in Rochester, NY: final analysis. *Haemophilia* 2000; **6**: 244.

89 Philipp CS, Dilley A, Miller CH, et al. Platelet functional defects in women with unexplained menorrhagia. *J Thromb Haemost* 2003; **1**: 477–484.

90 Larsson G, Milsom I, Jonasson K, et al. The long-term effects of copper surface area on menstrual blood loss and iron status in women fitted with an IUD. *Contraception* 1993; **48**: 471–480.

91 Hagenfeldt K. The role of prostaglandins and allied substances in uterine haemostasis. *Contraception* 1987; **36**: 23–35.

92 Willman EA, Collins WP, Clayton SG. Studies in the involvement of prostaglandins in uterine symptomatology and pathology. *Br J Obstet Gynaecol* 1976; **83**: 337–341.

93 Smith SK, Abel MH, Kelly RW, Baird DT. Prostaglandin synthesis in the endometrium of women with ovular dysfunctional uterine bleeding. *Br J Obstet Gynaecol* 1981; **88**: 434–442.

94 Makarainen L, Ylikorkala O. Primary and myoma-associated menorrhagia: role of prostaglandins and effects of ibuprofen. *Br J Obstet Gynaecol* 1986; **93**: 974–978.

95 Bonnar J, Sheppard BL, Dockeray CJ. The haemostatic system and dysfunctional uterine bleeding. *Res Clin Forum* 1983; **5**: 27–36.

96 Rybo G. Plasminogen activators in the endometrium. I. Methodological aspects. *Acta Obstet Gynecol Scand* 1966; **45**: 411–428.

97 Gleeson N, Devitt M, Sheppard BL, Bonnar J. Endometrial fibrinolytic enzymes in women with normal menstruation and dysfunctional uterine bleeding. *Br J Obstet Gynaecol* 1993; **100**: 768–771.

98 Bayer SR, DeCherney AH. Clinical manifestations and treatment of dysfunctional uterine bleeding. *JAMA* 1993; **269**: 1823–1828.

99 Munro MG. Dysfunctional uterine bleeding: advances in diagnosis and treatment. *Curr Opin Obstet Gynecol* 2001; **13**: 475–489.

100 Rees MC, Dunnill MS, Anderson AB, Turnbull AC. Quantitative uterine histology during the menstrual cycle in relation to measured menstrual blood loss. *Br J Obstet Gynaecol* 1984; **91**: 662–666.

101 Critchley HO, Abberton KM, Taylor NH, *et al.* Endometrial sex steroid receptor expression in women with menorrhagia. *Br J Obstet Gynaecol* 1994; **101**: 428–434.

102 Siegbahn A, Odlind V, Hedner U, Venge P. Coagulation and fibrinolysis during the normal menstrual cycle. *Ups J Med Sci* 1989; **94** (2): 137–152.

103 Middeldorp S, Meijers JC, van den Ende AE, *et al.* Effects on coagulation of levonorgestrel- and desogestrel-containing low dose oral contraceptives: a cross-over study. *Thromb Haemost* 2000; **84** (1): 4–8.

104 Salamonsen LA, Marsh MM, Findlay JK. Endometrial endothelin: regulator of uterine bleeding and endometrial repair. *Clin Exp Pharmacol Physiol* 1999; **26**: 154–157.

105 Emeis JJ, van den Eijnden-Schrauwen Y, van den Hoogen CM, *et al.* An endothelial storage granule for tissue-type plasminogen activator. *J Cell Biol* 1997; **139** (1): 245–256.

106 Casslén B, Åstedt B. Occurrence of both urokinase and tissue plasminogen activator in the human endometrium. *Contraception* 1983; **28**: 553–564.

107 Collen D. The plasminogen (fibrinolytic) system. *Thromb Haemost* 1999; **82** (2): 259–270.

108 Rybo G. Plasminogen activators in the endometrium. II. Clinical aspects. Variation in the concentration of plasminogen activators during the menstrual cycle and its relation to menstrual blood loss. *Acta Obstet Gynecol Scand* 1966; **45**: 429–450.

109 Hefnawi F, Saleh A, Kandil O, *et al.* Fibrinolytic activity of menstrual blood in normal and menorrhagic women and in women wearing the Lippes Loop and the Cu-T (200). *Int J Gynaecol Obstet* 1979; **16**: 400–407.

110 Casslén B, Åstedt B. Fibrinolytic activity of human uterine fluid. *Acta Obstet Gynecol Scand* 1981; **60** (1): 55–58.

111 Gleeson NC, Buggy F, Sheppard BL, Bonnar J. The effect of tranexamic acid on measured menstrual loss and endometrial fibrinolytic enzymes in dysfunctional uterine bleeding. *Acta Obstet Gynecol Scand* 1994; **73** (3): 274–277.

112 Azziz R. Adenomyosis: current perspectives. *Obstet Gynecol Clin North Am* 1989; **16** (1): 221–235.

113 Buttram VC, Jr., Reiter RC. Uterine leiomyomata: etiology, symptomatology, and management. *Fertil Steril* 1981; **36**: 433–445.

114 Fraser IS. Hysteroscopy and laparoscopy in women with menorrhagia. *Am J Obstet Gynecol* 1990; **162**: 1264–1269.

115 Edlund M, Blombäck M, He S. On the correlation between local fibrinolytic activity in menstrual fluid and total blood loss during menstruation and effects of desmopressin. *Blood Coagul Fibrinolysis* 2003; **14**: 593–598.

116 Blomback M, Konkle BA, Manco-Johnson MJ, *et al.* Preanalytical conditions that affect coagulation testing, including hormonal status and therapy. *J Thromb Haemost* 2007; **5**: 855–858.

117 Miller CH, Dilley AB, Drews C, *et al.* Changes in von Willebrand factor and factor VIII levels during the menstrual cycle. *Thromb Haemost* 2002; **87**: 1082–1083.

118 Lepine LA, Hillis SD, Marchbanks PA, *et al.* Hysterectomy surveillance – United States, 1980–1993. *MMWR CDC Surveill Summ* 1997; **46** (4): 1–15.

119 Makinen J, Johansson J, Tomas C, *et al.* Morbidity of 10 110 hysterectomies by type of approach. *Hum Reprod* 2001; **16**: 1473–1478.

120 Stirrat GM. Choice of treatment for menorrhagia. *Lancet* 1999; **353**: 2175–6.

121 Carlson KJ, Nichols DH, Schiff I. Indications for hysterectomy. *N Engl J Med* 1993; **328**: 856–860.

122 Wingo PA, Huezo CM, Rubin GL, *et al.* The mortality risk associated with hysterectomy. *Am J Obstet Gynecol* 1985; **152**: 803–808.

123 Lethaby A, Suckling J, Barlow D, *et al.* Hormone replacement therapy in postmenopausal women: endometrial hyperplasia and irregular bleeding. *Cochrane Database System Rev* 2004; (3): CD000402.

124 Marjoribanks J, Lethaby A, Farquhar C. Surgery versus medical therapy for heavy menstrual bleeding. *Cochrane Database System Rev* 2006; (2): CD003855.

125 Vercellini P, Zaina B, Yaylayan L, *et al.* Hysteroscopic myomectomy: long-term effects on menstrual pattern and fertility. *Obstet Gynecol* 1999; **94**: 341–347.

126 Emanuel MH, Wamsteker K, Hart AA, *et al.* Long-term results of hysteroscopic myomectomy for abnormal uterine bleeding. *Obstet Gynecol* 1999; **93**: 743–748.

127 Cheng L, Zhu H, Wang A, *et al.* Once a month administration of mifepristone improves bleeding patterns in women using subdermal contraceptive implants releasing levonorgestrel. *Hum Reprod* 2000; **15**: 1969–1972.

128 Gemzell-Danielsson K, van Heusden AM, Killick SR, *et al.* Improving cycle control in progestogen-only contraceptive pill users by intermittent treatment with a new anti-progestogen. *Hum Reprod* 2002; **17**: 2588–2593.

129 Lethaby AE, Cooke I, Rees M. Progesterone/progestogen releasing intrauterine systems versus either placebo or any other medication for heavy menstrual bleeding. *Cochrane Database System Rev* 2000; (2): CD002126.

130 Milsom I, Andersson K, Andersch B, Rybo G. A comparison of flurbiprofen, tranexamic acid, and a levonorgestrel-releasing intrauterine contraceptive device in the treatment of idiopathic menorrhagia. *Am J Obstet Gynecol* 1991; **164**: 879–883.

131 Crosignani PG, Vercellini P, Mosconi P, *et al.* Levonorgestrel-releasing intrauterine device versus hysteroscopic endometrial resection in the treatment of dysfunctional uterine bleeding. *Obstet Gynecol* 1997; **90**: 257–263.

132 Irvine GA, Campbell-Brown MB, Lumsden MA, *et al.* Randomised comparative trial of the levonorgestrel intrauterine system and norethisterone for treatment of idiopathic menorrhagia. *Br J Obstet Gynaecol* 1998; **105**: 592–598.

133 Andersson K. The levonorgestrel intrauterine system: more than a contraceptive. *Eur J Contracept Reprod Health Care* 2001; **6** (Suppl 1): 15–22.

134 Backman T, Huhtala S, Tuominen J, *et al.* Sixty thousand woman-years of experience on the levonorgestrel intrauterine system: an epidemiological survey in Finland. *Eur J Contracept Reprod Health Care* 2001; **6** (Suppl 1): 23–26.

135 Fraser IS, McCarron G. Randomized trial of 2 hormonal and 2 prostaglandin-inhibiting agents in women with a complaint of menorrhagia. *Aust N Z J Obstet Gynaecol* 1991; **31** (1): 66–70.

136 Rosendaal FR, Helmerhorst FM, Vandenbroucke JP. Oral contraceptives, hormone replacement therapy and thrombosis. *Thromb Haemost* 2001; **86**: 112–123.

137 Archer DF. Menstrual-cycle-related symptoms: a review of the rationale for continuous use of oral contraceptives. *Contraception* 2006; **74**: 359–366.

138 Thomas EJ, Okuda KJ, Thomas NM. The combination of a depot gonadotrophin releasing hormone agonist and cyclical hormone replacement therapy for dysfunctional uterine bleeding. *Br J Obstet Gynaecol* 1991; **98**: 1155–1159.

139 Dockeray CJ, Sheppard BL, Bonnar J. Comparison between mefenamic acid and danazol in the treatment of established menorrhagia. *Br J Obstet Gynaecol* 1989; **96**: 840–844.

140 Brown A, Cheng L, Lin S, Baird DT. Daily low-dose mifepristone has contraceptive potential by suppressing ovulation and menstruation: a double-blind randomized control trial of 2 and 5 mg per day for 120 days. *J Clin Endocrinol Metab* 2002; **87** (1): 63–70.

141 Wiman B, Lijnen HR, Collen D. On the specific interaction between the lysine-binding sites in plasmin and complementary sites in alpha2-antiplasmin and in fibrinogen. *Biochim Biophys Acta* 1979; **579**: 142–154.

142 Andersson L, Nilsson IM, Nilehn JE, *et al.* Experimental and clinical studies on AMCA, the antifibrinolytically active isomer of p-aminomethyl cyclohexane carboxylic acid. *Scand J Haematol* 1965; **2** (3): 230–247.

143 Andersch B, Milsom I, Rybo G. An objective evaluation of flurbiprofen and tranexamic acid in the treatment of idiopathic menorrhagia. *Acta Obstet Gynecol Scand* 1988; **67**: 645–648.

144 Higham JM, Shaw RW. Risk-benefit assessment of drugs used for the treatment of menstrual disorders. *Drug Saf* 1991; **6** (3): 183–191.

145 Rybo G. Tranexamic acid therapy effective treatment in heavy menstrual bleeding: Clinical update on safety. *TherAdv* 1991; **4**: 1–8.

146 Berntorp E, Follrud C, Lethagen S. No increased risk of venous thrombosis in women taking tranexamic acid. *Thromb Haemost* 2001; **86**: 714–715.

147 Mannucci PM. Hemostatic drugs. *N Engl J Med* 1998; **339**: 245–253.

148 Edlund M, Andersson K, Rybo G, *et al.* Reduction of menstrual blood loss in women suffering from idiopathic menorrhagia with a novel antifibrinolytic drug (Kabi 2161). *Br J Obstet Gynaecol* 1995; **102**: 913–917.

149 Fraser IS, McCarron G, Markham R, *et al*. Long-term treatment of menorrhagia with mefenamic acid. *Obstet Gynecol* 1983; **61** (1): 109–112.

150 Lethaby A, Farquhar C, Cooke I. Antifibrinolytics for heavy menstrual bleeding. *Cochrane Database System Rev* 2000; (4): CD000249.

151 Cash JD, Gader AM, da Costa J. Proceedings: The release of plasminogen activator and factor VIII to lysine vasopressin, arginine vasopressin, I-desamino-8-d-arginine vasopressin, angiotensin and oxytocin in man. *Br J Haematol* 1974; **27**: 363–364.

152 Lethagen S, Harris AS, Sjorin E, Nilsson IM. Intranasal and intravenous administration of desmopressin: effect on F VIII/vWF, pharmacokinetics and reproducibility. *Thromb Haemost* 1987; **58**: 1033–1036.

153 Mannucci PM, Åberg M, Nilsson IM, Robertsson B. Mechanism of plasminogen activator and factor VIII increase after vasoactive drugs. *Br J Haematol* 1975; **30**: 81–93.

154 Harris AS, Ohlin M, Lethagen S, Nilsson IM. Effects of concentration and volume on nasal bioavailability and biological response to desmopressin. *J Pharm Sci* 1988; **77**: 337–339.

155 Lethagen S, Rugarn P, Åberg M, Nilsson IM. Effects of desmopressin acetate (DDAVP) and dextran on hemostatic and thromboprophylactic mechanisms. *Acta Chir Scand* 1990; **156**: 597–602.

156 Edlund M, Blombäck M, Fried G. Desmopressin in the treatment of menorrhagia in women with no common coagulation factor deficiency but with prolonged bleeding time. *Blood Coagul Fibrinolysis* 2002; **13**: 225–231.

157 Mercorio F, De Simone R, Di Carlo C, *et al*. Effectiveness and mechanism of action of desmopressin in the treatment of copper intrauterine device-related menorrhagia: a pilot study. *Hum Reprod* 2003; **18**: 2319–2322.

3 Hemophilia A and hemophilia B

Christine A Lee

Inheritance

Hemophilia A and B are X-linked recessive bleeding disorders caused by a deficiency of factor VIII (FVIII) or IX (FIX) respectively. Hemophilia A and B mostly affect males, and females are carriers. Carriers have one affected chromosome and therefore the clotting factor is expected to be around 50% of normal (50–150 IU/dL). However, a wide range (22–116 IU/dL) of values has been reported [1] as a result of random inactivation of one of two X chromosomes, the process known as lyonization [2].

Carriers of hemophilia have a 50% chance of passing on the gene defect to their offspring; in each pregnancy there is a 50% chance of having an affected son or a 50% chance of having a daughter who will also be a carrier of the condition (Fig. 3.1).

The severity of the factor deficiency remains constant through generations of a kindred and thus carriers can be informed whether their risk is for severe (<1 IU/dL) or non-severe (>1 IU/dL) hemophilia according to the index case within the respective kindred.

There is a specific genetic defect or mutation causing the hemophilia in each family – this is discussed in detail in Chapter 8. Certain genetic defects carry a higher risk of inhibitor development [3] and this information can be provided for the potential carrier.

Laboratory diagnosis

Clotting factor level

The level of factor VIIIC (FVIIIC) or factor IXC (FIXC) can be measured in plasma. The normal range is 50–150 IU/dL in many laboratories, although the ISTH (International Society on Thrombosis and Haemostasis) has defined the lower limit of normal as 40 IU/dL [4].

In practice, elevation of FVIII can be caused by a number of factors including stress and exercise – this may be a complication of venipuncture in children. The proportion of females who can be diagnosed as carriers by a low clotting factor varies – an early (1962) study showed 60% [5]; in the previously quoted study it was 28% [1]; and in a more recent study 62 of 225 (35%) carriers had levels less than 40 IU/dL [6]. It is important to recognize that a carrier may have a normal clotting factor level, and the level does not correlate with the severity of hemophilia in the family.

The factor VIII activity to factor VIII-related antigen ratio

Until molecular diagnosis became possible, the mainstay of laboratory diagnosis of carriers of hemophilia A was the ratio of FVIII activity to FVIII-related antigen. This may be the only method available in less resourced countries. In a "blind" study designed to detect carriers of hemophilia, it was found that the lowest ratio in the control group was 0.61 and that 71% (24/34) of carriers had a ratio less than 0.61 [1] (Fig. 3.2). This is not applicable to carriers of hemophilia B.

Inherited Bleeding Disorders in Women, 1st edition. By CA Lee, RA Kadir and PA Kouides. Published 2009 by Blackwell Publishing, ISBN: 978-1-4051-6915-8.

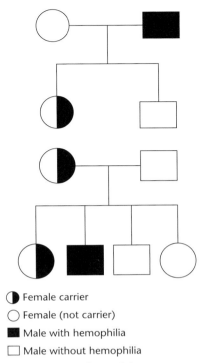

Fig. 3.1 The inheritance of hemophilia.

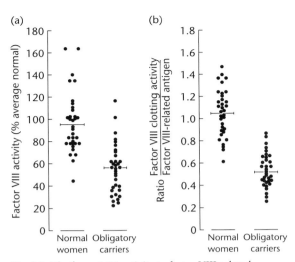

Fig. 3.2 The factor VIII activity to factor VIII-related antigen ratio. (a) Distribution of values of factor VIII activity in normal women and obligatory carriers of hemophilia. (b) Duration of values of the ratio of factor VIII activity to factor VIII-related antigen in normal women and obligatory carriers of hemophilia. Reproduced with permission from Rizza *et al.* [1].

Genetic diagnosis

It is now possible to perform genetic diagnosis (see Chapter 8). In severe hemophilia A, approximately 50% of families carry an inversion of intron 22 – a rearrangement of the long arm of the X chromosome [7] and thus it may be possible to confirm carriership without knowledge of the mutation in the index patient within a family. However, for most potential carriers it is necessary to know the mutation in the index family member and such mutations are listed on the HAMSTeRS database (http://europium.csc.mrc. ac.uk) for hemophilia A. In hemophilia B, almost every family has a unique mutation and in the UK most of these have been identified [8].

Bleeding in carriers of hemophilia

Women who are carriers of hemophilia and who have a low clotting factor level can be considered as having "mild hemophilia." It is therefore important to consider the bleeding risk of these individuals outside the context of pregnancy and the possible delivery of a hemophilic child.

The effect of heterozygous carriership on the occurrence of bleeding symptoms was investigated by use of a questionnaire in The Netherlands [6]. The median clotting factor level in carriers was 0.60 IU/mL (range 0.50–2.19) compared with 1.02 IU/mL (range 0.45–3.28) in non-carriers. It was found that the risk of bleeding from small wounds was two times higher in carriers (RR 2.2, 95% CI 1.4–3.5) and joint bleeds were reported by 8% of carriers compared with 5% of women not carrying hemophilia (RR 1.9, 95% CI 1.4–3.5). Tooth extraction had been performed in 228 carriers and 219 non-carriers, and the risk of bleeding was two times higher in the carriers (RR 2.3, 95% CI 1.5–3.40). A total of 123 carriers and 122 non-carriers underwent tonsillectomy or adenoidectomy: 24% of carriers and 13% of non-carriers reported bleeding for more than 3 hours after operation. Women with a clotting factor level <0.40 IU/mL had a three times (RR 3.3, 95% CI 0.7–5.7) increased risk of prolonged bleeding after operation compared with those with a clotting factor level of 0.60 or above.

Thus it is important that carriers of hemophilia with a lower than normal clotting factor should be issued with a card showing the level in order that appropriate treatment can be given prior to intraoperative intervention, including dental procedures. For carriers of hemophilia A treatments include tranexamic acid, DDAVP (desmopressin) and FVIII concentrate. For carriers of hemophilia B treatment includes tranexamic acid and FIX concentrate.

Genetic counseling and carrier detection

The purpose of genetic counseling is to provide the potential carrier and her parents or partner with adequate information to reach a decision regarding carrier testing and prenatal diagnosis and to provide support throughout the process [9]. Genetic counseling requires an empathetic, good communicator who has a detailed knowledge of hemophilia, genetics, molecular biology, and prenatal diagnostic procedures (Chapter 9). Counseling is a way of addressing the implication of the information that is given. It is a two-way process enabling a better understanding between the patient and healthcare worker about the full range of issues. Genetic counseling in hemophilia focuses on the medical condition (what it is, how it is treated, and how it is passed from generation to generation), personal and relationship concerns related to hemophilia, and beliefs and wishes about the person discussing possible inheritance, as well as on those who might be affected [9].

Ethical considerations include human rights, issues surrounding consent, and those relating to confidentiality. Sometimes the best interests of the person with hemophilia and the partner, sister, or child of a carrier can be in conflict – genetic counseling needs to address and consider these issues.

A framework for genetic service provision has been provided as a guideline by the UK Haemophilia Centre Doctors' Organisation (UKHCDO) [10] and this includes detailed guidance for carrier diagnosis and antenatal diagnosis which is summarized in Table 3.1.

The pedigree or family tree is the first step in carrier diagnosis. The daughter of a man with hemophilia is an obligate carrier and thus her sons have a 50% chance of having hemophilia and her daughters have a 50% chance of being a carrier. Within a family where an index patient with hemophilia has been identified, many of the females may be at risk of being carriers. However, in many countries, more than 50% of newly diagnosed cases are sporadic [11]. In the mother of a child with sporadic hemophilia there is the possibility of mosaicism, a mixture of normal and mutation-carrying cells. It is important to establish maternal carriership before pregnancy and certainly before embarking on prenatal diagnosis (Chapter 9).

Testing the carrier status of healthy children

The testing of carrier status of healthy children for recessively inherited conditions has recently been reviewed [12]. There are ethical issues about who can

Table 3.1 Counseling and consent for genetic testing in hemophilia

1	Establish that hemophilia is present in the family and determine the type and severity
2	Establish a family pedigree (tree) to exclude carriers and identify possible or definite (obligate) carriers
3	Provide a full explanation of the potential clinical effects of being a hemophilia carrier or affected male
4	Provide information about current treatment options and the implications of the condition
5	Provide a full explanation of the mode of inheritance of hemophilia
6	Discuss the rationale for identifying the genetic defect in patients with hemophilia
7	Outline the means by which carrier status is assessed
8	Discuss what is involved in genetic testing (consent, sample collection, transfer/storage of data, research projects on stored material, risk of error)
9	If appropriate, advise on the techniques for antenatal testing
10	Provide an opportunity to ask questions
11	Provide an opportunity for the individual being consulted to summarize the information that has been discussed
12	Provide a patient information sheet and an opportunity for a follow-up appointment

give consent and what is the earliest age testing should be offered.

In a statement by the United Nations Convention on the rights of the Child, it was held that any action or decision affecting this group should be in their "best interests" [13]. In the UK young people can give consent medically from the age of 16 years, but they can also give specific consent when under 16 if they are seen to have sufficient understanding and intelligence to allow them to fully understand what is being proposed – the "Gillick Competency Test" [14].

The World Health Organization (WHO) and professional organizations in the UK and the USA have largely agreed the reasons for genetically testing children. These should be to improve their medical care rather than to obtain reproductively significant information [10, 15–17]. A more flexible approach suggests that when thinking about the carrier testing of children, the health professional should recognize the dynamics and cohesion within the family [18]. A recent systematic review of guidelines and position papers has found an overall agreement in the recommendation to wait until children can give informed consent, but there were some exceptions [19].

One of the few papers to consider the age of testing by the hemophilia community itself was a survey on "the attitudes towards and beliefs about genetic testing in the hemophilia community" [20]. There were in-depth face to face interviews with 39 individuals, including men with hemophilia, female carriers, and family members. Most thought that testing was necessary for adolescent girls to determine carrier status to help prepare families for a child with hemophilia, rather than leading them to choose to terminate a pregnancy or not to have children.

Carrier diagnosis may be suggested by a low level of FVIII or FIX [1]. Clearly, because this is associated with an increased bleeding risk [6] it is recommended that the respective clotting factor is measured in young obligate carriers [10]. The ethical debate is redundant in these situations.

Diagnosis of carriership before pregnancy

It is important that carriership is diagnosed before pregnancy. The delay in diagnosis and subsequent morbidity was demonstrated in a study of 73 hemophilia patients and their mothers. Although a positive family history was present in 52 gravidae, 16 (31%), 15 of whom were carriers of non-severe hemophilia, were not aware of their carrier status at the time of delivery [21]. In the mothers who were unaware of carriership there was more frequent instrumental delivery, which is a significant risk factor for intra- or extracranial bleeding in newborn hemophilic babies [22].

Menorrhagia

Carriers of hemophilia may experience heavy menstruation with prolonged menstruation, episodes of flooding, and passage of clots [23].

Menorrhagia is defined as menstrual loss of more than 80 mL per period [24]. A pictorial blood assessment chart (PBAC) was developed to provide a practical way to assess menstrual blood loss [25] (Appendix ii).

Menstrual loss was assessed in 30 carriers of hemophilia using the PBAC. The median menstrual score was significantly higher in 113 carriers of hemophilia than in 73 age-matched control subjects. The incidence of menorrhagia was 57% compared with 29% in the age-matched control group [23].

Carriers of hemophilia may consider heavy menstruation as normal because the menorrhagia usually starts at the menarche. Other family members may also be carriers and have excessive menstrual loss; therefore, these women may not consider their menstrual loss to be greater than other women [26]. Furthermore, the issues relating to reproduction and having a hemophilic child are often of greater concern for these women. It is therefore important that women are asked about their periods, and an assessment is made using the PBAC and measuring hemoglobin and ferritin.

Heavy, prolonged, and irregular menstrual periods are frequent complaints in adolescent girls. This is likely to be due to immaturity of the hypothalamic–pituitary–ovarian axis [27]. Menstruation may be the first hemostatic challenge faced by girls who are carriers. It is therefore important to establish the clotting factor level before the onset of menarche in obligate carriers and girls with a positive family history. Plans should be made in anticipation of the possibility of acute menorrhagia at the onset of menarche if the FVIII or FIX are abnormal [28].

Treatment of menorrhagia in these patients with FVIII deficiency is discussed further in Chapter 4 (von Willebrand disease) and Chapter 7.

Treatment of menorrhagia in carriers of hemophilia A and B

Management of menorrhagia involves consideration of the age of the patient, childbearing status, and her need for contraception as well as preference in terms of perceived efficacy and side-effect profile. The therapeutic options in women who are carriers of hemophilia A and B include medical treatment, non-hormonal and hormonal, and surgical treatments.

Hemostatic therapy for carriers includes antifibrinolytic therapy (tranexamic acid), DDAVP (addressed in Chapters 2 and 7), and treatment with coagulation factors.

Clotting factor concentrate

Excessive menorrhagia in a carrier of hemophilia B (FIX deficiency) or hemophilia A (FVIII deficiency) where other therapeutic options are not possible can be controlled by monthly self-administration of the respective clotting factor concentrate. However, this is extremely rare but is more often used in severe von Willebrand disease (VWD) (Chapter 4).

Carriers of hemophilia A and B and pregnancy

Antenatal management

Serum FVIII levels have been shown to increase significantly in carriers of hemophilia A during pregnancy. Although the majority of patients will develop levels within the normal range, the rise is variable, and a small proportion may still have low levels at term [29–31]. In contrast, FIX levels do not rise in carriers of hemophilia B [29–31] (Fig. 3.3).

The risk of bleeding in early pregnancy and miscarriage is unknown in carriers of hemophilia, but there is evidence that the risk of antepartum hemorrhage – bleeding after 24 weeks' gestation – is not increased [29, 30].

Women may be exposed to various hemostatic challenges during pregnancy, including prenatal diagnostic techniques, termination of pregnancy, and spontaneous miscarriage. All of these may be complicated by excessive and prolonged hemorrhage. Therefore, prophylactic treatment with appropriate clotting factor concentrate should be considered.

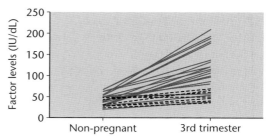

Fig. 3.3 Changes in the factor VIII (FVIII) and factor IX (FIX) levels during pregnancy in carriers of haemophilia. ———, FVIII; -------, FIX. Reproduced with permission from Chi *et al.* [31].

The FVIII level often rises to within the normal range at term, but the FIX level remains at the baseline level (Fig. 3.3); it is recommended that both FVIII and FIX levels are checked at booking in, and at 28 and 34 weeks of gestation [28]. This is particularly important in patients with low pre-pregnancy levels. Monitoring in the third trimester is essential in order to plan the management of labor and the provision of prophylactic treatment to decrease postpartum hemorrhage.

DDAVP

Administration of 1-deamino-8-arginine vasopressin (DDAVP) is generally useful for the prevention and treatment of bleeding in mild and moderate hemophilia A. However, the use during pregnancy is controversial because of the risk of DDAVP causing uterine contractions and preterm labor, but DDAVP is very specific to V2 receptors and has little effect on the uterine smooth muscle V1 receptors [32]. Desmopressin may cross the placenta and there is a potential risk of maternal and neonatal hyponatremia if given immediately before birth [33]. The use of antepartum DDAVP for the management of diabetes insipidus in a smaller dose than required for hemostatic purposes was reviewed in 53 cases and was not associated with prematurity, low birthweight, or any serious effect on maternal health or neonatal wellbeing [34]. A series of 30 women were treated safely early in the antenatal period using DDAVP [35].

DDAVP can be used in labor and the postpartum period

Clotting factor concentrates

Plasma-derived clotting factor concentrates, treated with the currently available virucidal methods, carry a negligible risk of transmitting the hepatitis B and C viruses and HIV [36]. However, they may not be effective against hepatitis A and parvovirus B19 [37] and emerging infections such as variant CJD. Parvovirus infection in pregnant women is of particular importance because it can cause severe fetal infection and hydrops fetalis. Therefore, it is recommended that recombinant FVIII and FIX should be used in pregnant carriers of hemophilia A and B [28].

Labor and delivery

A comprehensive review is given in Chapter 10.

Invasive monitoring using fetal scalp electrodes and fetal blood sampling are commonly used in labor and during delivery. Male fetuses affected with hemophilia are potentially at risk of scalp hemorrhage from the use of these techniques [38]. It is therefore recommended to avoid their use in fetuses at risk [28].

Babies with hemophilia are at risk of serious head bleeding, including cephalohematoma and intracranial hemorrhage, from the birth process (see Chapter 12). Thus, the safest method of delivery of fetuses at risk remains controversial. A survey in the USA reported that 11% of obstetricians preferred to deliver pregnant carriers of hemophilia by cesarean section [39]. In a review of 117 children with moderate to severe hemophilia born between 1970 and 1990, 23 neonatal bleedings were associated with delivery [40]. The risk of head bleeding was 3% with vaginal delivery, 64% with vacuum extraction and 15% with cesarean section. It was concluded that the risk of serious bleeding during normal vaginal delivery is small and that delivery of all fetuses at risk of hemophilia by cesarean section does not eliminate risk. In the USA it is being advised that pregnant carriers should undergo cesarean section because of the potential for litigation. However, the risk is significantly increased by the use of vacuum extraction or forceps, or after a prolonged second stage of labor and prolonged pushing [30, 40]. A recent review of the outcome of pregnancy in 53 carriers of hemophilia and 65 live births over a 10 year period showed a cesarean section rate of 47% [31]. However, there was also a rising cesarean rate in the general UK population – 10.4% in 1985, 15.5% in 1994/5, and 21.5% in 2000/01 [41]. It is inevitable that with the restrictions of the use of invasive monitoring the cesarean section rate will increase and also increasing patient demand may play a part.

Thus it is recommended that prolonged labor, especially prolonged second stage, and delivery by vacuum extraction and mid-cavity rotational forceps should be avoided in affected male fetuses whose coagulation status is unknown. Delivery should be achieved by the least traumatic method, and early recourse to cesarean section should be considered.

Third stage of labor and puerperium

Carriers of hemophilia, particularly those with low factor levels, are at risk of postpartum hemorrhage (PPH). Although the level of FVIIIC rises during pregnancy it falls to pre-pregnancy levels at an unpredictable rate postpartum. In one study there were five PPHs and a large perineal hematoma in 43% pregnancies in hemophilia carriers [33]. In a further study there was a significantly higher incidence of prolonged bleeding after delivery among hemophilia carriers (22%) than in the control group (6%) [6]. The risks of primary and secondary postpartum hemorrhage were respectively 22% and 11% in 82 pregnancies reviewed in the UK [30]. It is concluded that the maternal FVIII or FIX level has a significant influence on bleeding.

Therefore post-delivery factor levels should be checked daily and maintained above 50 U/dL for at least 3–4 days or 4–5 days if a cesarean section has been performed. Consideration should be given to treatment with tranexamic acid [28].

References

1 Rizza CR, Rhymes IL, Austen DEG, *et al*. Detection of carriers of haemophilia: a "blind" study. *Br J Haematol* 1975; **30**: 447–456.
2 Lyon MF. Sex chromatin and gene action in the mammalian X-chromosome. *Am J Hum Genet* 1962; **14**: 135–148.
3 Oldenburg J, Tuddenham EGT. Inhibitors to factor VIII-molecular basis In: Lee CA, Berntorp EE, Hoots WH (eds). *Textbook of hemophilia*. Oxford: Blackwell Science, 2005.
4 White GC, Rosendaal F, Aledort LM, *et al*. Definitions in haemophilia. Recommendation of the scientific

subcommittee on factor VIII and factor IX of the scientific and standardisation committee of the International Society on Thrombosis and Haemostasis. *Thromb Haemost* 2001; **85**: 560.

5 Nilsson IM, Blomback M, Ramgren O, von Franken I. Haemophilia in Sweden. II. Carriers of haemophilia A and B. *Acta Med Scand* 1962; **171**: 223.

6 Plug I, Mauser-Bunschoten EP, Brocker-Vriends AH, *et al.* Bleeding in carriers of hemophilia. *Blood* 2006; **108**: 52–56.

7 Antonarakis SE, Rossiter JP, Young M, *et al.* Factor VIII inversions in severe haemophilia A: results of an international consortium study. *Blood* 1995; **86**: 2206–2212.

8 Giannelli F, Green PM, Somner S. Haemophilia B. A database of point mutations and short editions and deletions. *Nucleic Acids Res* 1996; **24**: 103–118.

9 Miller R. *Genetic counselling for haemophilia.* WFH treatment monograph no 25. 2002.

10 Ludlam CA, Pasi KJ, Bolton-Maggs P, *et al.* A framework for genetic service provision for haemophilia and other inherited bleeding disorders. *Haemophilia* 2005; **11**: 145–163.

11 Ljund R, Petrini P, Nilsson IM. Diagnostic symptoms of severe and moderate haemophilia A and B – a survey of 140 cases. *Acta Paediatr Scand* 1990; **79**: 196–200.

12 Dunn NF, Miller R, Griffioen A, Lee CA. Carrier testing in haemophilia A and B: adult carriers and their partners experiences and their views on the testing of young females. *Haemophilia* 2008; **14**: 584–592.

13 The United Nations Convention on the Rights of the Child 20. xi.1989:TS 44:Cm 1976.

14 Gillick v West Norfolk and Wisbech AHA (1986).

15 World Health Organization. *Proposed international guidelines on ethical issues in medical genetics and genetic services.* Geneva: World Health Organization, 1998.

16 Working Party of the Clinical Genetics Society. The genetic testing of children. *J Med Genet* 1994; **31**: 785–797.

17 Committee on Bioethics American Academy of Pediatrics. Ethical issues with genetic testing. *Pediatrics* 2001; **107**: 1451–1455.

18 British Medical Association. *Consent, rights and choices in health care for children and young people.* London: BMJ Books, 2005.

19 Borry P, Fryns J-P, Schotsmans P, Dierickx K. Carrier testing in minors: a systematic review of guidelines position papers. *Eur J Hum Genet* 2006; **14**: 133–138.

20 Thomas S, Herbert D, Street A, *et al.* Attitudes towards beliefs about genetic testing in the haemophilia community: a qualitative study. *Haemophilia* 2007; **13**: 633–641.

21 MacLean PE, Fijnvandraat K, Beijlevelt M, Peters M. The impact of unaware carriership on the clinical presentation of haemophilia. *Haemophilia* 2004; **10**: 560–564.

22 Kulkarni R, Lusher JM, Henry RC, Kallen DJ. Current practices regarding newborn intracranial haemorrhage and obstetric care and mode of delivery of pregnant haemophilia carriers: a survey of obstetricians, neonatologists and haematologists in the United States, on behalf of National Haemophilia Foundation's Medical and Scientific Council. *Haemophilia* 1999; **5**: 410–415.

23 Kadir RA, Economides DL, Sabin CA, *et al.* Assessment of menstrual blood loss and gynaecological problems in patients with inherited bleeding disorders. *Haemophilia* 1999; **5**: 40–48.

24 Hallberg L, Hogdahl AM, Nilsson L, Rybo G. Menstrual blood loss and iron deficiency. *Acta Med Scand* 1966; **180**: 639–650.

25 Higham JM, O'Brien PM, Shaw RW. Assessment of menstrual blood loss using a pictorial chart. *Br J Obstet Gynaecol* 1990; **97**: 734–739.

26 Mauser Bunschoten MEP, van Houwelingen JC, Sjamsoedin Visser EJM, *et al.* Bleeding symptoms in carriers of haemophilia A and B. *Thromb Haemost* 1988; **59**: 349–352.

27 Falcone T, Desjardins C, Bourque J, *et al.* Dysfunctional uterine bleeding in adolescents. *J Reprod Med* 1994; **39**: 761–764.

28 Lee CA, Chi C, Pavord SR, *et al.* The obstetric and gynaecological management of women with inherited bleeding disorders – review with guidelines produced by a taskforce of UK Haemophilia Centre Doctors' Organisation. *Haemophilia* 2006; **12**: 301–336.

29 Greer IA, Lowe GD, Walker JJ, Forbes CD. Haemorrhagic problems in obstetrics and gynaecology in patients with congenital coagulopathies. *Br J Obstet Gynaecol* 1991; **98**: 909–918.

30 Kadir RA, Economides DL, Braithwaite J, *et al.* The obstetric experience of carriers of haemophilia. *Br J Obstet Gynaecol* 1997; **104**: 803–810.

31 Chi C, Lee CA, Shiltagh N, *et al.* Pregnancy in carriers of haemophilia. *Haemophilia* 2008; **14**: 56–64.

32 Mannucci PM. Desmopressin in the treatment of bleeding disorders: the first 20 years. *Blood* 1997; **90**: 2515–2521.

33 Chediak JR, Alban GM, Maxley B. von Willebrand's disease and pregnancy: management during delivery and outcome of offspring. *Am J Obstet Gynecol* 1986; **155**: 618–624.

34 Ray JG. DDAVP use during pregnancy: an analysis of its safety for mother and child. *Obstet Gynecol Surv* 1998; **53**: 450–455.

35 Mannucci PM. Use of desmopressin (DDAVP) during early pregnancy in factor-VIII deficient women. *Blood* 2005; **105**: 3382.

36 Mannucci PM. The choice of plasma-derived clotting factor concentrates. *Baillieres Clin Haematol* 1996; **9**: 273–290.

37 Yee TT, Cohen BJ, Pasi KJ, Lee CA. Transmission of symptomatic parvovirus B19 infection by clotting factor concentrate. *Br J Haematol* 1996; **93**: 457–459.

38 Kulkarni R, Lusher JM. Intracranial and extracranial hemorrhages in newborns with haemophilia: a review of the literature. *J Pediatr Hematol Oncol* 1999; **21**: 289–295.

39 Kulkarni R, Lusher JM, Henry RC, Kallen DJ. Current practices regarding newborn intracranial hemorrhage and obstetrical care and mode of delivery of pregnant haemophilia carriers: a survey of obstetricians neonatologists and haematologists in the United States, on behalf of the National Hemophilia Foundation's Medical Scientific Advisory Council. *Haemophilia* 1999; **5**: 410–415.

40 Ljund R, Lindgren AC, Petrini P, Tengborn L. Normal vaginal delivery is to be recommended haemophilia carrier gravidae. *Acta Paediatr* 1994; **83**: 609–611.

41 Royal College of Obstetricians and Gynaecologists Clinical Effectiveness Support Unit. *National sentinel audit report*. London: RCOG Press, 2001.

4 von Willebrand disease

Peter A Kouides

Introduction

In 1926, Erik von Willebrand [1] reported a kindred with mucocutaneous bleeding symptoms. The index case in the kindred was a female who had multiple mucocutaneous symptoms. She bled to death at the time of her fourth menstrual period. Furthermore, 16 of the 23 affected members of this kindred were females. More recently many studies have clearly documented the obstetrical and gynecological morbidity in females with von Willebrand disease (VWD). This is summarized in Fig. 4.1. The majority of these patients will develop menorrhagia (≥80%) and up to a half have undergone surgical intervention such as hysterectomy for control of the menorrhagia [2, 3]. In addition, persistent menorrhagia clearly impairs quality of life compared with women in the normal population [3–6]. This chapter will discuss the epidemiology and clinical presentation of VWD in women. Therapy with hemostatic agents will be discussed in this chapter whereas gynecological management will be discussed in Chapter 7. Postpartum hemorrhage related to VWD will be discussed in Chapter 10.

Epidemiology of von Willebrand disease in women

Menorrhagia is a public health challenge [7]. Insurance data and healthcare services research estimate

Inherited Bleeding Disorders in Women, 1st edition. By CA Lee, RA Kadir and PA Kouides. Published 2009 by Blackwell Publishing, ISBN: 978-1-4051-6915-8.

that at least 5–10% of women of reproductive age will seek medical attention for menorrhagia [8, 9]. The World Health Organization estimates that 18 million women worldwide have menorrhagia [10]. Within a year of seeking medical attention, such a patient has up to a 50% probability of undergoing a surgical intervention [11]. Historically, the causes of menorrhagia have focused on gynecological and endocrinological conditions in terms of organic pathology (primarily fibroids) and anovulation/hormonal imbalance with remaining etiologies being systemic disorders such as hypothyroidism [12] and iatrogenic causes including intrauterine devices and use of anticoagulants [9]. It has only been in the past decade that underlying disorders of hemostasis such as VWD have been clearly recognized as an important etiologic/contributory factor [7].

A systematic review [13] has summarized the overall prevalence of the laboratory diagnosis of VWD in women presenting with menorrhagia to be 13% (95% CI 11–15.6%) of a total of 988 women in 11 studies (see Fig. 4.2). However, this does not represent a worldwide prevalence of VWD since these studies have been primarily from Europe and North America. Recently, though, a well-conducted prevalence study for VWD and other hemostatic disorders in women presenting with menorrhagia ($n = 120$) in India reported a similar prevalence of 11.6% [14].

Only two studies [15, 16] necessitated the "gold standard" measurement of increased menstrual flow, spectrophotometric measurement of menstrual blood loss being defined as more than 80 mL, whereas the largest study [17] employed a pictorial blood assessment chart (PBAC) measurement of menstrual blood

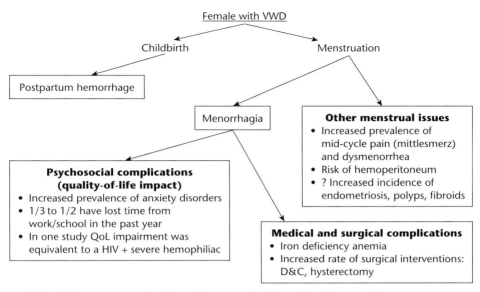

Fig. 4.1 von Willebrand disease (VWD)-related complications in females. D&C, dilation and curettage.

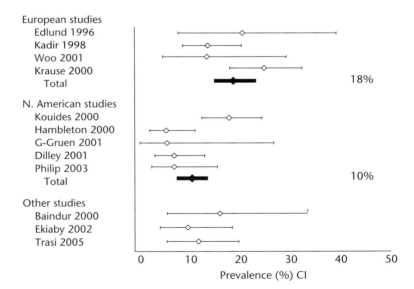

Fig. 4.2 Prevalence of von Willebrand disease in women presenting with menorrhagia.

loss that has been shown to have a sensitivity and specificity of approximately 85% for a score of ≥100 [18]. Furthermore, there have been numerous differences in the design of laboratory testing in these various studies wherein two of the studies did not adjust for the ABO type [15, 16]. There were also differences between these studies in terms of when testing for VWD was carried out in relation to the menstrual cycle [17]. In both the Swedish [16] and the London [17] studies, testing was done no later than day 7 of menses. The least interindividual variation may occur on days 5–7 as reported in the Swedish study [16]. Despite these numerous differences in clinical design and laboratory testing, these studies have established

Table 4.1 Prevalence of published studies of von Willebrand disease in adolescent menorrhagia

Study	n	Setting	von Willebrand factor deficiency (%)
Mikhail et al. 2007 [25]	61	Outpatient hematology clinic	36
Jayasinghe et al. 2005 [24]	106	Inpatient and outpatient gynecology department	5
Philipp et al. 2005 [89]	25	Outpatient primary care clinic	4
Bevan et al. 2001 [21]	71	Emergency department, urgent care and inpatient	8
Oral et al. 2002 [23]	25	Inpatient	8
Smith et al. 1998 [22]	46	Inpatient	11
Claessens et al. 1981 [20]	59	Inpatient	5

that a substantial proportion of women presenting with menorrhagia without an obvious gynecological abnormality had a laboratory diagnosis of VWD. However, screening of all women with menorrhagia is not feasible. In general, the probability of VWD in a woman with menorrhagia would be highest the younger the patient and if there are multiple mucocutaneous bleeding symptoms. It should be pointed out that the prevalence studies of VWD and menorrhagia have involved a relatively "older" population of women with the mean age of the diagnosis of VWD being approximately 38 years. However, VWF levels rise with increasing age [19] as discussed further in this chapter under "Other laboratory issues."

There have been few prevalence studies for an underlying bleeding disorder in the adolescent menorrhagia population [20–24] and most of these studies have focused on the inpatient and emergency setting. Three studies included adolescents admitted to the hospital for acute menorrhagia [21, 23, 24]. In another study the records of adolescent females with menorrhagia presenting to the emergency department for urgent care or who were admitted to the medical wards were retrospectively reviewed [22]. A larger cross-sectional prevalence study of 25 adolescent women aged 13–55 years presenting in the primary care setting with the diagnosis of menorrhagia has been reported [26]. A further study included 106 adolescents in an inpatient and outpatient gynecology tertiary care setting [24]. The mean prevalence of VWD was 8% from a total of 332 adolescents. In 61 adolescents referred for hemostasis evaluation to a hemophilia treatment center, a prevalence of VWD of 36% (22/61) (95% CI 24–49%) was found [25].

Table 4.1 reports the prevalence of VWD in the adolescent population.

The VWF level increases approximately 15 IU (international units) per decade [20] and therefore bleeding symptoms, including menorrhagia, may be less prevalent in older women. Anovulation is common, particularly at the start (menarche) and at the end of the reproductive lifespan (menopause). It is possible that women with VWD are more susceptible to menorrhagia at those times [26].

A bleeding score [27] and a screening tool [28] have been used as a surrogate instead of the assessment of VWF analysis in women presenting with menorrhagia.

Diagnostic aspects of von Willebrand disease in women

The results of the epidemiological studies reviewed above has led to relatively widespread VWD testing in the female population [29], but there are important factors that could significantly affect the laboratory diagnosis of VWD [30]:

1 Do VWF levels significantly decrease during menstruation such that the laboratory diagnosis of VWD could be "missed" if testing is not done during menstruation?

2 Do estrogen-based medications (for contraception, for hormone replacement) raise the VWF levels such that the laboratory diagnosis of VWD could be "missed"?

3 Do VWF levels vary in relation to the reproductive cycle such that the laboratory diagnosis of VWD may

be more likely after menopause if VWF levels fall in relation to falling estrogen levels?

4 Does race affect the VWF levels in women and subsequent laboratory diagnosis?

Relationship of VWF levels in regard to the menstrual cycle

Table 4.2 summarizes relevant laboratory studies of VWF levels in relation to the menstrual cycle. Initial reports regarding fluctuation of coagulation protein levels were conflicting [19, 31]. No variation in factor VIII coagulant activity (FVIII:C) (VWF levels were not studied) was found during menses in 13 healthy women over 6 weeks during five phases (early follicular phase, late follicular phase, early luteal phase, late luteal phase, and menstrual period) [32]. Another study reported a statistically significant fall in the FVIII:C level at the end of menstruation in nine control subjects with the average FVIII:C level falling to $87.5\% \pm 31.5\%$ at day 5–7 of menses compared with a peak FVIII:C level of $117.0\% \pm 40.3\%$ at day 14 [27].

A cohort of 15 controls with 10–16 samples from each of 15 women sampled six times during a period of 30 days showed a mean coefficient of variation of 16.1 ± 5.9 for FVIII:C, 18.8 ± 9.4 for von Willebrand factor antigen (VWF:Ag) and 13.0 ± 4.9 for the VWF ristocetin cofactor activity (VWF:RCo) with an intraindividual variability in some subjects of ~40% [33, 34]. There was no direct relation between these levels and estradiol, progesterone, or testosterone levels and a similar degree of variation of VWF levels was found in male subjects, making it unlikely that there was fluctuation of the VWF levels primarily because of the menstrual cycle. It was speculated that factors of

physical and mental stress [28, 35] were operative in both sexes, accounting for intraindividual variation. It was found that days 5–7 of the menstrual cycle were associated with the least intraindividual variation and the "most" representative sample of the menstrual cycle [33, 34].

A longitudinal study of 39 normal menstruating volunteers showed a statistically significant decrease in fibrinogen, VWF:Ag, and VWF:RCo concentrations during the first 3 days of menses with peak values in the luteal phase [19]. However by cross-sectional analysis, no difference was noted. Similarly no difference in VWF levels was found in another cross-sectional study of 93 patients sampled at days 4–7, 11–15, and 21–28 [31]. There was no association between hormonal levels of estradiol, progesterone, or testosterone with VWF or FVIII:C levels [36].

However, a more recent cross-sectional study showed that the lowest VWF level (VWF:Ag and VWF:RCo) was during the first 4 days of menses and the highest levels were on days 9 and 10 [32]. Given these conflicting results, it is most logical to advise the clinician that, in the case of normal or borderline VWF levels, repeat testing should be carried out during the first 4 days of the menstrual cycle. Furthermore, this would be a practical approach, as it is during those initial 3 days that the patient would be a candidate for intranasal or subcutaneous desmopressin (DDAVP) in raising the VWF levels [33, 37].

The studies noted above of possible menstrual variation of the VWF levels have involved controls. Whether there is variation specific to the menstrual cycle in women with documented VWD has been less extensively studied, although, in general, relatively significant fluctuation had been reported in both male and female VWD patients [34].

Table 4.2 Summary of FVIII:C and von Willebrand factor levels in relation to the menstrual cycle in normal menstruating women

Lead author	Methodological study	Decrease in levels during menses
Siegbahn [90]	Cross-sectional	No (no change in FVIII:C level, VWF levels not studied)
Mandalaki [27]	Cross-sectional	Yes (decrease in FVIII:C but not VWF:Ag)
Kadir [19]	Longitudinal	Yes
Onundarson [31]	Cross-sectional	No
Miller [32]	Cross-sectional	Yes

Relationship of von Willebrand factor levels in regard to hormonal therapy

Regarding oral contraceptive (OC) use, based on an initial report over 20 years ago, showing that three women with VWD had elevation of their levels when prescribed conjugated estrogen (which is >10 times the dose in present-day oral contraceptives) [38], there has been a general reluctance of hematologists to test for VWD in women taking OC. The assumption has been that hormonal therapy might "mask" the diagnosis [39]. Certainly at supra-physiological doses, VWF levels can rise significantly as reported in three particular clinical situations: (a) women receiving supra-physiological dosing for ovarian stimulation in the setting of infertility [36]; (b) post-menopausal women deliberately taking high does of estrogen [40]; and (c) pregnancy in a type 1 VWD patient [41, 42]. On the other hand, in normal women exposed to much lower doses of estrogen as contained in the second- and third-generation OC preparations, the majority of studies have shown no significant increase in the VWF levels [19, 43–46] with only a few exceptions [47]. Interestingly, in two of these studies there was a decrease noted in the VWF levels [19, 45], although this was not statistically significant. As for studies of VWF levels in women diagnosed with VWD, there have been no studies of the impact of OC on the sub-normal VWF levels. Intuitively, it is unlikely that OCs significantly raise VWF levels in women with VWD as present third-generation OCs do not raise VWF levels in control subjects. However, a beneficial effect of estrogen in the treatment of VWD-related menorrhagia in type 3 VWD patients has been reported [48, 49].

Other laboratory issues

Other factors that may have an impact on the laboratory diagnosis of VWD in women are race and age. Recent studies have demonstrated higher VWF levels in black women [19, 50, 51] with significantly higher VWF:Ag and VWF:RCo [20] or VWF:Ag [52, 53] levels even after adjusting for the blood group. An age-dependent increase in the VWF level independent of race has also been shown, with an increase by an average of 0.17 and 0.15 U/mL VWF:Ag and VWF:RCo, respectively, for each 10 year increase in age [19]. However, the mean age of this study group was 26 ± 5.5 years, so it is not known if this increase in VWF

levels continues towards menopause. Whether there is a change in VWF levels at menopause affecting the laboratory diagnosis of VWD is unknown, but it is possible that VWF levels fall as endogenous hormone production falls. However, published data contradict this assumption [52, 54].

Clinical characteristics of VWD in women

Women with VWD certainly have a very high relative risk of menorrhagia compared with the general population and the prevalence of menorrhagia by subjective report has been between 78% and 97% in women primarily with type 1 VWD [2, 3, 55]. Using the more objective PBAC [18] it has been reported that 78% of patients with VWD (primarily type 1) had evidence of menorrhagia [2]. Conversely, the relative risk of a low VWF in a woman with menorrhagia has been estimated at approximately fourfold [56].

Women with VWD use more tampons and pads than non-VWD menstruating women and have frequent staining of under clothes [3] and a higher prevalence of anemia (28–66% [3, 4, 55]). These women also have a much higher frequency of other mucocutaneous bleeding symptoms. In a study of 81 menstruating type 1 VWD patients registered in four upstate New York hemophilia treatment centers (HTCs), a comparison of various bleeding symptoms was carried out with a control cohort of 150 menstruating normal volunteers. A series of multiple logistic regression analyses were performed using variables from an administered questionnaire. After three successive analyses, the following variables were statistically significant: age (the younger the age, the higher the probability of VWD), history of dental work-related bleeding, past or present history of anemia and a diminished quality of life during menses in relation to family activities [3]. In a study carried out by the Centers for Disease Control (CDC) of Atlanta, USA, in a group of 102 women with VWD registered at HTCs, after multiple logistic regression analysis, surgical-related bleeding, excessive gum bleeding, and bleeding after minor injuries retained statistical significance [6]. However, epistaxis and bruising did not appear to be significantly more common in the VWD cohorts. Indeed, in one study, 24% of the normal menstruating control group (compared with 78% in the VWD cohort)

Table 4.3 Significant bleeding symptoms in women with von Willebrand disease (VWD)

Study	Study population	Symptoms more common in VWD patients than in non-VWD patients
Royal Free London 1998 [17]	26/150 women presenting with menorrhagia subsequently diagnosed with VWD (*n* = 26, presumed all type 1)	Bruising Dental-related bleeding Surgical-related bleeding Postpartum hemorrhage Menorrhagia since menarche Multiple bleeding symptoms
Upstate NY Hemophilia Treatment Centers study 2000 [3]	81 menstruating women registered at hemophilia treatment centers, all type 1 VWD compared with a cohort of 150 menstruating volunteers	Age (the younger the age, the higher the probability of VWD) History of dental work-related bleeding Past or present history of anemia A diminished quality of life during menses in relation to family activities.
Centers for Disease Control – Atlanta 2002 [6]	102 women with VWD registered at hemophilia treatment centers compared with 88 control subjects	Surgical-related bleeding Excessive gum bleeding Bleeding after minor injuries

reported easy bruising, defined as bruises greater than at least 5 cm in diameter at least once a month [3]. Table 4.3 summarizes the prevalence of these bleeding symptoms compared with a control group of non-VWD women from several recent studies [3, 6, 17].

Women with type 2 and type 3 VWD have not been so extensively studied as the women with type 1 VWD, but a study on behalf of the International Society of Thrombosis and Haemostasis (ISTH) von Willebrand Factor Subcommittee reported a high prevalence of menorrhagia and one-quarter of the patients required hysterectomy [48]. Subsequent studies have focused on the more common type 1 patient, and even in this population with milder depression of the VWF level there is a relatively high rate of hysterectomy for control of menorrhagia. A relatively significant proportion (~8–26%) of type 1 VWD patients historically have undergone surgical interventions such as hysterectomy for control of menorrhagia [2–4, 6, 55, 57]. In a case–control study of 102 women with VWD carried out by the CDC, 26% had undergone hysterectomy compared with 9% of controls [6]. In two studies, there was also underlying uterine pathology noted in the hysterectomy specimen, where it can be postulated that mild VWD may "unmask" a uterine fibroid [2, 3]. In the CDC study, a statistically higher rate of fibroids compared with age-matched controls (32% vs 17%) was noted [6]. There may also be a higher prevalence of endometriosis (30% vs 10%), endometrial hyperplasia (10% vs 1%) and endometrial polyps (8% vs 1%) in VWD women than in controls [6]. It has been hypothesized that VWD may exacerbate the presumed retrograde menstrual flow implicated in the pathophysiology of endometriosis [26]. The higher prevalence of endometrial hyperplasia and polyps in VWD women has been explained in terms of the VWD "unmasking" these lesions [26].

In patients with type 1 VWD, the menstrual bleeding will not be as dramatic as Erik von Willebrand's index case, who exsanguinated at the time of her fourth period and has ultimately been found to be a type 3 [58]. Nevertheless, the morbidity of menorrhagia in type 1 VWD is significant in terms of the proportion of these patients undergoing an unnecessary hysterectomy prior to the diagnosis of VWD (estimated to be 10% of all women with VWD [3, 55]), and also in terms of the cumulative morbidity of impairment of quality of life because of monthly heavy menstruation.

Regarding psychosocial aspects, four studies comprising over 300 patients with VWD compared with non-VWD women has shown unequivocally that these women do have impaired quality of life [3, 4, 6]. Two very similar studies from London [4] and upstate New York [3] had almost identical results in terms of decreased quality of life and its effect on numerous activities of daily living. Approximately 40% of women with VWD from a group of 180 patients reported losing time from work or school in the last year [4, 5]. Dysmenorrhea was also reported in approximately half the patients in both studies [4, 5]. In a Canadian study using a standardized quality of life tool, women with VWD assessed their own health status as being compromised to an extent similar to that reported by HIV-positive severe hemophilic patients and even greater than that experienced by adult survivors of brain tumors [5]. Furthermore, there was also a negative impact in terms of cognition. The authors hypothesize that this may be a result of chronic iron deficiency anemia related to menorrhagia. However, the sample size was small ($n = 12$), so further study is needed to confirm these provocative findings [6]. A report from Germany showed that women with VWD had a significantly higher prevalence of anxiety than the general baseline German population [57]. However, it should be emphasized that it had not been well established at this time if the impaired quality of life during menses in VWD women is any more pronounced than in the general menorrhagia population.

A high rate of mid-cycle pain, termed "mittlesmerz," has also been noted in women with VWD [3], and these patients can develop an acute surgical abdomen from hemoperitoneum due to bleeding into the corpus luteum with subsequent rupture [59]. A report from Sweden showed that nine of 136 women with VWD (6.8%) experienced hemorrhagic ovarian cysts [52]. There have also been reports of bleeding into the broad ligament with the patient presenting with a positive iliopsoas sign [60].

Management of von Willebrand disease in women

Non-menstrual bleeding

For non-menstrual bleeding, the patient with type 1 VWD has several hemostatic options [53]: intranasal, subcutaneous or intravenous, or antifibrinolytic therapy [60], either tranexamic acid (TA) or epsilon-amino caproic acid (EACA). EACA is approximately five times less potent then TA [61] but is prescribed in lieu

of TA in the USA as TA is not approved by the Food and Drug Administration. Combined DDAVP and antifibrinolytic therapy is also an option. Patients are educated beforehand that intranasal DDAVP carries a risk of fluid retention as well as symptomatic hyponatremia [62] if free water intake is not moderately restricted for up to 24 hours postoperatively. The patient is also informed that DDAVP can cause mild facial flushing, headache, palpitations, and hypotension; these are all attributable to its vasomotor effects [61, 63]. A trial is usually advised before prescribing intranasal DDAVP for several reasons: (a) to give instruction about proper intranasal administration; (b) to review potential side-effects; and (c) document a biological response defined as at least a twofold doubling of the VWF level.

Regarding antifibrinolytic therapy, the patient should be warned of possible gastrointestinal complaints such as nausea, vomiting, dyspepsia, or diarrhea. Symptoms usually disappear with dose reduction. Hypersensitivity reactions such as rash occur occasionally [64] and anaphylaxis to TA has been reported [65]. Uncommon (<1%) adverse events include change in mood, giddiness, low blood pressure/orthostatic reactions, myalgias, muscle tenderness, skin rash, and alteration in color vision [61, 66]. We also inform patients that both treatments carry a theoretical risk of thrombosis [61]. There have been several reports of acute myocardial infarction or cerebral thrombosis associated with DDAVP use [67–69]. Consequently, DDAVP should be used with caution in patients with coronary heart disease and in those with coexisting genetic prothrombotic conditions, such as factor V Leiden and/or coexisting acquired prothrombotic conditions, including the postoperative setting, hormone use, and smoking. A recent example is a case of a transient ischemic event in a female smoker using intranasal DDAVP for heavy menstrual bleeding in the setting of mild VWD [69]. There have been isolated reports of venous or arterial thrombosis or embolism associated with the use of TA [70, 71] but a causal relationship has not been established [66, 72]. Of interest, a review of the Swedish national registry of venous thromboembolism events did not show an increased rate after oral TA became available over the counter for the management of heavy menstrual bleeding [73]. On the basis of 10 years' experience in Sweden, oral TA is currently under consideration for reclassification from prescription-only medicine to pharmacy availability in the UK for this indication [61].

Menorrhagia

An algorithm for the management of menorrhagia is shown in Chapter 7 and gynecological management will also be discussed in detail in Chapter 7. This chapter will focus on hemostatic therapy of VWD-related menorrhagia.

Antifibrinolytic therapy

The rationale for this type of therapy is well founded as several studies have demonstrated increased fibrinolysis in uterine fluid in women with menorrhagia [74]. The seminal study was a three-arm randomized comparison of oral tranexamic acid (1 g p.o. qid) versus ethamsylate – a general hemostatic agent – and mefenamic acid – a prostaglandin synthetase inhibitor. There were approximately 25 patients in each arm, each with prior documented heavy menstrual blood flow by the spectrophotometric method. There was a statistically significant 54% decrease in menstrual flow compared with baseline in the tranexamic acid arm, compared with no statistically significant decrease with the other agents [75]. Further supportive evidence for TA in menorrhagia has been through the evidence-based database of the Cochrane review updated in 2007. It concludes that TA is an efficacious agent in general for menorrhagia [76]. Despite the widespread use of TA for decades for the general menorrhagia population, there is a paucity of adequate objective data on the efficacy of this treatment to reduce MBL in women with VWD. There have only been small case series specifically addressing the efficacy and tolerability of TA [77–79]. In a study from London, TA was successful as a first line therapy in 40% of 37 women with bleeding disorder-related menorrhagia by reducing MBL to a PBAC score of <100 or to a woman's satisfaction [80]. The actual effective dose and frequency, however, remain unclear at this time with a total of four women with VWD reported in the literature who received once daily dosing of 5 g for three consecutive days [31, 78]. However, this may be associated with severe gastrointestinal symptoms. There is also a new sustained-release formulation (XP12B) of TA that could be dosed only 2 or 3 times a day. This is currently under study in the USA [81].

DDAVP Historically, data in VWD-related menorrhagia have level C evidence (case series), with the subcutaneous form being rated very effective in 65% of 14 women using it throughout 43 periods; it was rated effective in 86% and rated no effect in 14% [82]. Another similar cohort study using the intranasal form with 721 daily uses in 90 women reported 64% as excellent, 28% as good, and 8% as no response [37]. In both studies, assessment was by patient report and not by the PBAC or the spectrophotometric method. The efficacy of intranasal DDAVP in 39 women with inherited bleeding disorders, 30 with VWD, was assessed using the PBAC in a randomized control crossover study [83]. Women were studied for two menstrual periods with one spray in each nostril (either placebo or 300 µg of DDAVP on days 2 and 3 of the period). Regardless of whether the first treatment period involved the placebo or the intranasal DDAVP, there was a reduction in the PBAC score that was statistically significant ($P = 0.01$). There was a trend towards a lower score if it was intranasal DDAVP, but this was not statistically significant with no significant difference in quality of life in terms of absence from work or school or avoidance of social activities or use of other medications. Similar results were noted in a related study of 20 women with menorrhagia and a prolonged bleeding time comparing 300 µg of IN-DDAVP with placebo [84]. There was no statistically significant decrease in menstrual blood flow spectrophotometrically with DDAVP compared with placebo. However, there was a statistically significant decrease when DDAVP was combined with TA.

In both studies, fluid intake was restricted to ~1.5 L/day, but nevertheless weight gain was reported in 12% of women using DDAVP compared with none using the placebo [83].

In summary, more objective measurements of efficacy have not shown as great a benefit of intranasal DDAVP for VWD-related menorrhagia compared with prior studies using subjective assessment as the endpoint of efficacy. However, a recent multicenter US trial comparing crossover intranasal DDAVP and TA using the PBAC for assessment of menstrual blood loss (MBL) and four previously validated quality of life measures has been completed [85]. The question remains whether the efficacy of DDAVP can be improved without an increase in the adverse event rate in terms of altering the schedule from the standard use of one puff to each nostril on days 2 and 3 of menses to twice a day dosing on the first 2 days, daily for three days, or one puff to each nostril on days 2–7 [86]. Further study of the efficacy and safety of combined therapy of IN-DDAVP and antifibrinolytic therapy or hormonal therapy is also needed.

Plasma-derived von Willebrand factor containing FVIII concentrates

Approximately 10–15% of women with VWD will not respond to DDAVP because they have either severe type 1 VWD or type 2 or type 3 VWD [87]. In those patients, for severe intractable menorrhagia refractory to antifibrinolytic therapy and/or hormonal therapy or for prophylaxis before surgery, a plasma-derived von Willebrand factor containing FVIII concentrate can be administered [53, 88, 89]. The dosing is typically 40–60 units/kg of VWF:RCo units for major surgery and 20–40 units/kg of VWF:RCo units for menorrhagia.

Preliminary data from the Swedish type 3 VWD prophylaxis registry shows there are patients requiring prophylaxis for control of menorrhagia [90]. To accrue further data and test a strategy of escalated prophylaxis, an international prophylaxis study is to be initiated in 2008 in women with types 2 and 3 VWD-related menorrhagia, with dosing initially at 50 units/kg VWF:RCo units weekly, which in non-responders in terms of the PBAC remaining >100 will be escalated to twice a week then three times a week.

References

1 von Willebrand EA. Hereditar pseudohemofili. *Finska Lakarsallskapets Handl* 1926; **67**: 7–112.

2 Kadir RA, Economides DL, Sabin CA, *et al.* Assessment of menstrual blood loss and gynaecological problems in patients with inherited bleeding disorders. *Haemophilia* 1999; **5**: 40–48.

3 Kouides PA, Burkhart P, Phatak P, *et al.* Gynecological and obstetrical morbidity in women with Type I von Willebrand disease: results of a patient survey. *Haemophilia* 2000; **6**: 643–648.

4 Kadir RA, Sabin CA, Pollard D, *et al.* Quality of life during menstruation in patients with inherited bleeding disorders. *Haemophilia* 1998; **4**: 836–841.

5 Barr RD, Sek J, Horsman J, *et al.* Health status and health-related quality of life associated with von Willebrand disease. *Am J Hematol* 2003; **73**: 108–114.

6 Kirtava A, Drews C, Lally C, *et al.* Medical, reproductive and psychosocial experiences of women diagnosed with von Willebrand's disease receiving care in haemophilia treatment centres: a case-control study. *Haemophilia* 2003; **9**: 292–297.

7 James AH, Ragni MV, Picozzi VJ. Bleeding disorders in premenopausal women: (another) public health crisis for hematology? *Hematology (Am Soc Hematol Educ Program)* 2006; 474–485.

8 Vessey MP, Villard-Mackintosh L, McPherson K, *et al.* The epidemiology of hysterectomy: findings in a large cohort study. *Br J Obstet Gynaecol* 1992; **99**: 402–407.

9 Oehler MK, Rees MC. Menorrhagia: an update. *Acta Obstet Gynecol Scand* 2003; **82**: 405–422.

10 Shaw JA, Shaw HA. Menorrhagia. (Emedicine). 2007.

11 Doherty L, Harper A, Russell M. Menorrhagia management options. *Ulster Med J* 1995; **64**: 64–71.

12 Krassas GE, Pontikides N, Kaltsas T, *et al.* Disturbances of menstruation in hypothyroidism. *Clin Endocrinol* 1999; **50**: 655–659.

13 Shankar M, Lee CA, Sabin CA, *et al.* von Willebrand disease in women with menorrhagia: a systematic review. *Br J Obstet Gynaecol* 2004; **111**: 734–740.

14 Trasi S, Pathare AV, Shetty S, *et al.* The spectrum of bleeding disorders in women with menorrhagia; a report from Western India. *Ann Hematol* 2005; **84**: 339–342.

15 Woo YL, White B, Corbally R, *et al.* von Willebrand's disease: an important cause of dysfunctional uterine bleeding. *Blood Coag Fibrinol* 2002; **13**: 89–93.

16 Edlund M, Blomback M, von Schoultz B, Andersson O. On the value of menorrhagia as a predictor for coagulation disorders. *Am J Hematol* 1996; **53**: 234–238.

17 Kadir RA, Economides DL, Sabin CA, *et al.* Frequency of inherited bleeding disorders in women with menorrhagia. *Lancet* 1998; **351**: 485–489.

18 Higham JM, O'Brien PM, Shaw RW. Assessment of menstrual blood loss using a pictorial chart. *Br J Obstet Gynaecol* 1990; **97**: 734–739.

19 Kadir RA, Economides DL, Sabin CA, *et al.* Variations in coagulation factors in women: effects of age, ethnicity, menstrual cycle and combined oral contraceptive. *Thromb Haemost* 1999; **82**: 1456–1461.

20 Claessens EA, Cowell CA. Acute adolescent menorrhagia. *Am J Obstet Gynecol* 1981; **139**: 277–280.

21 Bevan JA, Maloney KW, Hillery CA, *et al.* Bleeding disorders: a common cause of menorrhagia in adolescents. *J Pediatr* 2001; **138**: 856–861.

22 Smith YR, Quint EH, Hertzberg RB. Menorrhagia in adolescents requiring hospitalization. *J Pediatr Adolesc Gynecol* 1998; **11**: 13–15.

23 Oral E, Cada A, Gezer A, *et al.* Hematological abnormalities in adolescent menorrhagia. *Arch Gynecol Obstet* 2002; **266**: 72–74.

24 Jayasinghe Y, Moore P, Donath S, *et al.* Bleeding disorders in teenagers presenting with menorrhagia. *Aust N Z J Obstet Gynaecol* 2005; **45**: 439–443.

25 Mikhail S, Varadarajan R, Kouides PA. The prevalence of disorders of haemostasis in adolescents with menorrhagia referred to a haemophilia treatment centre. *Haemophilia* 2007; **13**: 627–632.

26 James AH. More than menorrhagia: a review of the obstetric and gynaecological manifestations of bleeding disorders. *Haemophilia* 2005; **11**: 295–307.

27 Mandalaki T, Louizou C, Dimitriadou C, Symeonidis P. Variations in factor VIII during the menstrual cycle in normal women [Letter]. *N Engl J Med* 1980; **302**: 1093–1094.

28 Jern C, Eriksson E, Tengborn L, *et al.* Changes in plasma coagulation and fibrinolysis in response to mental stress. *Thromb Haemost* 1989; **62**: 767.

29 Dilley A, Crudder S. von Willebrand disease in women: the need for recognition and understanding. *J Womens Health Gender-Based Med* 1999; **8**: 443–445.

30 Kouides PA. Aspects of the laboratory identification of von Willebrand disease in women. *Semin Thromb Hemost* 2006; **32**: 480–484.

31 Onundarson PT, Gumundsdottir BR, Arnfinnsdottir AV, *et al.* Von Willebrand factor does not vary during the normal menstrual cycle [Letter]. *Thromb Haemost* 2001; **85**: 183–184.

32 Miller CH, Dilley A, Drews C, *et al.* Changes in von Willebrand factor and Factor VIII levels during the menstrual cycle [Letter]. *Thromb Haemost* 2002; **87**: 1082–1083.

33 Lethagen S. Desmopressin in the treatment of women's bleeding disorders [Review]. *Haemophilia* 1999; **5**: 233–237.

34 Abildgaard CF, Suzuki Z, Harrison J, *et al.* Serial studies in von Willebrand's disease: variability versus "variants". *Blood* 1980; **56**: 712–716.

35 Prentice CRM, Forbes D, Smith SM. Rise of Factor VIII after exercise and adrenaline infusion, measured by immunological and biological techniques. *Thromb Res* 1972; **1**: 493.

36 Bremme K, Wramsby H, Andersson O, *et al.* Do lowered factor VII levels at extremely high endogenous oestradiol levels protect against thrombin formation? *Blood Coagul Fibrinolysis* 1994; **5**: 205–210.

37 Leissinger C, Becton D, Cornell C, Gill JC. High-dose DDAVP intranasal spray (Stimate) for the prevention and treatment of bleeding in patients with mild haemophilia A, mild or moderate type 1 von Willebrand disease and symptomatic carriers of haemophilia A. *Haemophilia* 2001; **7**: 258–266.

38 Alperin JB. Estrogens and surgery in women with von Willebrand's disease. *Am J Med* 1982; **73**: 367–371.

39 Mangal AK, Naiman SC. Oral contraceptives and von Willebrand's disease [Letter]. *Can Med Assoc J* 1983; **128**: 1274.

40 He S, Bremme K, Silveira A, *et al.* Hypercoagulation in surgical postmenopausal women having hormone replacement with overdose estradiol. *Blood Coagul Fibrinolysis* 2001; **12**: 677–681.

41 Kadir RA, Lee CA, Sabin CA, *et al.* Pregnancy in women with von Willebrands disease or Factor XI deficiency. *Br J Obstet Gynaecol* 1998; **105**: 314–321.

42 Ramsahoye BH, Davies SV, Dasani H, Pearson JF. Pregnancy in von Willebrand's disease [letter; comment]. *J Clin Pathol* 1994; **47**: 569–570.

43 Prasad RN, Koh SC, Viegas OA, Ratnam SS. Effects on hemostasis after two-year use of low dose combined oral contraceptives with gestodene or levonorgestrel. *Clin Appl Thromb Hemost* 1999; **5**: 60–70.

44 Solerte SB, Fioravanti M, Spinillo A, *et al.* Influence of triphasic oral contraceptives on blood rheology and hemostatic and metabolic patterns in young women. Results of a three-year study. *J Reprod Med* 1992; **37**: 725–732.

45 Gevers Leuven JA, Kluft C, Bertina RM, Hessel LW. Effects of two low-dose oral contraceptives on circulating components of the coagulation and fibrinolytic systems. *J Lab Clin Med* 1987; **109**: 631–636.

46 Hall G, Blomback M, Landgren BM, Bremme K. Effects of vaginally administered high estradiol doses on hormonal pharmacokinetics and hemostasis in postmenopausal women. *Fertil Steril* 2002; **78**: 1172–1177.

47 David JL, Gaspard UJ, Gillain D, *et al.* Hemostasis profile in women taking low-dose oral contraceptives. *Am J Obstet Gynecol* 1990; **163**: Pt 2): 420–423.

48 Foster PA. The reproductive health of women with von Willebrand Disease unresponsive to DDAVP: results of an international survey. On behalf of the Subcommittee on von Willebrand Factor of the Scientific and Standardization Committee of the ISTH. *Thromb Haemost* 1995; **74**: 784–790.

49 Lak M, Peyvandi F, Mannucci PM. Clinical manifestations and complications of childbirth and replacement therapy in 385 Iranian patients with type 3 von Willebrand disease. *Br J Haematol* 2000; **111**: 1236–1239.

50 Miller CH, Dilley A, Richardson L, *et al.* Population differences in von Willebrand factor levels affect the diagnosis of von Willebrand disease in African-American women. *Am J Hematol* 2001; **67**: 125–129.

51 Miller CH, Haff E, Platt SJ, *et al.* Measurement of von Willebrand factor activity: relative effects of ABO blood type and race. *J Thromb Haemost* 2003; **1**: 2191–2197.

52 Silwer J. Von Willebrand's disease in Sweden. *Acta Paediatr Scand* 1973; **238**: 1–159.

53 Federici AB, Mannucci PM. Management of inherited von Willebrand disease in 2007. *Ann Med* 2007; **39**: 346–358.

54 Rainsford SG, Jouhar AJ, Hall A. Tranexamic acid in the control of spontaneous bleeding in severe haemophilia. *Thromb Diath Haemorrh* 1973; **30**: 272–279.

55 Ragni MV, Bontempo FA, Cortese Hassett A. von Willebrand disease and bleeding in women. *Haemophilia* 1999; **5**: 313–317.

56 Sadler JE. Von Willebrand disease type 1: a diagnosis in search of a disease. *Blood* 2003; **101**: 2089–2093.

57 Rozeik C, Scharrer I. Gynecological disorders and psychological problems in 184 women with von Willebrand disease [Abstract]. *Haemophilia* 1998; **4**: 293.

58 Zhang ZP, Blomback M, Nyman D, Anvret M. Mutations of von Willebrand factor gene in families with von Willebrand disease in the Aland Islands. *Proc Natl Acad Sci USA* 1993; **90**: 7937–7940.

59 Jarvis RR, Olsen ME. Type I von Willebrand's disease presenting as recurrent corpus hemorrhagicum. *Obstet Gynecol* 2002; **99**: t-8.

60 Greer IA, Lowe GD, Walker JJ, Forbes CD. Haemorrhagic problems in obstetrics and gynaecology in patients with congenital coagulopathies. *Br J Obstet Gynaecol* 1991; **98**: 909–918.

61 Fraser IS, Lukes AS, Kouides PAA. Benefit-risk review of systemic haemostatic agents in surgery and gynaecology. *Drug Saf* 2008; **31**: 217–230.

62 Bertholini DM, Butler CS. Severe hyponatraemia secondary to desmopressin therapy in von Willebrand's disease. *Anaesth Intensive Care* 2000; **28**: 199–201.

63 Prescribing information, intranasal DDAVP (1.5 mg/mL). CSL Behring Inc. 2007.

64 Kavanagh GM, Sansom JE, Harrison P, *et al.* Tranexamic acid (Cyklokapron)-induced fixed-drug eruption. *Br J Dermatol* 1993; **128**: 229–230.

65 Lucas-Polomeni MM, Delaval Y, Menestret P, *et al.* [A case of anaphylactic shock with tranexamique acid (Exacyl)]. *Ann Fr Anesth Reanim* 2004; **23**: 607–609.

66 Cyclokapron® (tranexamic acid tablets and tranexamic acid injection). Prescribing information. Pharmacia and Upjohn Company. 2005.

67 Mannucci PM, Lusher JM. Desmopressin and thrombosis. *Lancet* 1989; **2**: 675–676.

68 Byrnes JJ, Larcada A, Moake JL. Thrombosis following desmopressin for uremic bleeding. *Am J Hematol* 1988; **28**: 63–65.

69 Grainge C, Nokes T. Cerebral arterial thrombosis in a young woman following vasopressin for von Willebrand's disease. *Thromb Haemost* 2005; **93**: 380.

70 Taparia M, Cordingley FT, Leahy MF. Pulmonary embolism associated with tranexamic acid in severe acquired haemophilia. *Eur J Haematol* 2002; **68**: 307–309.

71 Woo KS, Tse LK, Woo JL, Vallance-Owen J. Massive pulmonary thromboembolism after tranexamic acid antifibrinolytic therapy. *Br J Clin Pract* 1989; **43**: 465–466.

72 Lindoff C, Rybo G, Astedt B. Treatment with tranexamic acid during pregnancy, and the risk of thromboembolic complications. *Thromb Haemost* 1993; **70**: 238–240.

73 Berntorp E, Follrud C, Lethagen S. No increased risk of venous thrombosis in women taking tranexamic acid. *Thromb Haemost* 2001; **86**: 714–715.

74 Winkler UH. Menstruation: extravascular fibrinolytic activity and reduced fibrinolytic capacity. *Ann NY Acad Sci* 1992; **667**: 289–290.

75 Bonnar J, Sheppard BL. Treatment of menorrhagia during menstruation: randomised controlled trial of ethamsylate, mefenamic acid, and tranexamic acid. *BMJ* 1996; **313**: 579–582.

76 Lethaby A, Farquhar C, Cooke I. Antifibrinolytics for heavy menstrual bleeding. *Cochrane Database Syst Rev* 2007; CD000249.

77 Mohri H. High dose of tranexamic acid for treatment of severe menorrhagia in patients with von Willebrand disease. *J Thromb Thrombolys* 2002; **14**: 255–257.

78 Ong YL, Hull DR, Mayne EE. Menorrhagia in von-Willebrand disease successfully treated with single daily dose tranexamic acid. *Haemophilia* 1998; **4**: 63–65.

79 Onundarson PT. Treatment of menorrhagia in von Willebrand's disease [Letter]. *Haemophilia* 1999; **5**: 76.

80 Kadir RA, Lukes AS, Kouides PA, *et al.* Management of excessive menstrual bleeding in women with hemostatic disorders. *Fertil Steril* 2005; **84**: 1352–1359.

81 ClinicalTrials.gov. Efficacy and safety study of XP12B in women with menorrhagia. http://clinicaltrials.gov/ct/show/NCT00386308. 2007.

82 Rodeghiero F, Castaman G, Mannucci PM. Prospective multicenter study on subcutaneous concentrated desmopressin for home treatment of patients with von Willebrand disease and mild or moderate hemophilia A. *Thromb Haemost* 1996; **76**: 692–696.

83 Kadir RA, Lee CA, Sabin CA, *et al.* DDAVP nasal spray for treatment of menorrhagia in women with inherited bleeding disorders: a randomized placebo-controlled crossover study. *Haemophilia* 2002; **8**: 787–793.

84 Edlund M, Blomback M, Fried G. Desmopressin in the treatment of menorrhagia in women with no common coagulation factor deficiency but with prolonged bleeding time. *Blood Coag Fibrinolys* 2002; **13**: 225–231.

85 Kouides PA, Heit J, Philipp CS, *et al.* The effect of intranasal desmopressin vs. oral tranexamic acid on menstrual

blood loss among women with menorrhagia and abnormal laboratory hemostasis: a multicenter, randomized cross-over study [Abstract]. *J Thromb Haemost* 2007.

86 Edlund, M. Once daily dosing of intranasal DDAVP on days 2–7. 2007 [Personal communication].

87 Michiels JJ, van Vliet HH, Berneman Z, *et al.* Intravenous DDAVP and factor VIII-von Willebrand factor concentrate for the treatment and prophylaxis of bleedings in patients with von Willebrand disease type 1, 2 and 3. *Clin Appl Thromb Hemost* 2007; **13**: 14–34.

88 Michiels JJ, Gadisseur A, Budde U, *et al.* Characterization, classification, and treatment of von Willebrand diseases: a critical appraisal of the literature and personal experiences. *Semin Thromb Hemost* 2005; **31**: 577–601.

89 Berntorp E. Plasma product treatment in various types of von Willebrand's disease [Review]. *Haemostasis* 1994; **24**: 289–297.

90 Berntorp E, Abshire T. The von Willebrand disease prophylaxis network: exploring a treatment concept. *J Thromb Haemost* 2006; **4**: 2511–2512.

Rare bleeding disorders

Flora Peyvandi

Introduction

The intrinsic and extrinsic coagulation pathways involve a complex cascade of reactions leading ultimately to the cleavage of fibrinogen to fibrin and formation of a fibrin clot by covalent cross-linking. Abnormal activities of the enzymes or cofactors of this pathway are predicted or known to lead to various forms of coagulation disorders, the most common and best documented of these being hemophilia A and hemophilia B, due to mutations in the genes for coagulation factors VIII (FVIII) and IX (FIX) [1]. Hemophilia A and B together with von Willebrand disease (VWD), a defect of primary hemostasis associated with a secondary defect in coagulation FVIII, include 95–97% of all the inherited deficiencies of coagulation factors [2, 3]. The remaining so-called "rare bleeding disorders" (RBDs), including deficiency of fibrinogen, factor II (FII), FV, combined FV + FVIII, FVII, FX, FXI, and FXIII, represent 3–5% of all the inherited coagulation disorders with a prevalence of the presumably homozygous forms in the general population ranging from approximately 1 in 500 000 for FVII deficiency to 1 in 2 million for FII and FXIII deficiency [1, 4]. Exceptions to these low prevalences are countries with large Jewish communities (where FXI deficiency is much more prevalent) [5], Middle Eastern countries, and Southern India [1]; in the last two cases, consanguineous marriages are relatively common, so that autosomal recessive traits occur more frequently in homozygosity.

An indication of the worldwide prevalence of RBDs compared with other rare bleeding disorders comes from two available global surveys, performed by the World Federation of Hemophilia (WFH, http://www.wfh.org/2/7/7_0_Link7_GlobalSurvey2005.htm) and the Rare Bleeding Disorders Database (RBDD, www.rbdd.org). Although collected data are not homogeneous and information from a number of countries is still lacking, because of the limited number of reliable national registries, especially in developing countries, a picture of the global distribution of RBDs is emerging. According to these data, patients affected by RBDs around the world seem to number approximately 7000 (Fig. 5.1).

Since RBDs are autosomal recessive disorders, roughly about 50% of patients are women. This implies that the global distribution of RBDs reflects also the global distribution of affected women, posing important social and medical problems linked to the women's quality of life – these women have to face excessive menstrual bleeding or menorrhagia, bleeding complications during pregnancy and after delivery, and the related complication of chronic anemia.

In the developed world, a good quality of life is assured for patients with bleeding disorders with the availability of prophylactic clotting factor support and health insurance. However, in developing countries, where the frequency of RBDs is significantly higher (eight- to tenfold), the socioeconomical conditions are poor. Apart from economic constraints, there are limited laboratory resources and scarce availability of safe therapeutic products because factor concentrates

Inherited Bleeding Disorders in Women, 1st edition. By CA Lee, RA Kadir and PA Kouides. Published 2009 by Blackwell Publishing, ISBN: 978-1-4051-6915-8.

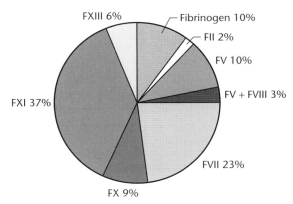

Fig. 5.1 Rare bleeding disorder distribution. For the derived global frequency of each rare bleeding disorder, factor XI (37%) and factor VII (23%) seem to be the most frequent disorders followed by fibrinogen and factor V deficiency (10%), factor X (9%), factor XIII (6%), and combined factor V + factor VIII deficiency and factor II deficiency as the rarest deficiencies (3% and 2%, respectively).

usually cannot be made locally and imported products are too expensive. This makes it particularly difficult to achieve the appropriate level of treatment for women living in developing countries.

Improvements in these countries requires an increase in public sector spending [6, 7]. Thus because the care for bleeding disorders in these countries is not optimal, preventive strategies are necessary for families at risk [8]. The availability of reliable antenatal diagnostic facilities for bleeding disorders using molecular genetic techniques is important, particularly if we are to reduce the economic burden of these disorders.

Clinical symptoms

Patients affected by RBDs present a wide spectrum of clinical symptoms that vary from a mild or moderate bleeding tendency to potentially serious or life-threatening hemorrhages. As a consequence of the rarity of RBDs, the actual management of bleeding episodes is not well established; however, knowledge of the spectrum of clinical manifestations of RBDs is much greater after the description of three large national registries from Iran, Italy, and North America [9–16].

Some general conclusions can be drawn about the spectrum of clinical manifestations. RBDs appear generally less severe than hemophilia A and B, life- and limb-threatening symptoms such as central nervous system and gastrointestinal tract bleeding, hemarthroses and hematomas are definitely less frequent but are more common in patients with afibrinogenemia, FII and FX deficiency. Umbilical cord bleeding, typical of afibrinogenemia and factor XIII deficiency, is also relatively frequent in FII, FV, and FX deficiency [1]. The most typical symptom, common to all RBDs, is the occurrence of excessive bleeding at the time of invasive procedures and surgery. An unexplained common feature of these disorders is frequent mucosal bleeding such as epistaxis, which is relatively uncommon in the hemophilias [1].

Menorrhagia occurs in about 50% of women affected by RBDs. Recurrent miscarriages, frequently described in afibrinogenemic and FXIII-deficient women [10, 11], are not common in women with other RBDs. Postpartum bleeding often occurs if replacement therapy is not administered for 2–3 days after delivery [9–15]. Bleeding during pregnancy requires further study.

Menorrhagia or heavy menstrual bleeding

Normal menstruation occurs every 21–35 days, lasts 7 days or less, and results in 25–69 mL of blood loss per cycle. Menorrhagia is the medical term for excessive blood loss as heavy menses lasting more than 7 days; an objective definition is menstrual blood loss of more than 80 mL per menstruation [17]. Menstruation may be a source of inconvenience to women in general, but is significantly more so for women with excessive blood loss, having a major influence on their lifestyle and employment. Many women decide not to go out at all during their periods, avoiding activities such as working, shopping, taking part in sports, traveling, and studying. Menorrhagia is a frequent problem that afflicts women from menarche to menopause as well as in the postmenopausal period. It has an enormous impact on the lives of women and may affect 25–30% of women at some point during their childbearing years.

Potential causes of excessive menstrual bleeding

Healthcare providers consider local and systemic disorders as potential causes of menorrhagia. Local causes

Table 5.1 Prevalence of menorrhagia in women with rare blood disorders

Sample size and population	Type of study	Prevalence (%)	Reference
20 women with afibrinogenemia	Case series	70	Lak 1999 [10]
20 women with factor XI deficiency	Prospective cohort	59	Kadir 1999 [21]
11 women with factor XIII deficiency	Summary of case reports	64	Burrows 2000 [22]
20 women with factor XIII deficiency	Case series	35	Lak 2003 [11]
3 women with combined factor V and factor VIII deficiency	Case series	50	Shetty 2000 [23]

include uterine and ovarian pathology (benign and malignant), infections, and local endometrial defects. Systemic pathologies include endocrine disorders (hypothyroidism and diabetes mellitus), chronic cardiac and renal disease, liver disease, and obesity, which can all influence hemostasis [18]. In the last decade, studies have found that 5–32% of women with menorrhagia have a bleeding disorder [19] (see Chapter 7).

A total of 101 women with severe RBDs among 261 Iranian women of reproductive age showed that the highest rate of menorrhagia is seen in women with VWD (69%) and factor II deficiency (75%) [20]. Menorrhagia was found in 50% of women affected by factor V, VII, X, afibrinogenemia, and combined V + VIII deficiency [20]. There are other reports of the prevalence of menorrhagia in women with RBDs, but these prevalences are variable because of the small numbers analyzed, mostly case reports and small case series (Table 5.1). A more extensive analysis on a larger group of affected women is thus required to evaluate the real prevalence of menorrhagia and other gynecological problems [19].

Assessment of menstrual blood loss

The alkaline hematin technique has been shown to be very accurate and reproducible, but it is not in routine clinical use. It is difficult to quantify menstrual blood loss objectively because it involves techniques that are specialized, time-consuming, and require collection of sanitary material by women. As a result, assessment of menorrhagia in clinical practice is usually subjective and often relies on the description provided by the patient. This method is unfortunately inaccurate and there is lack of correlation between a patient's impression and the objective assessment of actual volume of blood loss. In an attempt to address this problem, a pictorial blood loss assessment chart (PBAC) was developed (see Appendix ii) [24, 25].

A PBAC score >185 is taken as a cut-off to indicate the presence of menorrhagia. However, this score needs to be re-evaluated because of discordant data in the literature. The PBAC is strongly influenced by subjective judgment and a definite cut-off is not established because some authors consider 100 and others 185 as the minimum score. Furthermore, the PBAC may not accurately reflect the hygiene products used, and women change hygiene products at a varying frequency whether saturation has occurred or not and there is a difference between types of pads and tampons used. This instrument could be useful for the primary screening of women, but a critical evaluation of this symptom in affected women should be implemented. The concomitant presence of anemia and reduced ferritin levels could be a more specific indicator to evaluate blood loss and the need of a prophylactic approach in those women affected by a bleeding disorder and anemia due to severe menorrhagia.

Other gynecological bleedings in women affected by bleeding disorders

This is comprehensively covered in Chapter 7.

Menorrhagia is not the only gynecological problem that women with bleeding disorders are more likely to experience. Women with bleeding disorders are at risk of obstetrical and gynecological problems, as well as healthy women, while they appear to be at a higher risk of developing ovarian cysts, endometriosis, hyperplasia, polyps, and fibroids [19].

Miscarriages

Miscarriage is common in the general population, with 12–13.5% of recognized pregnancies resulting in spontaneous miscarriage [26, 27]. An increased risk of miscarriage and placental abruption resulting in fetal loss or premature delivery has been reported among women with a deficiency of FXIII [22, 28] or fibrinogen [19]. It is generally believed that women with bleeding disorders are protected by the hypercoagulable state of pregnancy, but whether women with other bleeding disorders (VWD, hemophilia carriers) [19] have an increased risk of miscarriage is unclear. Further studies are needed to confirm whether inherited bleeding disorders, other than deficiency of FXIII or fibrinogen, are associated with a higher rate of miscarriage.

Bleeding during pregnancy

Pregnancy is accompanied by increased concentrations of fibrinogen, FVII, FVIII, FX, and von Willebrand factor (VWF). FVIII and VWF levels rise even in hemophilia carriers or women with VWD. FII, FV and FIX are relatively unchanged. Free protein S, the active, unbound form, is decreased during pregnancy secondary to increased levels of its binding protein, the complement component C4b. Plasminogen activator inhibitor type 1 (PAI-1) levels are increased. All of these changes contribute to the hypercoagulable state of pregnancy, and, in women with bleeding disorders, contribute to improved hemostasis. Despite improved hemostasis, however, women with factor deficiencies do not achieve the same factor levels as those of women without factor deficiencies [19]. Bleeding during pregnancy is a common symptom reported in women with bleeding disorders [29–31].

Postpartum hemorrhage (see also Chapter 10)

Postpartum hemorrhage (PPH) is an anticipated problem among women with bleeding disorders. At the end of a normal pregnancy, an estimated 10–15% of a woman's blood volume, or at least 750 mL/min, flows through the uterus [32]. Normally after delivery of the infant and placenta, the uterine musculature or myometrium contracts around the uterine vasculature and the vasculature constricts in order to prevent exsanguination. Retained placental fragments and lacerations of the reproductive tract may also cause heavy bleeding, but the single most important cause of PPH is uterine atony [33]. Despite the critical role of uterine contractility in controlling postpartum blood loss, women with bleeding disorders are at an increased risk of PPH. There are multiple case reports and several case series documenting the incidence of postpartum hemorrhage in women with bleeding disorders [19] but there are limited data that compare women with bleeding disorders and control subjects.

Delayed or secondary PPH is rare in the general population (0.7% more than 24 hours after delivery) [34]. However, a higher prevalence of delayed PPH was reported among women affected by VWD, FXI deficiency and hemophilia carriers [30, 35, 36], making delayed postpartum hemorrhage more than 10–25 times more common among women with bleeding disorders. Among all women, the median duration of bleeding after delivery is 21–27 days [37, 38], but coagulation factors, elevated during pregnancy, return to baseline within 14–21 days [39]. Therefore, there is a period of time, 2–3 weeks after delivery, when coagulation factors have returned to pre-pregnancy levels, but women are still bleeding. Women with bleeding disorders are particularly vulnerable to delayed or secondary PPH during this period of time. The implication is that women with bleeding disorders may require prophylaxis and/or close observation for several weeks.

Laboratory diagnosis

Phenotype (see also Chapter 1)

In the screening test citrated plasma is separated from cells and should be centrifuged at a speed and time which produces samples with low residual platelet counts well below 10×10^9/L (usually 1500 g for 15 minutes). Centrifugation at a temperature of 18–25°C is acceptable for most clotting tests. After centrifugation, prolonged storage at 4–8°C should be avoided as this can cause cold activation, increasing FVII activity [40] and shortening of the prothrombin time (PT) or activated partial thromboplastin time (APTT). To interpret the result of any clotting test it is important to have data on results of the test in healthy normal subjects. Samples from normal subjects should be collected, processed, and analyzed locally using identical techniques to those for patient samples.

In the phenotypic diagnosis of RBDs the results of laboratory tests can be affected by the collection and processing of blood samples. These effects have important diagnostic implications. Once the blood sample is collected, if there is any delay between collection and mixing with anticoagulant the blood must be discarded because of possible activation of coagulation.

The combined performance of the screening coagulation tests PT and APTT is usually needed to identify RBDs of clinically significant severity but not FXIII deficiency. A prolonged APTT contrasting with a normal PT is indicative of FXI deficiency, provided hemophilia A and B and the asymptomatic defects of the contact phase are ruled out. A normal APTT and prolonged PT is typical of FVII deficiency, whereas the prolongation of both tests directs further analysis on the possible deficiencies of FX, FV, prothrombin, or fibrinogen. This paradigm is not valid for RBDs due to combined deficiencies, which prolong both the PT and the APTT. The sensitivity of PT and APTT to the presence of clotting factor deficiencies is dependent on the test system used [41, 42]. The degree of prolongation in the presence of a clotting factor deficiency can vary dramatically between reagents. Variation of reagents will also influence the sensitivity of PT methods for detecting abnormalities, particularly of FVII or FX. Specific assays of factor coagulant activity are necessary when the degree of prolongation of the global tests suggests the presence of severe, clinically significant deficiencies. Factor antigen assays are not strictly necessary for diagnosis and treatment but are necessary to distinguish type I from type II deficiencies.

The standard laboratory clotting tests (PT, APTT, fibrinogen level, platelet counts, bleeding time) are normal in FXIII deficiency. The diagnosis of factor XIII deficiency is established by the demonstration of increased clot solubility in 5 M urea, dilute monochloroacetic acid, or acetic acid. It is a qualitative test and is positive only if FXIII activity in the patient's plasma is zero, or very close to zero. If clot solubility in these reagents is found, it is important to perform some simple mixing experiments with normal plasma to make sure that the observed clot solubility is the result of FXIII deficiency and not due to the presence of a FXIII inhibitor. FXIII activity may also be deter-

mined quantitatively by measuring the incorporation of fluorescent or radioactive amines into proteins [43]. Specific enzyme-linked immunosorbent assays (ELISAs) have been developed to establish FXIII-A and FXIII-B antigen levels [44]. These assays are routinely available in the average coagulation laboratory in Europe and North America but are seldom carried out, so that proficiency and standardization may be limited.

Molecular diagnosis

RBDs are usually due to DNA defects in the genes encoding the corresponding coagulation factors (Table 5.2). Exceptions are the combined deficiencies of coagulation FV and FVIII and of vitamin K-dependent proteins (FII, FVII, FIX, and FX) caused respectively by mutations in genes encoding proteins involved in the FV and FVIII intracellular transport and in genes that encode enzymes involved in post-translational modifications and in vitamin K metabolism [45–48]. RBDs are often due to mutations unique for each kindred and scattered throughout the genes [1].

The identification of gene defects in patients with RBDs could represent the basis to conduct prenatal diagnosis in families that already have one affected child with severe bleeding. The molecular characterization and subsequent prenatal diagnosis gain

Table 5.2 General characteristics of coagulation factors genes

Deficient factor	Gene	Chromosome location
Fibrinogen	FGA	4q31.3
	FGB	4q31.3
	FGG	4q32.1
Prothrombin	F2	11p11.2
Factor V	F5	1q24.2
Factor V + VIII	MCFD2	2p21
	LMAN1	18q21.32
Factor VII	F7	13q34
Factor X	F10	13q34
Factor XI	F11	4q35.2
Factor XIII	F13A	6p25.1
	F13B	1q31.3
Vitamin K dependent	GGCX	2p11.2
	VKORC1	16p11.2

importance, particularly in developing countries, where patients with these deficiencies rarely live beyond childhood and where management is still largely inadequate; therefore, prenatal diagnosis remains the key step for the prevention of the birth of children affected by RBDs and severe bleeding manifestations, particularly in regions with low economic resources.

In order to identify the mutation responsible for the deficiency, venous blood is collected in sodium citrate, centrifuged, usually at 1500 *g* for 15 minutes, and, after discarding the plasma, genomic DNA is extracted from peripheral blood leukocytes. Following DNA extraction, the coding region, intron/exon boundaries, and 5′ and 3′ untranslated regions of the deficient factor gene are amplified by polymerase chain reaction (PCR) using the correctly designed oligonucleotides in order to avoid coamplification of unwanted gene regions. PCR products are then screened by single-strand conformation polymorphism (SSCP) or denaturing gradient gel electrophoresis (DGGE), alternatively they could be directly sequenced with an automated sequencer. The alignment of the obtained sequence with the normal sequence available on online databases, such as GenBank on the National Center for Biotechnology Information website (NCBI, http://www.ncbi.nlm.nih.gov/) or Ensembl (http://www.ensembl.org/index.html), will identify the genetic variant causing the deficiency. To confirm that the identified variant, if not previously reported, is not a frequent polymorphism, it has to be investigated in an adequate number of alleles coming from a healthy control population. Nowadays, mutations are named in accordance with the standard international nomenclature guidelines recommended by the Human Genome Variation Society (HGVS, http://www.hgvs.org/mutnomen/recs.html). A number of databases reporting all identified mutations are available online:

- http://www.med.unc.edu/isth/mutations-databases/
- http://www.hgmd.cf.ac.uk/ac/index.php/
- http://www.geht.org/databaseang/fibrinogen/ (for fibrinogen)
- http://www.lumc.nl/4010/research/Factor_V_gene.html (for FV)
- http://www.med.unc.edu/isth/registries.htm (for FVIII)
- http://www.factorxi.org/
- factorxi.org/ (for FXI)
- http://www.f13-database.de/ (xhgmobrswxgori45zk5jre45)/index.aspx) (for FXIII).

However, they are not always updated. In approx-

imately 5–10% of patients, no putative mutations are found. These cases may be due to defects in noncoding regions or in genes coding for regulators of intracellular transport and post-translational modifications of coagulation factors.

Differential diagnosis of an underlying bleeding disorder in women with menorrhagia

Gynecological assessment

Gynecological causes of abnormal vaginal bleeding (e.g., endometrial polyps, submucosal fibroids, cervicitis, cervical and vaginal lesions, etc.) should be excluded. A complete personal and family history as well as a physical examination including a careful pelvic/vaginal examination should be done [49]. An in-depth coagulation investigation should be considered for the patient with menorrhagia in whom gynecologic causes have been ruled out. However, a high index of suspicion for a possible bleeding abnormality needs to be maintained in all patients with excessive bleeding, as the prevalence of uterine abnormalities in patients with bleeding disorders in whom the gynecologic abnormality is "unmasked" by the bleeding disorder is uncertain [50]. Thus, a coagulation screen may be appropriate as part of the initial assessment, even in the absence of a pelvic examination.

Testing for inherited bleeding disorders in women with menorrhagia

Bleeding history
A personal and family history on bleeding symptoms should be collected, including:
- presence of menorrhagia since menarche
- bleeding after haemostatic challenge (dental extraction, surgery, or parturition)
- presence of any type of mucosal and/or not mucosal bleeding (location, severity and prevalence of bleeding should be reported).

In women who have a personal history of other bleeding or a family history of bleeding, further investigation should be considered.

Laboratory testing
Testing should include:
1 General laboratory tests:

- cells blood count and ferritin (exclude thrombocytopenia and assess degree of anaemia)
- thyroid (T3, T4, TSH)
- liver functional screening (GOT, GPT, PA, γGT)
- serum prolactin level

2 Coagulation laboratory test:
- prothrombin time (PT)
- activated partial thromboplastin time (APTT)
- thrombin time (TT)
- fibrinogen and FXIII.

Further investigations are requested in order to define the underlying coagulation disorder:
- bleeding time or PFA-100
- von Willebrand studies (VWF antigen, VWF functional assay, FVIII, blood group)
- platelet function analysis (PFA-100, aggregation, and ATP-release with different agonists)
- if PT, APTT, or TT are prolonged and VWF and platelet function analysis are both normal, mixing studies and single coagulation factor assays should be performed in order to test activity levels of missing factor.

The interpretation of abnormal or borderline results usually requires referral to a hematologist (or an internal medicine) consultant. It is important to have a precise hematological diagnosis because the diagnosis may affect such clinical situations as the treatment of both gynecologic and non-gynecologic bleeding, the optimal drugs/therapeutic modalities recommended for the management of severe bleeding, guidelines for patient preparation for surgery, including preoperative and post-operative management, and information for family counseling.

Treatment

Replacement of the deficient coagulation factor is the mainstay of treatment for RBDs, but safe and efficacious products are fewer and experiences on their optimal use much more limited. Specific recommendations could be found in previously published reports [1, 51]. The level of evidence is III or IV, and the recommendation grade is C or D, based on opinions of respected authorities, clinical experience, descriptive studies, or reports of expert committees. The strength of these recommendations is limited by the fact that the size of the series of patients on which they are based is not as large as evidence level I requires. It should be noted that no sufficient data are available in the literatureon management of pregnancy and delivery in women affected by prothrombin, FV, FV + FVIII, and FVII deficiency to make any recommendation.

Available treatments of menorrhagia (see also Chapters 2 and 7)

Specific treatment for menorrhagia is based on a number of factors, including:
- the age of the woman
- the overall health and medical history
- the cause and extent of menorrhagia
- tolerance for specific medications, procedures, or therapies
- the effects of menorrhagia on the patient's lifestyle
- personal preference.

Therapeutic options for the control of menorrhagia in women with underlying RBDs include medical treatments (such as antifibrinolytics, combined hormonal contraceptives, intranasal and subcutaneous DDAVP, oral contraceptives, levonorgestrel intrauterine device, and clotting factor replacement) and surgical treatments (such as endometrial ablation and hysterectomy). They are similar to the treatment options for menorrhagia in general. However, management of women with RBDs requires additional monitoring of the hemostatic parameters and awareness of the increased risk of bleeding with any surgical interventions. Therefore management of menorrhagia in women affected by RBDs should be provided by a multidisciplinary team including a hematologist and gynecologist.

Medical treatment of menorrhagia

This includes antifibrinolytics, combined oral contraceptives (COCs), DDAVP, progesterone, non-steroidal anti-inflammatory drugs (NSAIDS), ethamsylate, and the levonorgestrel-releasing intrauterine system (LNG-IUS).

These are discussed in detail in Chapters 3, 4, and 7.

Clotting factor
Clotting factor replacement, with fresh-frozen plasma (FFP), plasma-derived factor concentrate, or recombinant products, will be required in some women with bleeding disorders, especially in adolescents [52],

Table 5.3 Recommended schedules of treatment of different clinical situations in patients with rare bleeding disorders (modified from Mannucci *et al.* [1] and Bolton Maggs [51])

Deficient factor Target half-life	Treatment				
	Major surgery	Minor surgery	Spontaneous	Prophylaxis	Pregnancy/delivery
Fibrinogen 50 mg/dL 3–5 days	Concentrate: 20–30 mg/kg FFP: 15–20 mL/kg Cryo: 1 bag/10 kg	FFP: 15–20 mL/kg	Concentrates: 50–100 mg/dL FFP: 15–20 mL/kg	Estrogen/ progesterone in menorrhagia	>100 mg/dL + anticoagulant if history of thrombosis
Prothrombin 20–30% 2–3 days	PCC: 20–30 U/kg FFP: 15–20 mL/kg	FFP: 15–20 mL/kg	As for major surgery	No data	No data
FV 15% 36 hours	FFP: 15–20 mL/kg	As for major surgery	As for major surgery	No data	No data
FV + FVIII 10–15%	FFP: 15–20 mL/kg FVIII concentrate: 30–50 IU/dL/12 hours	As for major surgery	FFP: 15–20 mL/kg FVIII concentrate: 30–50 IU/dL	No data	No data
FVII 10–15% 4–6 hours	rFVIIa: 15–30 μg/kg/6–12 hours Concentrate: 30–40 U/kg/6–12 hours	As for major surgery	As for major surgery	Concentrate: 10–50 U/kg 1–3 times a week despite the short half-life	No data
FX 10–20% 20–40 hours	PCC: 20–30 U/kg FFP: 15–20 mL/kg	As for major surgery	As for major surgery	PCC: 30 U/kg twice weekly	As for prophylaxis
FXI 15–20% 48–72 hours	Concentrate: >70 U/dL FFP: 15–20 mL/kg	Concentrate: >30 U/dL FFP: 15–20 mL/kg	Usually it does not occur	–	Moderate: tranexamic acid/3 days; severe: FXI concentrate during labor
FXIII 2–5% 10–15 days	Concentrate: 10–20 U/kg FFP: 15–20 mL/kg Cryo: 1 bag/10 kg	As for major surgery	As for major surgery	Severe FXIII (risk ICH): 10 U/kg once monthly	As for prophylaxis

FFP, fresh-frozen plasma; PCC, prothrombin complex concentrate; ICH, intracranial hemorrhage.

those with severe deficiency, and those presenting with acute bleeding.

Specific recommendations are based on the hemostatic levels of each factor, on its plasma half-life (which governs the frequency of dose administration) (Table 5.3), and, most importantly, on safety.

The treatment with single-donor FFP (which contains all coagulation factors) is relatively inexpensive and widely available. However, the risk of volume overload is real when repeated infusions are administered to raise and keep the deficient factor at hemostatic levels. Most importantly, infectious complications with such blood-borne viruses as the hepatitis viruses or human immunodeficiency virus (HIV) are still perceived as a threat of FFP. Plasma concentrates of some single coagulation factors (fibrinogen, FVII, FXI, FXIII) are also available for replacement therapy, licensed, or on an investigational basis, but these are not widely available (see www.rbdd.org/art.htm). However, the number of available specific concentrates for RBDs are not as many as for hemophilia A and B; furthermore FV and FX concentrates are still lacking, hence FFP or prothrombin complex concentrates (PCCs, see below) are used for the treatment of FV and FX deficiency, respectively. PCCs, licensed for the treatment of FIX deficiency but also containing large amounts of FII, FVII, and FX, can also be used to treat these deficiencies, even though not all the available products are labeled in terms of coagulation factors other than FIX.

Until now, only one recombinant product, recombinant factor VIIa (rFVIIa), has been available and has been licensed by the USA and European regulatory agencies (FDA and EMEA, respectively) for replacement therapy in FVII deficiency. rFVIIa is also used off-label in a limited number of patients with other hereditary bleeding disorders such as FV and FXI deficiencies. The recommended dosage for FVII deficiency is 15–30 μg/kg, given every 4–6 hours, which can be repeated according to the clinical situation with the goal to keep FVII levels above 15–20%. The PT is often used as a surrogate to monitor rFVIIa therapy together with clinical response.

A second recombinant product, rFXIII, is under investigation in order to verify its safety, pharmacokinetics, and immunogenicity. It was tested on both healthy and FXIII-deficient adult volunteers with no evidence of serious adverse events such as development of antibodies [53, 54].

Conclusion

The recent increased interest in RBDs has led us to improve our knowledge on laboratory testing, diagnosis, and treatment of patients affected by RBDs. However, this is not yet sufficient to diagnose or exclude an underlying coagulation defect in all women who present with menorrhagia or other gynecological bleeding. In fact, the prevalence of undiagnosed bleeding disorders among these women is high, with estimates ranging from 5% to 20% [17, 55, 56]. Although the prevalence of menorrhagia among women with RBDs is increasing, information regarding the management of menorrhagia and other gynecological problems in these women is limited. With the exception of one small randomized trial [57], because of the rarity of RBDs studies are limited to case reports

and small case series. Therefore, clinical studies are still required to draw up guidelines based on clinical evidence. The scarce information, in particular the lack of recognition of the coagulation deficiency, may lead to inappropriate treatment (unnecessary surgical interventions or uncontrolled bleeding) that could be avoided with appropriate diagnosis. Prompt diagnosis, prophylaxis, or treatment may significantly improve the quality of life, which is often poor and debilitating. This is particularly the case in developing countries, with limited facilities and low budget resources.

In conclusion, the ideal management of women with RBDs who suffer from menorrhagia is through multidisciplinary clinics. However, at the present time, very few of these clinics exist and they are all located in tertiary care centers. These clinics include a nurse, a clinical hematologist, and a gynecologist who meet with the patient and liaise with the family physician. The ideal multidisciplinary team would have an even broader representation of expertise, and would include a laboratory hematologist, an obstetrician–gynecologist, an anesthesiologist, a family physician, a social worker, a pharmacist, and a laboratory technician.

Acknowledgements

I would like to thank Roberta Palla, Marta Spreafico, Silvia Lavoretano, Isabella Garagiola, and Marzia Menegatti for assisting the preparation of the manuscript

References

1 Mannucci PM, Duga S, Peyvandi F. Recessively inherited coagulation disorders. *Blood* 2004; **104**: 1243–1252.
2 Mannucci PM, Tuddenham EG. The hemophilias – from royal genes to gene therapy. *N Engl J Med* 2001; **344**: 1773–1779.
3 Mannucci PM. Hemophilia: treatment options in the twenty-first century. *J Thromb Haemost* 2003; **1**: 1349–1255.
4 Peyvandi F, Duga S, Akhavan S, Mannucci PM. Rare coagulation deficiencies. *Haemophilia* 2002; **8**: 308–321.
5 Shpilberg O, Peretz H, Zivelin A, *et al.* One of the two common mutations causing factor XI deficiency in Ashkenazi Jews (type II) is also prevalent in Iraqi Jews who represent the ancient gene pool of Jews. *Blood* 1995; **85**: 429–432.

6 Rizvi JH, Zuberi NF. Women's health in developing countries. *Best Pract Res Clin Obstet Gynaecol* 2006; **20**: 907–922.

7 Walraven G, Zuberi N, Temmerman M. The silent burden of gynaecological disease in low income countries. *Br J Obstet Gynaecol* 2005; **112**: 1177–1179.

8 Karimi M, Peyvandi F, Siboni S, *et al.* Comparison of attitudes towards prenatal diagnosis and termination of pregnancy for haemophilia in Iran and Italy. *Haemophilia* 2004; **10**: 367–369.

9 Lak M, Sharifian R, Peyvandi F, Mannucci PM. Symptoms of inherited factor V deficiency in 35 Iranian patients. *Br J Haematol* 1998; **103**: 1067–1069.

10 Lak M, Keihani M, Elahi F, *et al.* Bleeding and thrombosis in 55 patients with inherited afibrinogenaemia. *Br J Haematol* 1999; **107**: 204–206.

11 Lak M, Peyvandi F, Ali Sharifian A, *et al.* Pattern of symptoms in 93 Iranian patients with severe factor XIII deficiency. *J Thromb Haemost* 2003; **1**: 1852–1853.

12 Peyvandi F, Mannucci PM, Asti D, *et al.* Clinical manifestations in 28 Italian and Iranian patients with severe factor VII deficiency. *Haemophilia* 1997; **3**: 242–246.

13 Peyvandi F, Mannucci PM, Lak M, *et al.* Congenital factor X deficiency: spectrum of bleeding symptoms in 32 Iranian patients. *Br J Haematol* 1998; **102**: 626–628.

14 Peyvandi F, Tuddenham EG, Akhtari AM, *et al.* Bleeding symptoms in 27 Iranian patients with the combined deficiency of factor V and factor VIII. *Br J Haematol* 1998; **100**: 773–776.

15 Peyvandi F, Lak M, Mannucci PM. Factor XI deficiency in Iranians: its clinical manifestations in comparison with those of classic hemophilia. *Haematologica* 2002; **87**: 512–514.

16 Acharya SS, Coughlin A, Dimichele DM. Rare Bleeding Disorder Registry: deficiencies of factors II, V, VII, X, XIII, fibrinogen and dysfibrinogenemias. *J Thromb Haemost* 2004; **2**: 248–256.

17 Kadir RA, Economides DL, Sabin CA, *et al.* Frequency of inherited bleeding disorders in women with menorrhagia. *Lancet* 1998; **351**: 485–489.

18 Hurskainen R, Grenman S, Komi I, *et al.* Diagnosis and treatment of menorrhagia. *Acta Obstet Gynecol Scand* 2007; **86**: 749–757.

19 James AH. More than menorrhagia: a review of the obstetric and gynaecological manifestations of bleeding disorders. *Haemophilia* 2005; **11**: 295–307.

20 Lukes AS, Kadir RA, Peyvandi F, Kouides PA. Disorders of hemostasis and excessive menstrual bleeding: prevalence and clinical impact. *Fertil Steril* 2005; **84**: 1338–1344.

21 Kadir RA, Economides DL, Sabin CA, *et al.* Assessment of menstrual blood loss and gynaecological problems in patients with inherited bleeding disorders. *Haemophilia* 1999; **5**: 40–48.

22 Burrows RF, Ray JG, Burrows EA. Bleeding risk and reproductive capacity among patients with factor XIII deficiency: a case presentation and review of the literature. *Obstet Gynecol Surv* 2000; **55**: 103–108.

23 Shetty S, Madkaikar M, Nair S, *et al.* Combined factor V and VIII deficiency in Indian population. *Haemophilia* 2000; **6**: 504–507.

24 Higham JM, O'Brien PM, Shaw RW. Assessment of menstrual blood loss using a pictorial chart. *Br J Obstet Gynaecol* 1990; **97**: 734–739.

25 Reid PC, Coker A, Coltart R. Assessment of menstrual blood loss using a pictorial chart: a validation study. *Br J Obstet Gynaecol* 2000; **107**: 320–322.

26 Everett C. Incidence and outcome of bleeding before the 20th week of pregnancy: prospective study from general practice. *BMJ* 1997; **315**: 32–34.

27 Nybo Andersen AM, Wohlfahrt J, Christens P, *et al.* Maternal age and fetal loss: population based register linkage study. *BMJ* 320: 1708–1712.

28 Inbal A, Kenet G. Pregnancy and surgical procedures in patients with factor XIII. deficiency. *Biomed Prog* 2003; **16**: 69–71.

29 Greer IA, Lowe GD, Walker JJ, Forbes CD. Haemorrhagic problems in obstetrics and gynaecology in patients with congenital coagulopathies. *Br J Obstet Gynaecol* 1991; **98**: 909–918.

30 Kadir RA, Lee CA, Sabin CA, *et al.* Pregnancy in women with von Willebrand's disease or factor XI deficiency. *Br J Obstet Gynaecol* 1998; **105**: 314–321.

31 Kumar M, Mehta P. Congenital coagulopathies and pregnancy: report of four pregnancies in a factor X deficient woman. *Am J Hematol* 1994; **46**: 241–244.

32 Ross M. Placental and fetal physiology. In: Gabbe S, Niebyl J, Simpson J, eds. Obstetrics: normal and problem pregnancies. New York: Churchill Livingstone, 2002: 37–62.

33 Benedetti T. Obstetrical hemorrhage. In: Gabbe S, Niebyl J, Simpson J, eds. *Obstetrics: normal and problem pregnancies.* New York: Churchill Livingstone, 2002: 503–538.

34 Hoveyda F, MacKenzie IZ. Secondary postpartum hemorrhage: incidence, morbidity and current management. *Br J Obstet Gynaecol* 2001; **108**: 927–930.

35 Ramsahoye BH, Davies SV, Dasani H, Pearson JF. Pregnancy in von Willebrand's disease. *J Clin Pathol* 1994; **47**: 569–570.

36 Kadir RA, Economides DL, Braithwaite J, *et al.* The obstetric experience of carriers of haemophilia. *Br J Obstet Gynaecol* 1997; **104**: 803–810.

37 Edwards A, Ellwood DA. Ultrasonographic evaluation of the postpartum uterus. *Ultrasound Obstet Gynecol* 2000; **16**: 640–643.

38 Visness CM, Kennedy KI, Ramos R. The duration and character of postpartum bleeding among breast-feeding women. *Obstet Gynecol* 1997; **89**: 159–163.

39 Dahlman T, Hellgren M, Blombäck M. Changes in blood coagulation and fibrinolysis in the normal puerperium. *Gynecol Obstet Invest* 1985; **20**: 37–44.

40 Kitchen S, Malia RG, Greaves M, Preston FE. A method for the determination of activated factor VII using bovine and rabbit brain thromboplastins: demonstration of increased levels in disseminated intravascular coagulation. *Thromb Res* 1988; **50**: 191–200.

41 Lawrie AS, Kitchen S, Purdy G, *et al.* Assessment of actin FS and actin FSL sensitivity to specific clotting factor deficiencies. *Clin Lab Haematol* 1998; **20**: 179–186.

42 Turi DC, Peerschke EI. Sensitivity of three activated partial thromboplastin time reagents to coagulation factor deficiencies. *Am J Clin Pathol* 1986; **85**: 43–49.

43 Fickenscher K, Aab A, Stuber W. A Photometric assay for blood coagulation factor XIII. *Thromb Haemost* 1991; **65**: 535–540.

44 Katona E, Haramura G, Karpati L, *et al.* A simple, quick one-step ELISA assay for the determination of complex plasma factor XIII (A2B2). *Thromb Haemost* 2000; **83**: 268–273.

45 Nichols WC, Seligsohn U, Zivelin A, *et al.* Mutations in the ER-Golgi intermediate compartment protein ERGIC-53 cause combined deficiency of coagulation factors V and VIII. *Cell* 1998; **93**: 61–70.

46 Zhang B, Cunningham MA, Nichols WC, *et al.* Bleeding due to disruption of a cargo-specific ER-to-Golgi transport complex. *Nat Genet* 2003; **34**: 220–225.

47 Mousallem M, Spronk HM, Sacy R, *et al.* Congenital combined deficiencies of all vitamin K-dependent coagulation factors. *Thromb Haemost* 2001; **86**: 1334–1336.

48 Rost S, Fregin A, Ivaskevicius V, *et al.* Mutations in VKORC1 cause warfarin resistance and multiple coagulation factor deficiency type 2. *Nature* 2004; **427**: 537–41.

49 SOGC Clinical Practice Guidelines: guidelines for the management of abnormal uterine bleeding. *J Obstet Gynaecol Can* 2001; **106**: 1–6.

50 Kouides PA, Phatak PD, Burkart P, *et al.* Gynaecological and obstetrical morbidity in women with type 1 von Willebrand disease: results of a patient survey. *Haemophilia* 2000; **6**: 643–648.

51 Bolton-Maggs PH, Perry DJ, Chalmers EA *et al.* The rare coagulation disorders–review with guidelines for management from the United Kingdom Haemophilia Centre Doctors' Organisation. *Haemophilia* 2004; **10**: 593–628.

52 Kadir RA, Lee CA. Menorrhagia in adolescents. *Pediatr Ann* 2001; **30**: 541–546.

53 Reynolds TC, Butine MD, Visich JE, *et al.* Safety, pharmacokinetics, and immunogenicity of single-dose rFXIII administration to healthy volunteers. *J Thromb Haemost* 2005; **3**: 922–928.

54 Lovejoy AE, Reynolds TC, Visich JE, *et al.* Safety and pharmacokinetics of recombinant factor XIII-A2 administration in patients with congenital factor XIII deficiency. *Blood* 2006; **108**: 57–62.

55 Dilley A, Drews C, Miller C, *et al.* von Willebrand disease and other inherited bleeding disorders in women with diagnosed menorrhagia. *Obstet Gynecol* 2001; **97**: 630–6.

56 Edlund M, Blombäck M, von Schoultz B, Andersson O. On the value of menorrhagia as a predictor for coagulation disorders. *Am J Hematol* 1996; **53**: 234–8.

57 Kadir RA, Lee CA, Sabin CA, Pollard D, Economides DL. DDAVP nasal spray for treatment of menorrhagia in women with inherited bleeding disorders: a randomized placebo-controlled crossover study. *Haemophilia* 2002; **8**: 787–793.

6 Platelet disorders

Claire Philipp

Prevalence of platelet dysfunction in women

Platelet dysfunction is the most frequently found inherited bleeding disorder in females presenting with symptoms of menorrhagia who undergo comprehensive hemostatic testing, including tests of platelet function [1–3]. Platelet dysfunction has been reported in approximately 50% of women presenting with menorrhagia and is more common than von Willebrand disease and coagulation factor deficiencies in this population [1–3] (Table 6.1). Racial differences have also been observed in multiracial US populations of women with menorrhagia, with black women having a significantly higher prevalence of platelet dysfunction than white women (approximately 70% vs 40%) [1, 3].

The prevalence of inherited platelet function disorders in the general population has not been studied. Although men and women are equally at risk for inherited platelet function disorders, reproductive age women are more likely to have bleeding symptoms because of the obstetric and gynecologic challenges women face. However, the role of congenital platelet function defects among women with obstetric- and gynecology-associated bleeding other than menorrhagia remains poorly studied beyond case reports [4–7]. Severe, clearly defined platelet disorders are usually recognized in early childhood [5, 7, 8]. However, mild platelet function abnormalities are likely to be underdiagnosed in the clinical setting because of the generally mild symptoms in the absence of surgical or other hemostatic challenges [9, 10], the complexity of testing, including the requirement for testing fresh specimens [11, 12], and the specialized expertise required for the performance and interpretation of platelet function testing [12, 13].

Classification of inherited platelet disorders

Inherited platelet function disorders can be characterized on the basis of function or structure [14–16]. Platelet-based abnormalities of platelet adhesion and aggregation include Bernard–Soulier syndrome (deficiency or defect in glycoprotein 1b) [5, 17–19], pseudo- or platelet-type von Willebrand disease (platelet glycoprotein 1bα gain of functional phenotype) [20, 21], and Glanzmann's thrombasthenia (deficiency or defect in glycoprotein IIb–IIIa) [7, 19, 22, 23]. Platelet granule disorders include storage pool deficiency with reductions in the number and/or content of dense granules, alpha granules, or both granules [24–28], and Quebec platelet disorder associated with platelet multimerin deficiency and abnormal proteolytic degradation of alpha granule proteins [29]. Disorders of platelet secretion and signal transduction are a heterogeneous group of disorders including receptor defects for agonists such as collagen, adenosine diphosphate (ADP) (P_2Y_{12} deficiency) and thromboxane A_2, defects

Inherited Bleeding Disorders in Women, 1st edition. By CA Lee, RA Kadir and PA Kouides. Published 2009 by Blackwell Publishing, ISBN: 978-1-4051-6915-8.

Table 6.1 Distribution of platelet function defects, von Willebrand factor deficiency and coagulation factor deficiencies in females with menorrhagia

Reference	n	Type of study	Platelet function defects (%)	von Willebrand factor deficiency (%)	Coagulation factor deficiency (%)
Philipp et al. [1]	74	Prospective single site	54.1	13.5	5.4
Bevan et al. [2]	12	Retrospective single site	50.0	16.7	NR
Miller et al. [3]	231	Prospective multisite	58.4	10.8	6.9

NR, not reported.

in arachidonic acid pathways and thromboxane synthetase deficiency, and defects in G-protein activation [30, 31]. Disorders of platelet procoagulant activity (Scott syndrome) have also been described [32, 33]. Defects of platelet secretion and signal transduction are presumed to be the most common of the inherited platelet dysfunction disorders [16, 34]. Glanzmann's thrombasthenia, platelet-type von Willebrand disease, and Bernard–Soulier syndrome are rare disorders [5, 7, 14]. The pattern of inheritance for many congenital platelet disorders is unknown [35]. In inherited platelet disorders with known inheritance patterns, autosomal dominant (Quebec platelet disorder, platelet type von Willebrand disease), autosomal recessive (Glanzmann's thrombasthenia, Bernard–Soulier syndrome), and X-linked disorders (Wiscott–Aldrich syndrome) have been reported [5, 7, 29, 35–37].

Clinical features

Spontaneous mucocutaneous bleeding, including menorrhagia, bruising, and epistaxis, and bleeding after delivery, surgery, trauma, and dental extraction are common presenting symptoms in women with inherited platelet disorders [10, 38–42]. Typically, bleeding symptoms occur with rapid onset after trauma or surgery [35], and bleeding symptoms may not occur with each hemostatic challenge [9]. Hemarthrosis, muscle bleeds, urinary bleeding, and gastrointestinal bleeding are not usual manifestations of inherited platelet disorders [38, 40]. Some of the symptoms, such as easy bruising, gum bleeds, and epistaxis, overlap with symptoms found in the normal population [9, 40, 41, 43]. A family history of a bleeding disorder is useful in screening for bleeding disorders, including platelet function disorders [40, 44].

Laboratory diagnosis of platelet dysfunction

Patients undergoing evaluation for platelet dysfunction should also undergo evaluation for other coagulation abnormalities including von Willebrand disease and factor deficiencies, as bleeding symptoms may overlap and may occur concurrently [38, 43, 45]. A reliable drug history and discontinuing of possible platelet function-impairing medications and other agents prior to platelet function testing is indicated [11]. An assessment of platelet count, platelet size, and review of the blood smear should be performed as part of the evaluation [9, 38, 45]. Neither the bleeding time nor the platelet function analyzer (PFA-100, Siemans Healthcare Diagnostics, Deerfield, IL) are sensitive or specific enough to be used as screening tests for platelet function disorders [46–48]. Tests of platelet aggregation, usually performed with platelet-rich plasma, are clinically used to assess platelet function. Agonists uniformly include collagen, ADP, and arachidonic acid and usually ristocetin and epinephrine as well [9–13]. Platelet adenosine triphosphate release, useful in diagnosing storage pool disease and secretion abnormalities, can be assessed using luminescence methodologies [13]. Flow cytometry is useful in the evaluation of Bernard–Soulier disease and Glanzmann's thrombasthenia [49].

Management of inherited platelet disorders

There are limited studies on the management of bleeding in women with inherited platelet dysfunction [10, 38]. In women, management is directed at the control of symptoms of menorrhagia, and the prevention of bleeding complications with major and minor hemostatic challenges, including delivery, surgery, and teeth extraction [38, 50]. Intravenous desmopressin (DDAVP) has been shown to shorten the bleeding time and to be clinically effective in treating and preventing excessive bleeding in individuals undergoing invasive procedures [51–54]. In women with menorrhagia and platelet dysfunction, intranasal desmopressin has been demonstrated to reduce menstrual blood flow [55–57], with the reduction in menstrual blood flow correlating with increases in von Willebrand factor levels [58]. Antifibrinolytic agents (ε-aminocaproic acid and tranexamic acid) are useful for mild or moderate bleeding, especially mucocutaneous bleeding following dental extractions and oral surgery [14, 38]. Tranexamic acid alone [55] and in combination with desmopressin [56] has been demonstrated to significantly reduce menstrual flow in women with platelet dysfunction. In patients with severe platelet function disorders such as Glanzmann's thrombasthenia, or when desmopressin and antifibrinolytics do not control bleeding, platelet transfusions may be needed [38]. Recombinant FVIIa has been used in individuals with severe platelet function disorders and excessive bleeding, especially in those unresponsive to platelet transfusions because of isoimmunization [59–62]. There are limited data on the management of pregnancy, delivery, and postpartum bleeding in women with inherited platelet disorders. Epidural anesthesia should be avoided [38]. In women with Bernard–Soulier syndrome and Glanzmann's thrombasthenia, severe early and delayed postpartum bleeding has been reported [7, 39, 63]. Platelet transfusions before and after delivery for up to 6 days postpartum have been reported to reduce the risk of bleeding in women with Glanzmann's thrombasthenia [7]. The use of recombinant VIIa has been proposed [38]. In women with mild congenital platelet function disorders, desmopressin, and, in the case of severe bleeding, platelet transfusions have been used for management of vaginal and cesarean deliveries [38, 64]. Antifibrinolytics can be used as an adjunctive measure or, in the case of vaginal deliveries, alone [38].

References

1 Philipp CS, Dilley A, Miller CH, *et al.* Platelet functional defects in women with unexplained menorrhagia. *J Thromb Haemost* 2003; **1**: 477–484.

2 Bevan JA, Maloney KW, Hillery CA, *et al.* Bleeding disorders: a common cause of menorrhagia in adolescents. *J Pediatr* 2001; **138**: 856–861.

3 Miller CH, Heit JA, Kouides PA, *et al.* Laboratory characteristics of women with menorrhagia: a multi-site US study. *J Thromb Haemost* 2007; **5** (Suppl 2); p-m-187.

4 James AH. More than menorrhagia: a review of the obstetric and gynaecological manifestations of bleeding disorders. *Haemophilia* 2005; **11**: 295–307.

5 Lopez JA, Andrews RK, Afshar-Kharghen V, Berndt MC. Bernard-Soulier syndrome. *Blood* 1998; **91**: 4397–4418.

6 Sherer DM, Lerner R. Glanzmann's thrombasthenia in pregnancy: a case and review of the literature. *Am J Perinatol* 1999; **16**: 297–301.

7 George JN, Caen JP, Nurden AT. Glanzmann's thrombasthenia: the spectrum of clinical disease. *Blood* 1990; **75**: 1383–1395.

8 Pinto da Costa N, Armari-Alle C, Plantaz D, Pagnier A. Bernard-Soulier syndrome revealed by major neonatal thrombocytopenia. *Arch Pediatr* 2003; **10**: 983–985.

9 Hayward CPM. Diagnosis and management of mild bleeding disorders. *Hematology (Am Soc Hematol Educ Program)* 2005; 423–428.

10 Greaves M, Watson HG. Approach to the diagnosis and management of mild bleeding disorders. *J Thromb Haemost* 2007; **5** (Suppl 1): 167–174.

11 Peerschke EIB. The laboratory evaluation of platelet dysfunction. *Clin Lab Med* 2002; **22**: 405–420.

12 Hayward CP. Platelet function testing: quality assurance. *Semin Thromb Hemost* 2007; **33**: 273–282.

13 Moffat KA, Ledford-Kraemer MR, Nichols WL, Hayward CPM. Variability in clinical laboratory practice in testing for disorders of platelet function: results of two surveys of the North American Specialized Coagulation Laboratory Association. *Thromb Haemost* 2005; **93**: 549–553.

14 Hayward CPM, Rao AK, Cattaneo M. Congenital platelet disorders: overview of their mechanisms, diagnostic evaluation, and treatment. *Haemophilia* 2006; **12** (Suppl 3): 128–136.

15 Handin RI. Inherited platelet disorders. *Hematology (Am Soc Hematology Educ Program)* 2005; 396–402.

16 Cattaneo M. Inherited platelet-based bleeding disorders. *J Thromb Haemost* 2003; **1**: 1628–1636.

17 Bernard J, Soulier JP. Sur une nouvele variete de dystrophie thrombocytaire-hemorragipare congenitale. *Semaine des Hospitaux de Paris* 1948; **244**: 159–160.

18 Ware J, Russel SR, Marchese P, *et al.* Point mutation in a leucine-rich repeat of platelet glycoprotein 1balpha resulting in the Bernard-Soulier syndrome. *J Clin Invest* 1993; **92** (3): 1213–1220.

19 Nurden AT, Caen JP. Specific roles for platelet surface glycoproteins in platelet function. *Nature* 1975; **255**: 720–722.

20 Russell SD, Roth GJ. Pseudo-von Willebrand disease: a mutation in the platelet glycoprotein Ib alpha gene associated with a hyperactive surface receptor. *Blood* 1993; **81**: 1787–1791.

21 Miller JL, Cunningham D, Lyle VA, Finch CN. Mutation in the gene encoding the alpha chain of platelet glycoprotein Ib in platelet-type von Willebrand disease. *Proc Natl Acad Sci USA* 1991; **88**: 4761–4765.

22 D'Andrea G, Colaizzio D, Vecchione G, *et al.* Glanzmann's thrombasthenia: identification of 19 mutations in 30 patients. *Thromb Haemost* 2002; **87**: 1034–1042.

23 Belluci S, Caen J. Molecular basis of Glanzmann's thrombasthenia and current strategies in treatment. *Blood Rev* 2002; **16**: 193–202.

24 Nieuwenhuis HK, Akkerman JW, Sixma JJ. Patients with a prolonged bleeding time and normal aggregation tests may have storage pool deficiency: studies on one hundred six patients. *Blood* 1987; **70**: 620–623.

25 Weiss HJ, Chevervenick PA, Zalusky R, Factor A. A familial defect in platelet function associated with impaired release of adenosine diphosphate. *N Engl J Med* 1969; **281**: 1264–1270.

26 Raccuglia G. Gray platelet syndrome. A variety of qualitative platelet disorder. *Am J Med* 1971; **51**: 818–828.

27 Weiss HJ, Witte LD, Kaplan KL, *et al.* Heterogeneity in storage pool deficiency: studies on granule-bound substances in 18 patients including variants deficient in alpha-granules, platelet factor 4, beta thromboglobulin, and platelet-derived growth factor. *Blood* 1979; **54**: 1296–1319.

28 Lages B, Shatil SJ, Bainton DF, Weiss HJ. Decreased content and surface expression of alpha-granule membrane protein GMP-140 in one of two types of platelet alpha delta storage pool deficiency. *J Clin Invest* 1991; **87**: 919–929.

29 Hayward CPM, Rivard GE, Kane WH, *et al.* An autosomal dominant qualitative platelet disorder associated with multimerin deficiency, abnormalities in platelet factor V, thrombospondin, Von Willebrand factor, and fibrinogen, and an epinephrine aggregation defect. *Blood* 1996; **87**: 4967–4978.

30 Rao AK. Congenital disorders of platelet function: disorder of signal transduction and secretion. *Am J Med Sci* 1998; **316**: 69–77.

31 Rao AK. Inherited defects in platelet signaling mechanisms. *J Thromb Haemost* 2003; **1**: 671–681.

32 Weiss HJ. Scott syndrome: a disorder of platelet coagulant activity. *Semin Hematol* 1994; **31**: 312–319.

33 Zwaal RF, Comfurius P, Bevers EM. Scott syndrome, a bleeding disorder caused by defective scrambling of membrane phospholipids. *Biochim Biophys Acta* 2004; **1636**: 119–128.

34 Rao AK, Gabbeta J. Congenital disorders of platelet signal transduction. *Arterioscler Thromb Vasc Biol* 2000; **20**: 285–289.

35 Hayward CPM. Inherited platelet disorders. *Curr Opin Hematol* 2003; **10**: 362–368.

36 Tracy PB, Giles AR, Mann KG, *et al.* Factor V (Quebec): a bleeding diathesis associated with a qualitative platelet Factor V deficiency. *J Clin Invest* 1984; **74**: 1221–1228.

37 Jin Y, Mazza C, Christie JR, *et al.* Mutations of the Wiskott-Aldrich Syndrome Protein (WASP): hotspots, effect on transcription, and translation and phenotype/genotype correlation. *Blood* 2004; **104**: 4010–4019.

38 Bolton-Maggs PHB, Chalmers EA, Collins PW, *et al.* A review of inherited platelet disorders with guidelines for their management on behalf of the UKHCDO. *Br J Haematol* 2006; **135**: 603–633.

39 Prabu P, Parapia LA. Bernard-Soulier syndrome in pregnancy. *Clin Lab Med* 2006; **28**: 198–201.

40 Sramek A, Eikenboom J, Briet E, *et al.* Usefulness of patient interview in bleeding disorder. *Arch Intern Med* 1995; **155**: 1409–1415.

41 McKay H, Derome F, Anwar Haq M, *et al.* Bleeding risks associated with inheritance of the Quebec Platelet Disorder. *Blood* 2004; **104** (1): 159–165.

42 Philipp CS, Faiz A, Dowling N, *et al.* Age and the prevalence of bleeding disorders in women with menorrhagia. *Obstet Gynecol* 2005; **105**: 61–66.

43 Gudmundsdottir BR, Marder VJ, Onundarson PT. Risk of excessive bleeding associated with marginally low von Willebrand factor and mild platelet dysfunction. *J Thromb Haemost* 2007; **5**: 274–281.

44 Philipp CS, Faiz A, Dowling NF, *et al.* Development of a screening tool for identifying women with menorrhagia for hemostatic evaluation. *Am J Obstet Gynecol* 2008; **198**: 163.e1–8.

45 Kouides PA, Jacqueline C, Peyvandi F, *et al.* Hemostasis and menstruation: appropriate investigation for underlying disorders of hemostasis in women with excessive menstrual bleeding. *Fertil Steril* 2005; **84**: 1345–1351.

46 Hayward CPM, Harrison P, Cattaneo M, *et al.* on behalf of ISTH-SSC Platelet Physiology Subcommittee. Platelet function analyzer (PFA-100) closure time in the evaluation of platelet disorders and platelet function. *J Thromb Haemost* 2006; **4**: 312–319.

47 Philipp CS, Miller CH, Faiz A, *et al.* Screening women with menorrhagia for underlying bleeding disorders: the utility of the platelet function analyzer and bleeding time. *Haemophilia* 2005; **11**: 497–503.

48 Quiroga T, Goycoolea M, Munoz B, *et al.* Template bleeding time and PFA-100 have low sensitivity to screen patients with hereditary mucocutaneous hemorrhages. *J Thromb Haemost* 2004; **2**: 892–898.

49 Linden MD, Frelinger AL III, Barnard MR, *et al*. Application of flow cytometry to platelet disorders. *Semin Thromb Hemost* 2004; **30**: 501–511.

50 Lee CA, Chi C, Pavord SR, *et al*. The obstetric and gynaecological management of women with inherited bleeding disorders – review with guidelines produced by a taskforce of UK Haemophilia Centre Doctors' Organization. *Haemophilia* 2006; **12**: 301–336.

51 Schulman S, Johnsson H, Egberg N, Blomback M. DDAVP-induced correction of prolonged bleeding time in patients with congenital platelet function defects. *Thromb Res* 1987; **45**: 165–174.

52 Kentro TB, Lottenberg R, Kitchens CS. Clinical efficacy of desmopressin acetate for hemostatic control in patients with primary platelet disorders undergoing surgery. *Am J Hematol* 1987; **24**: 215–219.

53 DiMichele DM, Hathaway WE. Use of DDAVP in inherited and acquired platelet dysfunction. *Am J Hematol* 1990; **33**: 39–45.

54 Rao AK, Ghosh S, Sun L, *et al*. Mechanisms of platelet dysfunction and response to DDAVP in patients with congenital platelet function defects. *Thromb Haemost* 1995; **74**: 1071–1078.

55 Kouides PA, Heit JA, Philipp CS, *et al*. A multisite prospective crossover study of intranasal desmopressin and oral tranexamic acid among women with menorrhagia and abnormal laboratory hemostasis [Abstract]. *Blood* 2007; **111**: 711.

56 Edlund M, Blomback M, Fried G. Desmopressin in the treatment of menorrhagia in women with no common coagulation factor deficiency but with prolonged bleeding time. *Blood Coag Fibrinol* 2002; **13**: 225–231.

57 Kadir RA, Lee CA, Sabin CA, *et al*. DDAVP nasal spray for treatment menorhagia in women with inherited bleeding disorders: a randomized placebo controlled cross-over study. *Haemophilia* 2002; **8**: 787–793.

58 Rose SS, Faiz A, Miller CH, *et al*. Laboratory response to intranasal desmopressin in women with menorrhagia and platelet dysfunction. *Haemophilia* **14**: 571–578.

59 Poon MC, d'Oiron R, Hann I, *et al*. Use of recombinant factor VIIa (Novoseven) in patients with Glanzmann thrombasthenia. *Semin Hemost* 2001; **38** (4 Suppl 12): 21–25.

60 d'Oiron R, Menart C, Trzeciak MC, *et al*. Use of recombinant factor VIIa in 3 patients with inherited type 1 Glanzmann's thrombasthenia undergoing invasive procedures. *Thromb Haemost* 2000; **83**: 644–647.

61 Kaleelrahman M, Minford A, Parapia LA. Use of recombinant factor VIIa in inherited platelet disorders. *Br J Haematol* 2004; **125**: 95–96.

62 Ozelo MC, Svirin P, Larina L. Use of recombinant factor VIIa in the management of severe bleeding episodes in patients with Bernard-Soulier syndrome. *Ann Hematol* 2005; **84**: 816–822.

63 Khalil A, Seoud M, Tannous R, *et al*. Bernard-Soulier syndrome in pregnancy. *Clin Lab Med* 1998; **20**: 125–128.

64 Fausett B, Silver R. Congenital disorders of platelet function. *Clin Obst Gynecol* 1999; **42** (2): 390–405.

7 Gynecology

Rezan A Kadir

Introduction

Inherited bleeding disorders are underestimated in women in terms of their frequency and severity. Because of the concept of carriership in hemophilia, women are expected to carry bleeding disorders but not to be symptomatic. Excessive bleeding during menstruation and childbirth is usually overlooked by the women and their care givers [1, 2] as bleeding is expected during these events. In addition, because of the inherited nature of these disorders many of their female family members also have abnormal bleeding symptoms. There may be social and cultural issues that prevent these women from seeking medical advice, especially in developing counties. Furthermore, assessment of blood loss during menstruation and delivery is very subjective and usually underestimated.

Menstruation is a unique, significant and frequent hemostatic challenge for women. Similarly, ovulation is another monthly event that requires an integral hemostatic system. Most gynecological conditions either present with bleeding, such as fibroids and polyps, or symptoms secondary to bleeding, such as endometriosis and some ovarian cysts. Therefore, women and especially those of reproductive age are more likely to suffer from bleeding disorders and can be symptomatic with even mild forms. Data from the United Kingdom Haemophilia Centre Doctors Organisation (UKHCDO) show that 62%, 67%, and 68%

of patients with von Willebrand disease (VWD), factor XI (FXI) deficiency, and platelet function disorders, respectively, are women, [3]. Data from an international registry of 200 families with less common bleeding disorders indicate that over 70% of women on the registry are of reproductive age, the majority with menorrhagia (Table 7.1) [4]. Women with bleeding disorders are more likely to suffer from and present with gynecological problems because of their inherited bleeding tendency. Therefore, obstetricians and gynecologists have a pivotal role in the identification of these women. However, there seems to be a lack of awareness among obstetricians and gynecologists of the high prevalence and the magnitude of bleeding disorders in women. In a survey in the UK, only 13% and 2% of gynecologists would consider clotting screen and testing for VWD, respectively, when managing menorrhagia [1]. Similarly, a US survey found that 17% of physicians would order bleeding time determination for reproductive age women with menorrhagia and only 4% would consider VWD as the cause of menorrhagia [2]. Increased awareness among obstetricians and gynecologists and hematologists as well as their combined expertise are crucial for optimal management of these women.

Assessment of menstrual blood loss and diagnosis of menorrhagia

Menorrhagia is the most common presenting symptom for women with bleeding disorders. However, menorrhagia is not easy to define. Subjectively, it is defined as excessive or prolonged menstrual loss that

Inherited Bleeding Disorders in Women, 1st edition. By CA Lee, RA Kadir and PA Kouides. Published 2009 by Blackwell Publishing, ISBN: 978-1-4051-6915-8.

Table 7.1 Women with rare bleeding disorders and proportion with excessive menstrual bleeding

Deficiency	Women/total patients	Reproductive age women (%)	Women with EMB/reproductive age women (%)
VWD type 3	182/385	130 (71)	90/130 (69)
Fibrinogen	28/55	20 (71)	10/20 (50)
F II	8/13	8 (100)	6/8 (75)
FV	10/35	10 (100)	5/10 (50)
FV + FVIII	12/27	12 (100)	7/12 (60)
FVII	10/28	10 (100)	6/10 (60)
FX	9/32	8 (90)	4/8 (60)
FXI	13/38	13 (100)	1/13 (10)
FXIII	37/93	20 (54)	7/20 (35)

EMB, excessive menstrual bleeding; F, factor; VWD, von Willebrand disease. From Lukes et al. [4].

occurs at regular intervals over several cycles. Based on a population study (476 women from Göleborg, Sweden) in 1966, average menstrual loss was shown to be 30–40 mL per cycle with the upper limit of normal loss 60–80 mL [5]. A reduction in hemoglobin concentration and plasma iron concentration were noted when menstrual loss was between 60 and 80 mL, with a more marked decrease with menstrual loss greater than 80 mL [5]. Thus the 80 mL criterion was adopted as the definition for menorrhagia. Subjective diagnosis relying on the women's descriptions can be inaccurate, and only 40–50% of women complaining of heavy menstrual loss have losses more than 80 mL [6, 7]. Objective assessment can only be performed by the alkaline hematin method [8]. This method is specialized, time-consuming, and costly. It involves the collection of used sanitary protection by the women. It is, therefore, neither suitable nor feasible for clinical practice. In addition, doubt has been cast on the validity and the clinical usefulness of the 80 mL criterion. In a recent study, the greatest proportion of women with low hemoglobin (<12 g/dL) and ferritin levels were those with menstrual blood loss (MBL) of >120 mL, and no differences were observed in women with a MBL above or below 80 mL [9]. Thus 40 years on, with changing reproductive patterns and dietary habits, the effect of menstrual loss on women's health may now be different. Women with heavy menstruation have many concerns other than the volume of their menstrual loss, such as pain, mood changes, and worries about health and quality of life. Therefore the exact assessment of menstrual loss may be of limited usefulness, and clinicians should focus on the impact of menstruation on the iron status, quality of life, and its associated symptoms when managing a woman with menorrhagia.

Clinical features associated most strongly with excessive menstrual loss are the frequency of changing sanitary protections and the passage and sizes of the clots during menstruation [10]. A low serum ferritin level correctly predicts 60% of women with losses of more than 80 mL [10]. Adding the presence of clots larger than a 50 pence piece (2.7 cm) and changing protection less than every 2 hours increases the sensitivity to 76% [10]. Therefore, subjective judgment can be improved by including these important clinical features. The pictorial blood assessment chart (PBAC, Appendix ii) is a semi-objective method that takes into account the number of towels and tampons used, the degree to which individual items are soiled with blood, the passage of clots, and flooding [11]. Using a special scoring system, a score of 100 or more was reported to have a sensitivity and specificity of >80% for the diagnosis of menorrhagia (menstrual blood loss of 80 mL or more with the alkaline hematin method) by Higham et al. [11]. Good acceptance and simplicity of use were also reported in the same study. This chart has been validated in another study by Janssen et al. [12]. However, this group suggested a cut-off score of 185 for the diagnosis of menorrhagia to achieve equally high predictive values for positive and negative tests. Clinicians may choose different cut-off levels depending on the desired sensitivity and negative predictive value of the test. In a population with a high prevalence of iron deficiency such as in women with bleeding disorders, a highly sensitive test is needed to avoid underestimation of menstrual blood loss. Thus, we use a lower score of 100 in our population. In identifying bleeding disorders in women with menorrhagia, a PBAC score >100 was also shown to be a useful parameter as part of a clinical screening tool developed recently by Philipp *et al.* [13] and it significantly increased the sensitivity of their tool.

Menorrhagia as a predictor for bleeding disorders

Menorrhagia is the most common symptom of bleeding disorders in women [4, 14, 15]. It is also the presenting symptom in the majority of them. Therefore, menorrhagia can be a valuable predictor for bleeding disorders in women. This concept has been long appreciated in adolescent girls presenting with acute menorrhagia. More recently, there is increasing evidence that menorrhagia can be due to an undiagnosed bleeding disorder in a significant proportion of women and screening for these disorders especially VWD has been suggested. Regarding VWD, a systematic review by Shankar *et al.* [16] showed an overall prevalence of 13% (95% CI 11–15.6%) among 988 women in 12 studies (see Fig. 4.2). This is significantly higher than the 1–2% prevalence in the general population [17, 18]. The prevalence was higher in European studies than in North American studies [18% (95% CI 15–23%) vs 10% (95% CI 7.5–13%) $P = 0.007$]. This may be due to the ethnic composition of study populations with a higher number of black women in the North American studies. Black people are known to have a higher von Willebrand factor (VWF) and lower prevalence of VWD. Further discussion on epidemiology of VWD in women is found in Chapter 4.

In addition to VWD, hemostatic abnormalities such as factor VIII [19], factor XI deficiency [19], disorders of fibrinolysis [20, 21], and platelet function [22] have also been identified in women presenting with menorrhagia. In a study by Philipp *et al.* [22], platelet aggregation abnormalities were noted in a high proportion of 74 women with idiopathic menorrhagia. The maximal percent platelet aggregation was decreased with one or more agonists in 35 (47%) women. Decreased adenosine triphosphate release was also noted in 58% of the patients compared with 23% in the control subjects. These abnormalities were far more prevalent in the black population. Further studies are required to assess the role of platelet aggregation and release in normal menstruation and the potential role of platelet function abnormalities as a cause of heavy menstruation. For further discussion on platelet disorders, see Chapter 6.

Screening for bleeding disorders in women with menorrhagia

The above data indicate that a high proportion (up to 50%) of women with idiopathic menorrhagia may have a laboratory abnormality of hemostasis. Extensive hemostatic testing in all women with menorrhagia is not feasible and is unnecessary. A screening tool is required to help clinicians identify those likely to have a bleeding disorder for appropriate referral to a hematologist and assessment of their hemostasis.

To date, there is no clear consensus or guidance on what should be used as a screening tool. The American College of Obstetricians and Gynecologists published a committee opinion in 2001 recommending testing in the following situations: all adolescents with severe menorrhagia, adult women with no identifiable cause for menorrhagia, and women undergoing hysterectomy for menorrhagia [23]. However, there is currently insufficient evidence to support these recommendations. The presence of a pelvic pathology does not eliminate the possibility of VWD and may even unmask the condition in previously asymptomatic women [24]. The National Institute for Health and Clinical Excellence in the UK recommends hemostatic testing for menorrhagia during the teenage years and in women with menorrhagia since menarche and those with a personal or a family history suggesting a coagulation disorder [25]. Menorrhagia since menarche is a strong predictor of a bleeding disorder. This was present in 65% of women with menorrhagia who were diagnosed with a bleeding disorder compared with 9% in those with normal hemostasis [26]. However, many women may present toward the end of their reproductive age because of increased anovulatory cycles and the appearance of pelvic pathologies. In addition, many women stop the use of hormonal contraception at this age, which may have controlled their menorrhagia for many years. A focused history, including family and personal history of bleeding symptoms, is useful in the identification of women who are more likely to be affected by a hemostatic disorder. Bleeding symptoms that are most predictive of a bleeding disorder are bleeding after dental extraction, postoperative bleeding, and postpartum bleeding [26]. However, many women and especially girls presenting with menorrhagia may not have been challenged by trauma or surgery, and menorrhagia may be their only bleeding symptom [26].

Recently, a standardized questionnaire with a bleeding score has been suggested as a useful screening tool for VWD [27]. In a study of 42 women with documented VWD at the Royal Free Hospital using a bleeding score >5, this tool had a sensitivity of 83% [28]. A recent screening tool by Philipp *et al.* [13] appears promising for identification of both VWD and platelet function disorders. Based on analysis of bleeding symptoms of 146 women with menorrhagia, they identified a combination of bleeding and menstrual symptoms with a sensitivity of 81% (95% CI 74–89%) and positive predictive value of 71% (95% CI 63–71%) for hemostatic abnormalities [13]. Furthermore, the addition of a PBAC score of >100 increased the sensitivity of the screening tool to 95% (95% CI 91–99%) [13].

Laboratory testing for the diagnosis bleeding disorders is addressed in Chapter 1.

Gynecological problems in women with bleeding disorders

Normal menstruation is a complex process. Hemostasis (including primary platelet aggregation, and subsequent secondary fibrin formation with concurrent fibrinolytic modeling of the fibrin clot) plays an important part in the control of bleeding (Fig. 7.1). Therefore, hemostatic abnormalities are commonly associated with excessive or prolonged menstruation. Furthermore, women with these disorders are more likely to be symptomatic and suffer from other gynecological problems, especially those who present with bleeding or symptoms secondary to bleeding.

Menorrhagia

Menorrhagia is a common and major health problem for women with inherited bleeding disorders. It usually starts at menarche and may persist throughout their reproductive life. In VWD, menorrhagia is the most common bleeding symptom with a reported prevalence of 74–93% [14, 29, 30]. An international survey of 44 women with severe VWD, mainly types 2 and 3, reported severe menorrhagia requiring blood product therapy at least once in 80% of the women [31]. Using a PBAC to assess menstrual blood loss, menorrhagia (PBAC score >100) was confirmed in

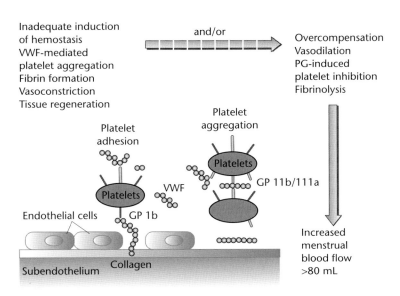

Fig. 7.1 Pathophysiology of hemostasis of menstruation resulting in menorrhagia. PG, prostaglandin.

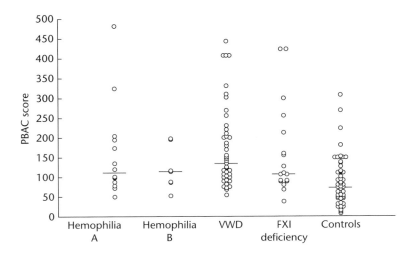

Fig. 7.2 Pictorial blood assessment chart (PBAC) scores in carriers of hemophilia, women with von Willebrand disease or factor XI deficiency.

74%, 59%, and 57% of women with VWD, FXI deficiency, and carriers of hemophilia, respectively (Fig. 7.2) [29]. The duration of menstruation was also found to be significantly longer, with more episodes of flooding in women with inherited bleeding disorders than in the control group. Excessive menstrual loss was more often reported by 105 menstruating carriers of hemophilia than by non-carriers, especially those with factor levels below 40 IU/µL [32]. Similarly, menorrhagia is reported in the majority of women with platelet dysfunction [33, 34] and rare bleeding disorders (Table 7.1) [4].

Heavy menstruation is a major cause of iron deficiency in women. A past or present history of anemia has been reported in 64% of 81 menstruating women with type 1 VWD [30]. Many women undergo unnecessary surgical interventions, including early hysterectomy for unexplained menorrhagia, often prior to the diagnosis of their bleeding disorders. In a recent survey, more women with VWD underwent hysterectomy (25% vs 9%) and at a younger age (33 vs 38 years of age) than the control subjects [15]. In a study by Woo *et al.* [35], four out of five women diagnosed with VWD had undergone hysterectomy for control of menorrhagia before VWD testing.

Menstruation has a major influence on a woman's lifestyle and employment. Quality of life during menstruation has been shown to be worse in women with bleeding disorders than in control subjects [36]. All scales of health-related quality of life are significantly affected in women with inherited bleeding disorders with pain, mental health, vitality, and social functioning the worst affected parameters [37]. Among individuals with VWD, women are less likely than men to undertake higher (college or university) education (5.5% vs 35%) [38]. It is possible that this burden of morbidity reflects the effect of menorrhagia directly, by physical and social limitations, or indirectly because of chronic iron deficiency secondary to menorrhagia. Early recognition, accurate diagnosis, and appropriate management of bleeding disorders should improve not only the quality of care for these women but also their quality of life.

Management of menorrhagia in women with inherited bleeding disorders

Ideally, women with bleeding disorders should be managed in a multidisciplinary clinic, including a hematologist and a gynecologist, within the network of hemophilia treatment centers (HTCs). This ensures the provision of comprehensive care with accurate on-site hemostasis testing and the availability of appropriate hemostatic agents when required. In a survey by the Centers for Disease Control and Prevention in the USA, 95% (71 out of 75) of women receiving care in HTCs reported a strong positive opinion and satisfaction [39]. Similar positive findings were also reported in the UK among women managed in a multidisciplinary clinic at the Royal Free Hospital in London [40].

Investigations

Once an underlying hemostatic abnormality is detected, the next question is what investigations, specifically gynecological investigations, are necessary for assessment of these women. Menorrhagia in women with disorders of hemostasis may be due to the underlying hematological problem, but not necessarily exclusively. Thus, menorrhagia may be multifactorial and other causes must be considered. In a survey of women with VWD, half of the women undergoing hysterectomy for menorrhagia had additional uterine pathology such as fibroids or endometriosis [30]. Local uterine causes must be evaluated, especially the possibility of malignancy in older women. Table 7.2 presents the investigations used for women with menorrhagia in general and the level of evidence to support their usefulness [25]. Most of these investigations have not been assessed in bleeding disorder-related menorrhagia. For clinical practice, the results of general menorrhagia patients can be extrapolated. However, the risk of bleeding complications and the need for blood products must always be assessed against the possible benefit prior to any invasive investigations.

Therapeutic options for menorrhagia

Management of menorrhagia involves consideration of the patient's age, childbearing status, and her need for contraception as well as preference in terms of perceived efficacy and side-effect profile. The therapeutic options in women with bleeding disorders include medical (non-hormonal and hormonal) and surgical treatments. They are similar to the treatment options for menorrhagia in general (this is addressed in Chapter 2). However, women with inherited bleeding disorders may also require of the use of hemostatic agents such as desmopressin (DDAVP) and clotting factor replacement for the control of menorrhagia, especially those with severe disorders. A management algorithm is presented in Fig. 7.3.

Medical treatment of menorrhagia

a. Non-hormonal treatment

Antifibrinolytic therapy Tranexamic acid an antifibrinolytic agent that reversibly blocks lysine binding sites on plasminogen and prevents fibrin degradation. Increased fibrinolysis is well documented in the endometrium with menorrhagia [20]. Tranexamic acid treatment was associated with a significant reduction in endometrial tissue plasminogen activator (t-PA) levels in 12 menorrhagic women [41]. In another study, tranexamic acid was also shown to significantly reduce t-PA and plasmin activity in the menstrual as well as in the peripheral blood of menorrhagic women compared with pre-treatment values [42].

In a systematic review by Lethaby *et al.* [43], two trials showed a significant reduction in mean menstrual blood loss (94 mL, 95% CI 36.5–151.4 mL)

Table 7.2 Summary of levels of evidence of menorrhagia investigations

Investigations	Level of evidence in menorrhagia in general [25]	Level of evidence of menorrhagia with bleeding disorders
PBAC	D – against	C – in favor
FBC/CBC	C – in favor	C – in favor
Serum ferritin	B – against	C – in favor
Female hormone testing	C – against	?
Thyroid function test	C – in favor (only when clinically indicated)	C – in favor
Pelvic scan	A – in favor	?
Saline sonography	A – against	?
Endometrial biopsy	D – in favor (only if persistent inter-menstrual bleeding, age >45 or failed medical treatment)	?
Hysteroscopy	A – in favor (only when only ultrasound outcomes are inconclusive)	?
Dilation and curettage	B – against	?

A, randomized trial; B, robust observational; C, case series; D, good practice point; ?, unknown – not studied; FBC/CBC, full blood count/complete blood count; PBAC, pictorial blood assessment chart.

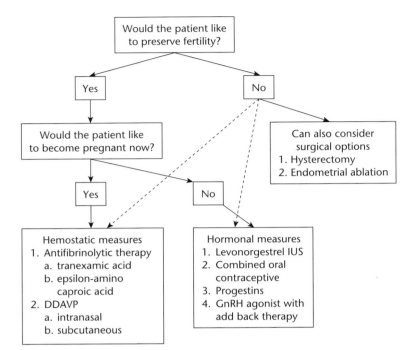

Fig. 7.3 Algorithm of management of menorrhagia. DDAVP, desmopressin; IUS, intrauterine System; GnRH, gonadotrophin-releasing hormone.

with antifibrinolytic therapy compared with placebo [44, 45]. Tranexamic acid was also superior to non-steroidal anti-inflammatory drugs (NSAIDs) in the reduction of menstrual loss; 54% versus 20% when compared with mefenamic acid [46], and 44% versus 20% when compared with flurbiprofen. However, none of them affected the duration of menses [46].

Oral tranexamic acid is generally well tolerated by women with menorrhagia. Nausea and diarrhea are the most common side-effects. Adverse events with tranexamic acid treatment for menorrhagia were not higher than with placebo, NSAIDs, cyclic progestogens, or ethamsylate in the Cochrane systematic review [43]. There have been isolated reports of thromboembolic complications with the use of tranexamic, which have led to a reluctance to use it. However, the incidence of thrombosis, over 19 years and 238 000 patient-years of treatment with tranexamic acid, was shown to be similar to the spontaneous frequency of thrombosis in women in the general population [47]. Nonetheless, the use of tranexamic acid is contraindicated in patients with a history of thromboembolic disease.

The Royal College of Obstetricians and Gynaecologists' guidelines in the UK recommend tranexamic acid for 3 months as a first-line medical treatment for menorrhagia [48]. If successful, tranexamic acid can be used indefinitely in patients not requiring contraception or who prefer non-hormonal treatment. In women with bleeding disorders, tranexamic acid is widely used (orally, intravenously, or topically, alone or as an adjuvant therapy) in the prevention and management of oral cavity bleeding, epistaxis, gastrointestinal bleeding as well as menorrhagia. However, there is a lack of objective data on its efficacy in reducing menstrual loss in these women. At the Royal Free Hospital in London, as a first-line therapy tranexamic acid 1 g 6 hourly was successful in 40% of 37 women with various causes of bleeding disorder-related menorrhagia by reducing menstrual loss to a PBAC score of <100 or to the woman's satisfaction [40].

The bioavailability of tranexamic acid is only about 35%; therefore, frequent administration (6 hourly) is necessary. This may reduce patient compliance. There have been reports of successful use of single, high-dose antifibrinolytic therapy (tranexamic acid at a dose of 4 g orally) in four VWD patients [49, 50]. However, this regime can be associated with severe nausea and vomiting. A new modified-release tranexamic acid formulation (XP12B) that allows less frequent dosing is currently being assessed for treatment of menorrhagia.

γ-Amino caproic acid is also an antifibrinolytic agent, but less potent than tranexamic acid. It can be used when tranexamic acid is not available.

Desmopressin (1-desamino-8-D-arginine vasopressin, DDAVP) is a synthetic analog of the antidiuretic hormone vasopressin. It increases the plasma concentration of FVIII and VWF through endogenous release [51, 52]. It is an important therapeutic alternative to plasma-derived coagulation products because it is effective in selected cases and avoids the risks of infection with blood-borne viruses. A test dose (as reviewed in Chapter 4) is recommended before treatment to assess its effectiveness as the response is not universal. DDAVP has been shown to be effective in the prevention and treatment of bleeding episodes in patients with mild VWD and hemophilia A. It can also be effective in some types of platelet disorders because of its effect on increasing platelet adhesiveness [53]. DDAVP is available in several formulations. It can be administered parenterally via intravenous or subcutaneous injection, or nasally as a spray. Intranasal administration of DDAVP is an attractive route because it allows patients to treat themselves at home without delay at the onset of menstruation, and without the use of needles [54, 55]. The effect of intranasal administration of 300 μg with a metered-dose spray is similar to that of a 0.2 μg/kg intravenous injection, with a similar reproducibility of the hemostatic effect [56].

Case series have shown subcutaneous [57] and intranasal DDAVP [58] to be effective in the management of menorrhagia in women with bleeding disorders who respond to DDAVP. Subjectively, the efficacy of DDAVP was reported as excellent or good in 86% and 92% of women treated with subcutaneous and intranasal DDAVP, respectively, in reducing their menstrual flow [57, 58]. However, in a randomized placebo-controlled crossover trial using a PBAC, intranasal DDAVP was not significantly ($P = 0.51$) different from placebo in reducing PBAC scores [59]. There was a statistically significant reduction in the PBAC score ($P = 0.0001$) in both groups compared with the pretreatment score and a trend towards a lower score when using intranasal DDAVP. It is possible that this difference did not reach statistical significance because of the small sample size. Similarly, intranasal DDAVP was not significantly different from placebo in reducing menstrual loss in 20 women with menorrhagia and prolonged bleeding [60]. However, there was a statistically significant decrease in menstrual blood loss when the DDAVP was combined with tranexamic acid. DDAVP has been shown to increase tissue t-PA in the circulation [52]. t-PA is the main physiological activator of the fibrinolytic system in blood and in the endometrium. It is possible that tranexamic acid counteracts the increased fibrinolytic activity induced by DDAVP, making the combination treatment more effective. In a recent US multicenter randomized crossover study of nasal DDAVP spray versus tranexamic acid, both treatments reduced PBAC scores and improved the quality of life in women with abnormal hemostasis. However, the reduction in menstrual scores was significantly greater with tranexamic acid treatment [61].

Common side-effects of DDAVP are mild tachycardia, headache, and flushing. These are related to its vasomotor effects. Owing to the antidiuretic effect of DDAVP, there is a small risk of hyponatremia and potentially water intoxication. This complication can be greatly reduced by restriction of fluid intake and avoidance of low-sodium drinks. In a small series by Dunn *et al.* [62], women had a much higher incidence of side-effects and the majority of the incidents coincided with the use of DDAVP nasal spray to control menorrhagia. The premenstrual phase is an antidiuretic phase due to the effect of progesterone. This may contribute to the increased risk of water retention of DDAVP when used for menorrhagia. Avoidance of treatment in the first day of the menses may help reduce the risk. We adopt this policy in our center and we have not had any serious side-effects.

Currently, there is no consensus regarding the optimum dose and duration of nasal DDAVP for treatment of menorrhagia in women with bleeding disorders. Most studies have used high-dose DDAVP intranasal spray 150–300 μg once or twice daily during the first 2–3 days of the menstrual period. This is based on the finding that 90% of all menstrual flow occurs during the first 3 days. However, the pattern of menstruation seems to be different in women with bleeding disorders. Women with bleeding disorders bleed heavily throughout their menstruation [29]. Therefore, it is essential to adjust the dose and duration of treatment according to the patient's menstrual pattern. Personal experience from our center indicates that a once-daily dose regime for a longer duration (4–5 days), especially in combination with tranexamic acid, can improve the efficacy of the treatment without an increase in adverse events.

Non-steroidal anti-inflammatory drugs (NSAIDs) have been shown to be more effective than placebo in reducing menstrual blood loss but less effective than tranexamic acid [63]. NSAIDs have the added advantage of reducing menstrual pain and menstrual migraine. However, their use is contraindicated in women with inherited bleeding disorders because of their antiaggregator effect on platelet function. This highlights the need for awareness of inherited bleeding disorders as a potential cause of menorrhagia in order to avoid the use of NSAIDs in such cases.

Ethamsylate is a hemostatic agent that maintains platelet and capillary integrity and affects prostaglandin synthesis. In the only randomized controlled trial in women with menorrhagia, ethamsylate showed no reduction in menstrual blood loss compared with 20% and 54% reduction found with mefenamic acid and tranexamic acid, respectively [46]. There are no data on the efficacy of this treatment in women with bleeding disorders. However, it may have a different effect on heavy menstrual loss in these women because of its positive effect on platelets. Further studies are warranted to assess its use in bleeding disorder-related menorrhagia.

b. Hormonal treatment

Combined hormonal contraceptive methods currently available include combined oral contraceptives (COCs), transdermal contraceptive patches and vaginal rings. Combined hormonal contraceptives (CHCs) are a highly reliable method of birth control. They are also useful for cycle regulation and to improve symptoms of dysmenorrhea and premenstrual tension. They inhibit the growth and development of the endometrium and reduce menstrual blood loss in women with or without menorrhagia [64, 65]. The COCs are the most commonly used method in clinical practice. In a trial of a 50 µg ethinylestradiol pill, menstrual loss was reduced by 52.6% in 68% of 164 women with objective menorrhagia [66]. The newer low-dose COCs are also shown to significantly reduce menstrual loss by 43% in a randomized controlled trial [67]. The efficacy of COCs in reducing menstrual blood loss in women with bleeding disorders is unknown. In a survey of women with VWD (types 2 and 3) unresponsive to DDAVP, the use of COCs was reported to be effective in controlling menorrhagia in 88% of the women [31]. On the other hand, in type I patients, a standard dose and a higher dose COC were effective in only 24%

and 37% of the cases, respectively [30]. COCs suppress ovulation. Therefore, in women with bleeding disorders, they have an added advantage of preventing ovulation bleedings that can be recurrent and potentially life-threatening, especially in those with severe disorders [68].

Traditionally, CHCs are used in a regimen of 21 hormonally active days, followed by 7 hormone-free days (21/7) during which uterine bleeding occurs. In recent years, the extended or continuous administration of CHCs (greater than 21 days of active hormones) has been reported as a successful regime in the treatment of endometriosis, dysmenorrhea, and other menstruation-association symptoms [69, 70]. Avoidance of menstruation through continuous dosing of CHCs has potential benefits, which include less interference with daily activities or special events and less menstruation-related absenteeism from work or school [71, 72]. The Cochrane systematic review of six randomized controlled trials of continuous (ranging from 49 days to 365 days) versus cyclical (28 days) use of COCs concluded that both regimes have similar patient satisfaction, compliance, pregnancy rate, and safety [73]. It also showed that continuous administration has a similar, if not better, effect on improving bleeding patterns and may improve menstruation-associated symptoms (headaches, genital irritation, tiredness, and menstrual pain). This regime could be very helpful in the management of menorrhagia in women with bleeding disorders as this regime allows women to control the timing and reduce the frequency of their menstruation. It may also be more effective than the cyclical regime in reducing menstrual blood loss.

Increased risk of thrombosis is the main concern associated with the use of CHCs. However, women with bleeding disorders have a low inherited thrombotic risk. Serious side-effects of CHCs include hypertension and, rarely, impaired liver function and hepatic tumors. Other less serious side-effects include nausea, vomiting, headache, breast tenderness, breakthrough bleeding, fluid retention, depression, and skin reactions.

Oral progestogens are one of the most commonly prescribed medications for menorrhagia. There are two different cyclical regimes of oral progestogens: a short luteal phase treatment (days 19–26 or days 15–25) or a longer 21 day course starting from day 5 of the cycle. A Cochrane systematic review, including six randomized controlled trials of the short luteal phase oral progestogen therapy, showed this regime to be significantly less effective in reducing menstrual blood loss than danazol, tranexamic acid, and the progesterone-releasing intrauterine system (IUS) [74]. A single trial comparing a long 21 day course (norethisterone 5 mg three times daily) with the levonorgestrel intrauterine system (LNG-IUS) showed a significant reduction in menstrual blood loss in both groups, but oral progestogen was less effective and acceptable by patients when compared with LNG-IUS [75].

Cyclical 21 day progesterone therapy can be considered as a second-line treatment for patients who do not respond to other medical therapies previously discussed or in whom such treatments are contraindicated. Owing to its side-effects and the long duration of treatment each cycle, the compliance with this regime is not usually good. The side-effects include fatigue, mood changes, weight gain, bloating, headaches, depression, irregular bleeding, and an adverse effect on bone density and lipid profile.

Oral progestogens in high doses alone, or in combination with DDAVP or clotting factor concentrate, may be useful in the treatment of acute menorrhagia in women with inherited bleeding disorders. Other forms of progestogens, injections or implants, have not been evaluated in women with menorrhagia, but studies in women without menorrhagia have shown that a considerable proportion of women experience amenorrhea with such therapies. More research is needed before recommendation can be made for women with menorrhagia with or without bleeding disorders. In addition, these modes of administration can be associated with a risk of excessive bruising and hematoma in women with bleeding disorders, especially severe forms.

Danazol and gonadotrophin-releasing hormone (GnRH) agonists are effective in reducing menstrual loss and duration of menstruation. Data on their effectiveness in the treatment of menorrhagia related to bleeding disorders are lacking. The profile of their side-effects and risks associated with a long-term hypoestrogenic state make them unacceptable for long-term use. Danazol may have a carry-over effect on reducing the menstrual loss [76]. Therefore, intermittent use of danazol has been suggested to increase acceptability and reduce side-effects. GnRH agonists with simultaneous hormone replacement therapy (add-back therapy) with combined estrogen/progesterone or tibolone may be an alternative option to surgery for women with severe bleeding disorders, such as type 3 VWD or

Glanzmann thrombasthenia, not responding to other treatments.

The **levonorgestrel-releasing intrauterine system** (LNG-IUS, Mirena, Schering, Germany) is an intrauterine system that steadily releases 20 µg of levonorgestrel into the endometrial cavity per 24 hours over a recommended duration of use of 5 years. It was originally developed as a contraceptive device. It suppresses endometrial growth causing the glands of the endometrium to become atrophic [77], thus reducing the menstrual loss. In a recent study the LNG-IUS was also shown to have antifibrinolytic properties within the endometrium, with significant increased plasminogen activator inhibitor levels and increased urokinase–plasminogen activator receptors levels after 6 months of use [78]. In terms of its clinical efficacy, in a systematic review by Stewart et al. [79], LNG-IUS was shown to reduce menstrual blood loss by 74% and 97% at 3 and 12 months in women with menorrhagia and normal coagulation. The Cochrane systematic review revealed LNG-IUS to be more effective in the treatment of menorrhagia than oral norethisterone given during days 5–26 of the menstrual cycle [80]. In another trial of women awaiting hysterectomy for the treatment of menorrhagia, 64% of women randomized to have the LNG-IUS decided to cancel the hysterectomy at 6 months compared with 14% for those who continued with their existing medical treatment (prostaglandin synthesis inhibitors or fibrinolysis inhibitors) [81]. All quality of life scores were significantly higher in the LNG-IUS group at 6 months.

When compared with endometrial ablation, LNG-IUS appears to be slightly less effective in reducing the menstrual loss [80]. A larger proportion of women with ablation (92%) had successful treatment (as measured by a PBAC score of less than 75) than those with LNG-IUS (75%). However, there was no significant difference in the rates of satisfaction with treatment or hemoglobin values after treatment [80]. Endometrial ablation may provide a quicker resolution to menstrual symptoms, but it is not suitable for women who want to preserve their fertility. The LNG-IUS is an effective reversible contraception. It is an attractive treatment option for women who require contraception and wish to preserve their fertility and for those who are unlikely to comply with drug treatments.

In a study by Kingman et al. [82], the use of LNG-IUS was evaluated in 16 women with inherited bleeding disorders (13 VWD, two FXI deficiency and one Hermansky–Pudlak syndrome) and menorrhagia not responding to various medical treatments. Nine months after the insertion of the IUS, the PBAC scores decreased significantly from a median of 213 (range 98–386) to 47 (range 24–75). Nine women became amenorrheic. The hemoglobin concentrations increased significantly from a median of 12.1 g/dL (range 8.0–13.2 g/dL) to 13.1 g/dL (range 12.3–14) (*P* = 0.0001). Quality of life was also improved with the treatment. No side-effects were reported except irregular spotting. The duration of spotting ranged from 30 to 90 days (median 42 days). In another study conducted in New York, the use of LNG-IUS was associated with a significant reduction in menstrual bleeding in 13 women with inherited bleeding disorders (11 VWD, one carrier of hemophilia A, one platelet function disorder) [83]. Similarly, there was a significant improvement in the quality of life in all women. The median duration of spotting after insertion was 12 weeks.

The long-term (5 years) efficacy of LNG-IUS for contraception is well established. However, data on its long-term efficacy in the treatment of menorrhagia are limited. The LNG-IUS was found to induce atrophy of the endometrial epithelium for more than 5 years [84], which provides a rationale for the reduction of menstrual blood loss for a prolonged period of time. An observational study has demonstrated a continuation rate of 50% after a mean 54 months of follow-up. Among these women, 57% had occasional bleeding and 35% had amenorrhea [85]. A significant reduction in menstrual blood loss and an increase in hemoglobin and serum ferritin levels were shown to last for as long as 36 months in women with idiopathic menorrhagia [86].

A recent study assessing the long-term effect of LNG-IUS in the management of menorrhagia in women with inherited bleeding disorders suggests that this treatment continues to be effective at a median duration of 53 months (range 24–60 months) after insertion [87]. The PBAC score decreased from a median of 286 (range 165–386) prior to insertion to a median of 8 (0–77). Six of 13 women in the study were amenorrheic (Fig. 7.4). Their mean hemoglobin concentration increased from 11.5 g/dL (range 10.6–12.9) to 13.1 g/dL (range 11.8–14.2). There is also a significant improvement in all aspects of quality of life compared with pre-LNG-IUS insertion. There was only

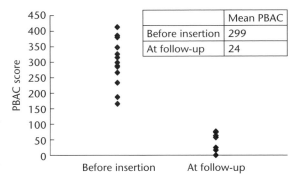

	Mean PBAC
Before insertion	299
At follow-up	24

Fig. 7.4 Mirena IUS and pictorial blood assessment chart scores (PBAC): long-term follow-up ≥24 months after insertion.

one discontinuation at 12 months in a woman who wanted to conceive. All of the women in this study had mild to moderate factor deficiencies and it would be interesting to see if this treatment is as effective in those with severe factor deficiencies.

The overall discontinuation rate for the LNG-IUS was shown to be 20% in randomized controlled trials and 17% in the case series [80]. The most common side-effect associated with LNG-IUS is irregular bleeding/spotting in the first 3–6 months after insertion. It usually resolves after 6–12 months in the majority of cases. Amenorrhea is also commonly reported; 44% of the women had no bleeding after 6 months in one study [88]. Therefore, appropriate counselling on the potential changes in the bleeding pattern may help to improve its acceptability. The expulsion rates (5–10%) are similar to other intrauterine devices [89, 90]. Other side-effects of LNG-IUS include those related to the systematic effects of progestogens, such as weight gain, bloating, breast tenderness, greasy hair or skin, acne, nausea, mood changes, and depression. On the other hand, LNG-IUS has the advantage of also being a very effective contraceptive, not requiring patient compliance, and of being better tolerated than systemic progestogens. It may also help menstrual pain. A 66% reduction in pain score has been reported with this system [91].

Women with bleeding disorders could potentially be at risk of bleeding at the time of insertion. Adequate hemostatic coverage is recommended, especially in women with severe forms of bleeding disorders. LNG-IUS suppresses ovulation in only 20% of the cycles; therefore, it may be necessary to continue the use of the combined oral contraceptive pill in women with recurrent or severe ovulation bleedings. The use of the LNG-IUS has been reported to be associated with an increased occurrence of ovarian cysts [92–94]. Using transvaginal ultrasound examination, ovarian cysts have been found in 17.5% and 21.5% of women after 6 and 12 months, respectively, of LNG-IUS use [94]. The cysts are asymptomatic and relatively small. The majority of these cysts are functional with a high rate of spontaneous resolution. However, there is a potential risk of hemorrhage into the cyst in women with severe hemostatic disorders. Therefore, ultrasound screening may be indicated in selected women with a high bleeding tendency to allow early detection and appropriate follow-up of the cyst. Future studies are required to assess the incidence and the resolution rate of ovarian cysts in these women.

Clotting factors Clotting factor replacement, with either recombinant or plasma-derived factor concentrate, will be required in some women with severe bleeding disorders when they present acutely with menorrhagia or as regular prophylaxis during menstruation for those not responding to other treatments. Prophylaxis may also be required in women planning conception to prevent ovulation bleeding that is otherwise controlled by COCs. A multidisciplinary assessment approach by hematologists and gynecologists is crucial in the management of these women. Further discussion is found in Chapter 4.

Surgical treatment for menorrhagia

Surgical intervention may be required in some women who do not tolerate medical treatments or where such treatments have failed. An underlying bleeding disorder can potentially be the reason for failed medical therapy [95]. Surgery may also be indicated in the presence of pelvic pathology. Women with a late-onset diagnosis of VWD may prefer a surgical option because of suffering for decades from the morbidity of heavy menstruation [96].

Women with inherited bleeding disorders are at greater risk of bleeding complications from surgery, including increased perioperative and delayed (7–10 days after surgery) bleeding. Prophylactic treatment is recommended in women with bleeding disorders.

Close follow-up for at least 10 days after surgery is also recommended to monitor specific factor levels and to assess for delayed bleeding complications. Multidisciplinary care by hematological, gynecological/surgical and anesthetic teams is essential to ensure an optimal outcome. Any surgical intervention in women with bleeding disorders should be carried out by experienced professionals. A surgical method with least risk of bleeding should be chosen. Extra care should be taken to ensure adequate hemostasis. Bleeding points should be ligated rather than cauterized and the use of surgical drains should be considered.

Hysterectomy Hysterectomy is an established, effective, and definitive treatment for menorrhagia associated with high patient satisfaction. However, hysterectomy is a major surgical procedure with significant physical and emotional complications and social and economic costs. A large cohort study evaluated 37 298 hysterectomies performed for benign indications in the UK in 1994 and 1995 with a 6 week post-surgery follow-up and found the associated mortality rate to be 0.38 per 1000 (95% CI 0.25–0.64) [97]. The overall operative complication rate was 3.5% (3% severe) and post-operative complication rate was 9% (1% severe) [97, 98]. Hysterectomy also has a risk of long-term complications, including early ovarian failure, and urinary and sexual problems. For these reasons, less invasive alternatives (e.g., endometrial resection and ablation) have been developed for the treatment of menorrhagia. However, hysterectomy may remain the only choice for some women with certain pelvic pathologies.

Endometrial ablation Endometrial ablative techniques are increasingly used today as an effective alternative to hysterectomy for the management of heavy menstrual bleeding. They have a shorter operating time and hospital stay, quicker recovery, and fewer complications than hysterectomy [99]. In recent years various endometrial ablative techniques have evolved. The first-generation techniques (resection, laser, and roller-ball) were introduced in the 1980s. They are performed under direct vision and require specialized surgical skills. The second-generation techniques are designed to ablate the full thickness of the endometrium by the controlled application of heat, cold, microwave, or other forms of energy. They require sophisticated equipment and are mostly performed blindly. A systematic review reported that, in general, they are technically simpler and quicker to perform than first-generation techniques, and satisfaction rates and reduction in menstrual blood loss are similar [100]. Second-generation techniques may be a safer option for women with bleeding disorders because of less risk of bleeding. The need for fluid distension media and its risks is avoided. This complication can be serious if DDAVP is used as a hemostatic cover for the procedure.

One study evaluated thermal balloon ablation in 70 women with severe menorrhagia and severe systematic disease, including 25 with "coagulopathy" [101]. The procedure was performed under local anesthesia and the success rate was over 90% at 3 year follow-up. The findings of a smaller retrospective study, which assessed the efficacy of endometrial ablation in seven women with VWD-related menorrhagia, were less favorable [102]. Four women experienced recurrence of menorrhagia after a median of 8 months after ablation, and three of them eventually underwent hysterectomy at a median of 11 months after ablation.

Consideration for the presence of an underlying bleeding disorder may be warranted in women who "fail" endometrial ablations or continue to have excessive menstrual bleeding after an ablation. Prophylactic treatment should always be considered to prevent bleeding complications. Guidance regarding the selection and use of therapeutic products for surgery in patients with VWD and other hereditary bleeding disorders can be obtained from the United Kingdom Haemophilia Centre Doctors' Organisation (UKHCDO) guidelines [103, 104].

Adolescent menorrhagia

Heavy, prolonged, and irregular menstrual periods are frequent complaints in adolescent girls. This is most likely to be due to immaturity of the hypothalamic–pituitary–ovarian axis resulting in anovulatory cycles. In these girls, only 14% and 56% of the cycles are ovulatory 1 and 4 years after menarche, respectively [105]. However, in a significant proportion of these cases, an underlying bleeding disorder may be identified [106–111]. Menorrhagia since menarche [108], positive family history of bleeding symptoms, and clinical anemia [107] are predictive of a bleeding disorder as an underlying cause for heavy menstruation in these young girls. Acute adolescent menorrhagia requiring hospital admission is also a strong predictor

of a bleeding disorder [108, 109]. Further discussion on the prevalence of bleeding disorders in adolescents with menorrhagia is found in Chapter 4. Menstruation may be the first hemostatic challenge faced by girls with an inherited bleeding disorder. With anovulatory cycles and prolonged shedding of the endometrium, it is possible that even mild disorders lead to disproportionately heavy menstrual loss. As VWF and FVIII levels increase with age and many of these girls start using hormonal contraception, menstrual symptoms are resolved and their bleeding disorders remain undiagnosed.

Menorrhagia in adolescent girls is associated with a significant morbidity and affects their quality of life as well as educational achievements. Unfortunately, there is a lack of evidence and guidance for the optimal management especially for acute menorrhagia. Clinicians are either unaware or reluctant to use many effective treatment options such as systemic hormonal therapy and Mirena IUS, leading to hysterectomy in girls as young as 14 years [112]. Nasal DDAVP spray together with tranexamic acid provides a good option as a first choice for very young girls and can be administered in a community setting [113]. These hemostatic agents can also be used in combination with hormonal therapies during the period or breakthrough bleedings. Combined oral contraceptives are a safe option for these girls with no adverse effects on their future fertility or attainment of their peak bone mass [114]. In a prospective study of young girls (12–21 years), oral contraceptive use was associated with a 1.5% increase in bone mineral density after 1 year [115]. Extended or continuous administration of COCs can be a very good option for these young girls to reduce the frequency and severity of their bleeding episodes. Mirena IUS has been used successfully in adolescents [116] and should be considered as an option when patients do not respond to other hormonal therapies. In severe cases, regular prophylaxis with an appropriate hemostatic agent may be necessary. A GnRH analogue with add-back therapy is also another option for girls with severe disorders not responding to other measures. These girls should be managed by a multidisciplinary team with close collaboration between hematologists and gynecologists to ensure consideration and optimal use of different treatment strategies and avoidance of hysterectomy.

In cases of acute menorrhagia, after resuscitation and volume replacement, the replacement of an appropriate hemostatic agent and the use of a high dose of hormonal therapy is sufficient to control the bleeding in the majority of cases. There are no data on the best hormonal option in these circumstances. Progestagens (medroxy progesterone acetate or norethisterone) in high doses are commonly used. Large doses of intravenous estrogen (e.g., Premarin Wyeth, USA, 25–40 mg intravenously, repeated 4 hourly to a maximum of 48 hours) promotes regeneration of the endometrium. Estrogen in high doses also increases coagulation factors including FVIII and VWF [117, 118] and promotes platelet aggregation [119]. Therefore, it can be effective in controlling severe menstrual bleeding. This should be used concurrently with a COC pill and antiemetics if necessary. In a recent randomized controlled trial, Premarin was more effective than placebo in controlling blood loss, and 64% of the Premarin-treated group stopped bleeding after the second dose compared with 11% of the control group [120]. However, this treatment is not commonly used and may not be available. GnRH analogs may also be useful in these situations. Examination under general anesthesia and evacuation of the blood clots from the uterine cavity and endometrial curetting should be considered in intractable cases. The use of a Foley catheter inserted transcervically and the balloon inflated can also be used to tamponade the bleeding within the uterine cavity. Uterine artery embolization has been successfully used in a 12 year old girl with plasminogen activator inhibitor deficiency and life-threatening menorrhagia at menarche [121]. This should be considered only as a life-saving measure and a last resort to obviate hysterectomy. The long-term effect of this procedure on fertility is not clearly known. Embolic agents with a high chance of recanalization of the uterine artery may be a better option for these girls to preserve their future fertility. Further experience/studies are required to determine the best embolic agents as well as the long-term effect and outcome of pregnancies following this procedure.

Dysmenorrhea

Dysmenorrhea is a common gynecological complaint. It has been classified into primary or secondary dysmenorrhea. Primary dysmenorrhea occurs in the absence of organic pathology and usually begins during adolescence. The prevalence of dysmenorrhea is highest among adolescent women, with estimates ranging from 60% to 93%, depending on the measurement method used [122, 123]. Secondary dysmenorrhea is caused by pelvic pathology (e.g., endometriosis, adenomyosis, and fibroids). Women with bleeding disorders commonly experience dysmenorrhea. This could be secondary to their heavy menstruation or possibly because they have a higher prevalence of pelvic pathologies such as endometriosis. The severity of dysmenorrhea has been shown to be significantly greater in women with bleeding disorders than in a control group [36]; 51% of women with bleeding disorders reported moderate, severe, or very severe pain during their period compared with 28% in the control group. In another study, 86% (70/81) of women with type 1 VWD reported menstrual pain rated at a median score of 4 on a Likert scale of 1–10 [30].

NSAIDs are commonly used and effective in the treatment of dysmenorrhea. Their use, however, is contraindicated in women with bleeding disorders because of the antiplatelet aggregating effect, making the management of dysmenorrhea in these women difficult. Treatment options for these women include other types of analgesia such as paracetamol and codeine or cyclo-oxygenase-2 inhibitors. Combined oral contraceptives and Mirena IUS are also useful for the control of menstrual pain. Surgery may be indicated in the presence of pelvic pathologies.

Ovulation bleeding

Ovulation may be associated with some degree of bleeding. In women with normal hemostasis, this is of little clinical significance and occasionally may be associated with some degree of mid-cycle (mittelschmerz) pain. In a survey of 81 menstruating women with type I VWD, 60 reported mid-cycle mittelschmerz pain at a median intensity of 4 on a Likert scale of 1–10, similar to the pain that accompanied their menstrual period [34]. Two-thirds of the cycles associated with mid-cycle pain have ultrasonically demonstrated pelvic fluid [124]. This suggests that mittelschmerz is associated with bleeding at ovulation and could explain the large proportion of women with VWD suffering from it.

In women with severe forms of bleeding disorders, the bleeding may continue into the corpus luteum and lead to hemorrhagic ovarian cysts. Rupture of these cysts may occur and lead to a life-threatening hemoperitoneum or broad ligament/retroperitoneal hematomas. A recent review identified 15 studies, mostly case reports and case series, reporting one or more hemorrhagic ovarian cysts in women with inherited bleeding disorders [24]. In one study, the prevalence was found to be 6.8% (9 of 136 women with VWD) [125].

A conservative approach with clotting factor replacement is advisable for the management of these complications in women with bleeding disorders [126]. Surgery can lead to further damage, especially in cases with broad ligament hematoma. Surgical intervention, however, may be necessary in some cases and it is important to give appropriate prophylaxis to cover the surgery and postoperative period. Recurrences of hemorrhagic ovarian cysts can also be a manifestation of a bleeding disorder [127]. Combined oral contraceptives have been shown to inhibit ovulation [128] and have been used successfully to prevent recurrences of such complications [126, 129, 130]. In women with recurrent ovulation bleeding who wish to conceive, prophylactic replacement therapy may be indicated. Alternatively, follicular tracking by serial ultrasound examination of the ovaries during the follicular phase and timing the replacement therapy with ovulation should be considered.

Other gynecological problems

Several studies have demonstrated increased rates of endometriosis in women with heavy menstruation [131]. This is probably due to the increased rate of retrograde menstruation, a possible etiology for endometriosis. Thus women with bleeding disorders may be at increased risk because of their heavy menstruation. In a survey of 102 women with VWD, 30% reported a history of endometriosis compared with 13% in the control group [15]. In the same survey, a higher prevalence of endometrial hyperplasia (10% vs 1%), endometrial polyps (8% vs 1%) and fibroids (32% vs 17%) were also reported among women with VWD compared with control subjects [15]. Since these conditions can manifest with bleeding symptoms, it is likely that more women with bleeding disorders become symptomatic. However, there is currently insufficient evidence to support these findings. Further studies are required to assess the prevalence and course of gynecological conditions in women with bleeding disorders.

Uterine fibroids are the most common benign gynecological tumors and affect 25% of women of reproductive age [132]. They cause numerous symptoms and can negatively affect health and quality of life of women. In addition to menorrhagia, large fibroids can also cause pelvic pain, dysparunia, and pressure symptoms, leading to urinary and defecation disorders. They can also be associated with infertility and adverse pregnancy outcome. Traditional treatment for large and symptomatic fibroids is surgery (abdominal, vaginal, or laparoscopic hysterectomy or myomectomy). Uterine artery embolization is an alternative option especially for women who no longer desire fertility and wish to avoid surgery. This is a minimally invasive, percutaneous, image-guided procedure and is ideal for women with high operative risk such as obesity, cardiac and pulmonary conditions, as well as women with hemostatic disorders [133]. It has a low complication rate and high patient satisfaction rate. The majority of women report marked reduction in the severity of fibroid-specific symptoms and improvement in quality of life [134]. This option should be considered in women with bleeding disorders, especially if they have other operative risk factors. This procedure may also have a role in management of acute gynecological bleeding such as acute menorrhagia (see "Adolescent menorrhagia") and operative and postoperative bleeding not responding to other measures.

References

1 Chi C, Shiltagh N, Kingman CE, et al. Identification and management of women with inherited bleeding disorders: a survey of obstetricians and gynaecologists in the United Kingdom. Haemophilia 2006; **12**: 405–412.
2 Dilley A, Drews C, Lally C, et al. A survey of gynecologists concerning menorrhagia: perceptions of bleeding disorders as a possible cause. J Women's Health Gend Based Med 2002; **11**: 39–44.
3 United Kingdom Haemophilia Centres Doctors Organisation. Annual Report 2007 Annual Returns 2006. A report from UKHCDO and NHD. Manchester: UKHCDO, 2007.
4 Lukes A, Kadir RA, Peyvandi F, Kouides PA. Disorders of hemostasis and excessive menstrual bleeding: prevalence and clinical impact. Fertil Steril 2005; **84**: 1338–1344.
5 Hallberg L, Hogdahl AM, Nilsson L, Rybo G. Menstrual blood loss: a population study. Variation at

different ages and attempts to define normality. *Acta Obstet Gynecol Scand* 1966; **45**: 320–351.

6 Fraser IS, McCarron G, Markham R. A preliminary study of factors influencing perception of menstrual blood loss volume. *Am J Obstet Gynecol* 1984; **149**: 788–793.

7 Chimbira TH, Anderson AB, Turnbull A. Relation between measured menstrual blood loss and patient's subjective assessment of loss, duration of bleeding, number of sanitary towels used, uterine weight and endometrial surface area. *Br J Obstet Gynaecol* 1980; **87**: 603–609.

8 Hallberg L, Nilsson L. Determination of menstrual blood loss. *Scand J Clin Lab Invest* 1964; **16**: 244–248.

9 Warner PE, Critchley HO, Lumsden MA, *et al.* Menorrhagia II: is the 80-mL blood loss criterion useful in management of complaint of menorrhagia? *Am J Obstet Gynecol* 2004; **190**: 1224–1229.

10 Warner PE, Critchley HO, Lumsden MA, *et al.* Menorrhagia I: measured blood loss, clinical features, and outcome in women with heavy periods: a survey with follow-up data. *Am J Obstet Gynecol* 2004; **190**: 1216–1223.

11 Higham JM, O'Brien PM, Shaw RW. Assessment of menstrual blood loss using a pictorial chart. *Br J Obstet Gynaecol* 1990; **97**: 734–739.

12 Janssen CA, Scholten PC, Heintz AP. A simple visual assessment technique to discriminate between menorrhagia and normal menstrual blood loss. *Obstet Gynecol* 1995; **85**: 977–982.

13 Philipp CS, Faiz A, Dowling NF, *et al.* Development of a screening tool for indentifying women with menorrhagia for hemostatic evaluation. *Am J Obstet Gynecol* 2008; **198**: 163–168.

14 Ragni MV, Bontempo FA, Hassett AC. von Willebrand disease and bleeding in women. *Haemophilia* 1999; **5**: 313–517.

15 Kirtava A, Drews C, Lally C, *et al.* Medical, reproductive and psychosocial experiences of women diagnosed with von Willebrand's disease receiving care in haemophilia treatment centres: a case-control study. *Haemophilia* 2003; **9**: 292–297.

16 Shankar M, Lee CA, Sabin CA, *et al.* von Willebrand disease in women with menorrhagia: a systematic review. *Br J Obstet Gynaecol* 2004; **111**: 734–740.

17 Rodeghiero F, Castaman G, Dini E. Epidemiological investigation of the prevalence of von Willebrand's disease. *Blood* 1987; **69**: 454–459.

18 Werner EJ, Broxson EH, Tucker EL, *et al.* Prevalence of von Willebrand disease in children: a multiethnic study. *J Pediatr* 1993; **123**: 893–898.

19 Kadir RA, Economides DL, Sabin CA, *et al.* Frequency of inherited bleeding disorders in women with menorrhagia. *Lancet* 1998; **351**: 485–489.

20 Winkler UH. Menstruation: extravascular fibrinolytic activity and reduced fibrinolytic capacity. *Ann NY Acad Sci* 1992; **667**: 289–290.

21 Edlund M, Blomback M, He S. On the correlation between local fibrinolytic activity in menstrual fluid and total blood loss during menstruation and effects of desmopressin. *Blood Coagul Fibrinolysis* 2003; **14**: 593–598.

22 Philipp CS, Dilley A, Miller CH, *et al.* Platelet functional defects in women with unexplained menorrhagia. *J Thromb Haemost* 2003; **1**: 477–484.

23 ACOG committee on Gynecologic Practice. von Willebrand's disease in gynecologic practice. ACOG Committee Opinion No. 263. *Obstet Gynecol* 2001; **98**: 1185–1186.

24 James AH. More than menorrhagia: a review of the obstetric and gynaecological manifestations of bleeding disorders. *Haemophilia* 2005; **11**: 295–307.

25 National Institute for Health and Clinical Excellence. *Heavy menstrual bleeding. Clinical Guideline.* London: RCOG, 2007.

26 Kadir RA, Economides DL, Sabin CA, *et al.* Frequency of inherited bleeding disorders in women with menorrhagia. *Lancet* 1998; **351**: 485–489.

27 Rodeghiero F, Castaman G, Tosetto A, *et al.* The discriminant power of bleeding history for the diagnosis of type 1 von Willebrand disease: an international, multicenter study. *J Thromb Haemost* 2005; **3**: 2619–2626.

28 Chi C, Chase A, Riddell A, *et al.* Bleeding score as a screening tool for identification and assessment of VWD in women [Abstract]. *Thromb Res* 2007; **119** (Suppl 1): S101.

29 Kadir RA, Economides DL, Sabin CA, *et al.* Assessment of menstrual blood loss and gynaecological problems in patients with inherited bleeding disorders. *Haemophilia* 1999; **5**: 40–48.

30 Kouides PA, Phatak PD, Burkart P, *et al.* Gynaecological and obstetrical morbidity in women with type I von Willebrand disease: results of a patient survey. *Haemophilia* 2000; **6**: 643–648.

31 Foster PA. The reproductive health of women with von Willebrand disease unresponsive to DDAVP: results of an international survey. On behalf of the Subcommittee on von Willebrand Factor of the Scientific and Standardization Committee of the ISTH. *Thromb Haemost* 1995; **74**: 784–790.

32 Plug I, Mauser-Bunschoten EP, Broker-Vriends AH, *et al.* Bleeding in carriers of hemophilia. *Blood* 2006; **108**: 52–56.

33 George JN, Caen JP, Nurden AT. Glanzmann's thrombasthenia: the spectrum of clinical disease. *Blood* 1990; **75**: 1383–1393.

34 Lopez JA, Andrews RK, Afshar-Kharghan V, Berndt MC. Bernand-Soulier syndrome. *Blood* 1998; **91**: 4397–4418.

35 Woo YL, White B, Corbally R, *et al*. von Willebrand's disease: an important cause of dysfunctional uterine bleeding. *Blood Coagul Fibrinolysis* 2002; **13**: 89–93.

36 Kadir RA, Sabin CA, Pollard D, *et al*. Quality of life during menstruation in patients with inherited bleeding disorders. *Haemophilia* 1998; **4**: 836–841.

37 Shanker M, Chi C, Kadir RA. Review of quality of life: menorrhagia in women with or without inherited bleeding disorders. *Haemophilia* 2008; **14**: 15–20.

38 Barr RD, Sek J, Horsman J, *et al*. Health status and health-related quality of life associated with von Willebrand disease. *Am J Hematol* 2003; **73**: 108–114.

39 Kirtava A, Crudder S, Dilley A, *et al*. Trends in clinical management of women with von Willebrand disease: a survey of 75 women enrolled in haemophilia treatment centres in the United States. *Haemophilia* 2004; **10**: 158–161.

40 Lee CA, Chi C, Shiltagh N, *et al*. Review of a multidisciplinary clinic for women with inherited bleeding disorders. *Haemophilia* 2008; published online..

41 Gleeson NC, Buggy F, Sheppard BL, Bonnar J. The effect of tranexamic acid on measured menstrual loss and endometrial fibrinolytic enzymes in dysfunctional uterine bleeding. *Acta Obstet Gynecol Scand* 1994; **73**: 274–277.

42 Dockeray CJ, Sheppard BL, Daly L, Bonnar J. The fibrinolytic enzyme system in normal menstruation and excessive uterine bleeding and the effect of tranexamic acid. *Eur J Obstet Gynecol Reprod Biol* 1987; **24**: 309–318.

43 Lethaby A, Farquhar C, Cooke I. Antifibrinolytics for heavy menstrual bleeding. *Cochrane Database Syst Rev* 2000; CD000249.

44 Edlund M, Andersson K, Rybo G, *et al*. Reduction of menstrual blood loss in women suffering from idiopathic menorrhagia with a novel antifibrinolytic drug (Kabi 2161). *Br J Obstet Gynaecol* 1995; **102**: 913–917.

45 Callender ST, Warner GT, Cope E. Treatment of menorrhagia with tranexamic acid. A double-blind trial. *BMJ* 1970; **4**: 214–216.

46 Bonnar J, Sheppard BL. Treatment of menorrhagia during menstruation: randomised controlled trial of ethamsylate, mefenamic acid, and tranexamic acid. *BMJ* 1996; **313**: 579–582.

47 Rybo G. Tranexamic acid therapy: effective treatment in heavy menstrual bleeding: clinical update on safety. *Adv Ther* 1991; **4**: 1–8.

48 Royal College of Obstetricians and Gynaecologists. *The initial management of menorrhagia – national evidence-based clinical guidelines No. 1. 1998*. London: RCOG Press; 1998.

49 Ong YL, Hull DR, Mayne EE. Menorrhagia in von Willebrand disease successfully treated with single daily dose tranexamic acid. *Haemophilia* 1998; **4**: 63–65.

50 Onundarson PT. Treatment of menorrhagia in von Willebrand's disease [Letter]. *Haemophilia* 1999; **5**: 76.

51 Lethagen S, Harris AS, Sjorin E, Nilsson IM. Intranasal and intravenous administration of desmopressin: effect on F VIII/vWF, pharmacokinetics and reproducibility. *Thromb Haemost* 1987; **58**: 1033–1036.

52 Cash JD, Gader AM, da Costa J. Proceedings: The release of plasminogen activator and factor VIII to lysine vasopressin, arginine vasopressin, I-desamino-8-d-arginine vasopressin, angiotensin and oxytocin in man. *Br J Haematol* 1974; **27**: 363–364.

53 Sakariassen KS, Cattaneo M, Berg A, *et al*. DDAVP enhances platelet adherence and platelet aggregate growth on human artery subendothelium. *Blood* 1984; **64**: 229–236.

54 Rose EH, Aledort LM. Nasal spray desmopressin (DDAVP) for mild hemophilia A and von Willebrand disease. *Ann Intern Med* 1991; **114**: 563–568.

55 Lethagen S, Ragnarson Tennvall G. Self-treatment with desmopressin intranasal spray in patients with bleeding disorders: effect on bleeding symptoms and socioeconomic factors. *Ann Hematol* 1993; **66**: 257–260.

56 Lethagen S, Harris AS, Nilsson IM. Intranasal desmopressin (DDAVP) by spray in mild hemophilia A and von Willebrand's disease type I. *Blut* 1990; **60**: 187–191.

57 Rodeghiero F, Castaman G, Mannucci PM. Prospective multicenter study on subcutaneous concentrated desmopressin for home treatment of patients with von Willebrand disease and mild or moderate hemophilia A. *Thromb Haemost* 1996; **76**: 692–696.

58 Leissinger C, Becton D, Cornell C, Jr., Cox Gill J. High-dose DDAVP intranasal spray (Stimate) for the prevention and treatment of bleeding in patients with mild haemophilia A, mild or moderate type 1 von Willebrand disease and symptomatic carriers of haemophilia A. *Haemophilia* 2001; **7**: 258–266.

59 Kadir RA, Lee CA, Sabin CA, *et al*. DDAVP nasal spray for treatment of menorrhagia in women with inherited bleeding disorders: a randomized placebo-controlled crossover study. *Haemophilia* 2002; **8**: 787–793.

60 Edlund M, Blomback M, Fried G. Desmopressin in the treatment of menorrhagia in women with no common coagulation factor deficiency but with prolonged bleeding time. *Blood Coagul Fibrinolysis* 2002; **13**: 225–231.

61 Kouides PA, Heit JA, Philipp CS, *et al*. The effect of intranasal desmopressin vs. oral tranexamic acid on

menstrual blood loss among women with menorrhagia and abnormal laboratory hemostasis: a multicentre, randomized cross-over study [Abstract]. *J Thomb Haemost* 2007; **5** (Suppl 2); p-m-183.

62 Dunn AL, Powers JR, Ribeiro MJ, *et al.* Adverse events during use of intransal desmopressin acetate for haemophilia A and von Willebrand disease: a case report and review of 40 patients. *Haemophilia* 2000; **6**: 11–14.

63 Lethaby A, Augood C, Duckitt K, Farquhar C. Nonsteroidal anti-inflammatory drugs for heavy menstrual bleeding. *Cochrane Database Syst Rev* 2007; CD000400.

64 Callard GV, Litofsky FS, DeMerre LJ. Menstruation in women with normal or artificially controlled cycles. *Fertil Steril* 1966; **17**: 684–688.

65 Ramcharan S, Pellegrin FA, Ray RM, Hsu JP. The Walnut Creek Contraceptive Drug Study. A prospective study of the side effects of oral contraceptives. Volume III, an interim report: a comparison of disease occurrence leading to hospitalization or death in users and nonusers of oral contraceptives. *J Reprod Med* 1980; **25** (6 Suppl): 345–372.

66 Nilsson L, Rybo G. Treatment of menorrhagia. *Am J Obstet Gynecol* 1971; **110**: 713–720.

67 Fraser IS, McCarron G. Randomized trial of 2 hormonal and 2 prostaglandin-inhibiting agents in women with a complaint of menorrhagia. *Aust N Z J Obstet Gynaecol* 1991; **31**: 66–70.

68 Jarvis RR, Olsen ME. Type I von Willebrand's disease presenting as recurrent corpus hemorrhagicum. *Obstet Gynecol* 2002; **99**: 887–888.

69 Vercellini P, De Giorgi O, Mosconi P, *et al.* Cyproterone acetate versus a continuous monophasic oral contraceptive in the treatment of recurrent pelvic pain after conservative surgery for symptomatic endometriosis. *Fertil Steril* 2002; **77**: 52–61.

70 Sulak PJ, Cressman BE, Waldrop E, *et al.* Extending the duration of active oral contraceptive pills to manage hormone withdrawal symptoms. *Obstet Gynecol* 1997; **89**: 179–183.

71 Miller L, Notter KM. Menstrual reduction with extended use of combination oral contraceptive pills: randomized controlled trial. *Obstet Gynecol* 2001; **98**: 771–778.

72 Miller L, Hughes JP. Continuous combination oral contraceptive pills to eliminate withdrawal bleeding: a randomized trial. *Obstet Gynecol* 2003; **101**: 653–661.

73 Edelman AB, Gallo MF, Jensen JT, *et al.* Continuous or extended cycle versus cyclic use of combined oral contraceptives for contraception. *Cochrane Database Syst Rev* 2005; CD004695.

74 Lethaby A, Irvine G, Cameron I. Cyclical progestogens for heavy menstrual bleeding. *Cochrane Database Syst Rev* 1998; CD001016.

75 Irvine GA, Campbell-Brown MB, Lumsden MA, *et al.* Randomised comparative trial of the levonorgestrel intrauterine system and norethisterone for treatment of idiopathic menorrhagia. *Br J Obstet Gynaecol* 1998; **105**: 592–598.

76 Shaw RW. Treating the patient with menorrhagia. *Br J Obstet Gynaecol* 1994; 101 Suppl **11**: 1–2.

77 Silverberg SG, Haukkamaa M, Arko H, *et al.* Endometrial morphology during long-term use of levonorgestrel-releasing intrauterine devices. *Int J Gynecol Pathol* 1986; **5**: 235–241.

78 Koh SC, Singh K. The effect of levonorgestrel-releasing intrauterine system use on menstrual blood loss and the haemostatic, fibrinolytic/inhibitor systems in women with menorrhagia. *J Thromb Haemost* 2007; **5**: 133–138.

79 Stewart A, Cummins C, Gold L, *et al.* The effectiveness of the levonorgestrel-releasing intrauterine system in menorrhagia: a systematic review. *Br J Obstet Gynaecol* 2001; **108**: 74–86.

80 Lethaby AE, Cooke I, Rees M. Progesterone or progestogen releasing intrauterine systems for heavy menstrual bleeding. *Cochrane Database Syst Rev* 2005; CD002126.

81 Lahteenmaki P, Haukkamaa M, Puolakka J, *et al.* Open randomised study of use of levonorgestrel releasing intrauterine system as alternative to hysterectomy. *BMJ* 1998; **316**: 1122–1126.

82 Kingman CE, Kadir RA, Lee CA, Economides DL. The use of levonorgestrel-releasing intrauterine system for treatment of menorrhagia in women with inherited bleeding disorders. *Br J Obstet Gynaecol* 2004; **111**: 1425–1428.

83 Kouides P, Phatak P, Sham R, *et al.* The efficacy and safety of the levonorgestrel intrauterine device (Mirena) for bleeding disorder-related menorrhagia in an American cohort [Abstract]. *Hemophilia* 2006; **12** (Suppl 2): 146.

84 Silverberg SG, Haukkamaa M, Arko H, *et al.* Endometrial morphology during long-term use of levonorgestrel-releasing intrauterine devices. *Int J Gynecol Pathol* 1986; **5**: 235–241.

85 Nagrani R, Bowen-Simpkins P, Barrington JW. Can the levonorgestrel intrauterine system replace surgical treatment for the management of menorrhagia? *Br J Obstet Gynaecol* 2002; **109**: 345–347.

86 Xiao B, Wu SC, Chong J, *et al.* Therapeutic effects of the levonorgestrel-releasing intrauterine system in the treatment of idiopathic menorrhagia. *Fertil Steril* 2003; **79**: 963–969.

87 Chi C, Chase A, Kadir R. Levonorgestrel-releasing intrauterine system for the management of menorrhagia in women with inherited bleeding disorders: longterm follow-up [Abstract]. *Thromb Res* 2007; **119** (Suppl 1): S101.

88 Hidalgo M, Bahamondes L, Perrotti M, *et al*. Bleeding patterns and clinical performance of the levonorgestrel-releasing intrauterine system (Mirena) up to two years. *Contraception* 2002; **65**: 129–132.

89 Andersson K, Odlind V, Rybo G. Levonorgestrel-releasing and copper-releasing (Nova T) IUDs during five years of use: a randomized comparative trial. *Contraception* 1994; **49**: 56–72.

90 Sivin I, el Mahgoub S, McCarthy T, *et al*. Long-term contraception with the levonorgestrel 20 mcg/day (LNg 20) and the copper T 380Ag intrauterine devices: a five-year randomized study. *Contraception* 1990; **42**: 361–378.

91 Hurskainen R, Teperi J, Rissanen P, *et al*. Clinical outcomes and costs with the levonorgestrel-releasing intrauterine system or hysterectomy for treatment of menorrhagia: randomized trial 5-year follow-up. *JAMA* 2004; **291**: 1456–1463.

92 Pakarinen PI, Suvisaari J, Luukkainen T, Lahteenmaki P. Intracervical and fundal administration of levonorgestrel for contraception: endometrial thickness, patterns of bleeding, and persisting ovarian follicles. *Fertil Steril* 1997; **68**: 59–64.

93 Jarvela I, Tekay A, Jouppila P. The effect of a levonorgestrel-releasing intrauterine system on uterine artery blood flow, hormone concentrations and ovarian cyst formation in fertile women. *Hum Reprod* 1998; **13**: 3379–3383.

94 Inki P, Hurskainen R, Palo P, *et al*. Comparison of ovarian cyst formation in women using the levonorgestrel-releasing intrauterine system vs. hysterectomy. *Ultra-sound Obstet Gynecol* 2002; **20**: 381–385.

95 Lukes AS, Kouides PA. Hysterectomy versus expanded medical treatment for abnormal uterine bleeding: clinical outcomes in the medicine or surgery trial. *Obstet Gynecol* 2004; **104**: 864–865.

96 Howard F, Phatak P, Braggins C, *et al*. Patient preferences/outcomes for the treatment of menorrhagia from a prospective study of the prevalence of von Willebrand disease-related menorrhagia [Abstract]. *Haemophilia* 2000; **6**: 242.

97 Maresh MJ, Metcalfe MA, McPherson K, *et al*. The VALUE national hysterectomy study: description of the patients and their surgery. *Br J Obstet Gynaecol* 2002; **109**: 302–312.

98 McPherson K, Metcalfe MA, Herbert A, *et al*. Severe complications of hysterectomy: the VALUE study. *Br J Obstet Gynaecol* 2004; **111**: 688–694.

99 Lethaby A, Shepperd S, Cooke I, Farquhar C. Endometrial resection and ablation versus hysterectomy for heavy menstrual bleeding. *Cochrane Database Syst Rev* 1999; CD000329.

100 Lethaby A, Hickey M. Endometrial destruction techniques for heavy menstrual bleeding: a Cochrane review. *Hum Reprod* 2002; **17**: 2795–2806.

101 Toth D, Gervaise A, Kuzel D, Fernandez H. Thermal balloon ablation in patients with multiple morbidity: 3-year follow-up. *J Am Assoc Gynecol Laparosc* 2004; **11**: 236–239.

102 Rubin G, Wortman M, Kouides PA. Endometrial ablation for von Willebrand disease-related menorrhagia – experience with seven cases. *Haemophilia* 2004; **10**: 477–482.

103 Pasi KJ, Collins PW, Keeling DM, *et al*. Management of von Willebrand disease: a guideline from the UK Haemophilia Centre Doctors' Organization. *Haemophilia* 2004; **10**: 218–231.

104 Keeling D, Tait C, Maknis M. Guidelines on the selection and use of therapeutic products to treat haemophilia and other hereditary bleeding disorders. *Haemophilia* 2008; **14**: 671–684.

105 Read GF, Wilsonn DW, Hughes IA, Griffith SK. The use of salivary progesterone assays in the assessment of ovarian function in postmenarcheal girls. *J Endocrinol* 1984; **102**: 265–268.

106 Bevan JA, Maloney KW, Hillery CA, *et al*. Bleeding disorders: a common cause of menorrhagia in adolescents. *J Pediatr* 2001; **138**: 856–861.

107 Jayasinghe Y, Moore P, Donath S, *et al*. Bleeding disorders in teenagers presenting with menorrhagia. *Aust N Z J Obstet Gynaecol* 2005; **45**: 439–443.

108 Claessens EA, Cowell CA. Acute adolescent menorrhagia. *Am J Obstet Gynecol* 1981; **139**: 277–80.

109 Smith YR, Quint EH, Hertzberg RB. Menorrhagia in adolescents requiring hospitalization. *J Pediatr Adolesc Gynecol* 1998; **11**: 13–15.

110 Philipp CS, Faiz A, Dowling N, *et al*. Age and the prevalence of bleeding disorders in women with menorrhagia. *Obstet Gynecol* 2005; **105**: 61–66.

111 Mikhail S, Varadarajan R, Kouides P. The prevalence of disorders of haemostasis in adolescents with menorrhagia referred to a haemophilia treatment centre. *Haemophilia* 2007; **13**: 627–632.

112 Leung PL, Ng PS, Lok IH, Yuen PM. Puberty menorrhagia secondary to inherited bleeding disorders. *Acta Obstet Gynecol Scand* 2005; **84**: 921–922.

113 Khair K, Baker K, Mathias M, *et al*. Intranasal desmopressin: a safe and efficacious treatment option for children with bleeding disorders. *Haemophilia* 2007; **13**: 548–551.

114 Faculty of Family Planning and Reproductive Health Care Clinical Effectiveness Unit. FFPRHC Guideline (October 2004). Contraceptive choices for young people. *J Fam Plan Reprod Health Care* 2004; **30**: 237–251.

115 Cromer BA, Blair JM, Mahan JD, *et al*. A prospective comparison of bone density in adolescent girls receiving

depot medroxyprogesterone acetate (Depo-Provera), levonorgestrel (Noeplant), or oral contraceptives. *J Pediatr* 1996; **129**: 671–676.

116 Jayasinghe K, Moore P, Jayasinghe Y, Grover S. The use of levonorgestrel intrauterine system in adolescents. *North American Society Pediatric and Adolescent Gynecology, 20th Annual Clinical meeting*, 18–20 May 2006. Orlando, FL: NASPAG, 2006.

117 Alperine JE. Estrogens and surgery in women with von Willebrand disease. *Am J Med* 1982; **73**: 367–371.

118 Glueck HI, Flessa HC. Control of hemorrhage in with von Willebrand disease and haemophilic carrier with norethynordrelmestranol. *Thromb Res* 1972; **1**: 253–266.

119 Elkeles RS, Hampton JR, Mitchell JRA. Effect of oestrogen on human platelet behaviour, *Lancet* 1968; **2**: 315–317.

120 DeVore GR, Owens O, Kase N. Use of intravenous Premarin in the treatment of dysfunctional uterine bleeding: a double-blind randomized control study. *Obstet Gynecol* 1982; **59**: 285–291.

121 Bowkley CW, Dubel GJ, Haas RA, *et al.* Uterine artery embolization for control of life-threatening haemorrhage at menarche: Brief report. *J Vasc Interv Radiol* 2007; **18**: 127–131.

122 Klein JR, Litt IF. Epidemiology of adolescent dysmenorrhea. *Pediatrics* 1981; **68**: 661–664.

123 Banikarim C, Chacko MR, Kelder SH. Prevalence and impact of dysmenorrhea on Hispanic female adolescents. *Arch Pediatr Adolesc Med* 2000; **154**: 1226–1229.

124 Hann LE, Hall DA, Black EB, Ferrucci JT, Jr. Mittelschmerz. Sonographic demonstration. *JAMA* 1979; **241**: 2731–2732.

125 Silwer J. von Willebrand's disease in Sweden. *Acta Paediatr Scand Suppl* 1973; **238**: 1–159.

126 O'Brien PM, DiMichele DM, Walterhouse DO. Management of an acute hemorrhagic ovarian cyst in a female patient with hemophilia A. *J Pediatr Hematol Oncol* 1996; **18**: 233–236.

127 Jarvis RR, Olsen ME. Type I von Willebrand's disease presenting as recurrent corpus hemorrhagicum. *Obstet Gynecol* 2002; **99**: 887–888.

128 Mishell DR, Jr. Noncontraceptive health benefits of oral steroidal contraceptives. *Am J Obstet Gynecol* 1982; **142**: 809–816.

129 Bottini E, Pareti FI, Mari D, *et al.* Prevention of hemoperitoneum during ovulation by oral contraceptives in women with type III von Willebrand disease and afibrinogenemia. Case reports. *Haematologica* 1991; **76**: 431–433.

130 Ghosh K, Mohanty D, Pathare AV, Jijina F. Recurrent haemoperitoneum in a female patient with type III von Willebrand's disease responded to administration of oral contraceptive. *Haemophilia* 1998; **4**: 767–768.

131 Vercellini P, De Giorgi O, Aimi G, *et al.* Menstrual characteristics in women with and without endometriosis. *Obstet Gynecol* 1997; **90**: 264–268.

132 Stewart EA. Uterine fibroids. *Lancet* 2001; **357**: 293–298.

133 Lund N, Justesen P, Elle B, *et al.* Fibroids treated by uterine artery embolization. *Acta Obstet Gynecol Scand* 2000; **79**: 905–910.

134 Seals JG, Jones PA, Wolfe C. Uterine artery embolization as a treatment for symptomatic fibroids: a review of literature and case report. *J Am Acad Nurse Pract* 2006; **18**: 361–367.

8 Genetic and laboratory diagnosis

Edward Tuddenham

Introduction

This chapter will cover the integrated genetic and laboratory diagnosis of the most prevalent bleeding disorders, hemophilia A, hemophilia B, and von Willebrand disease (VWD), as applied to women. The first two being sex-linked recessive disorders rarely affect women in a severe form and then only for specific genetic reasons that will be discussed. However, women in families segregating hemophilia A or B should always be offered carrier status determination and milder degrees of clinically significant factor deficiency are common in carriers, a fact that is not widely appreciated. VWD, being autosomal (dominant or recessive depending on the underlying mutation type), should affect both sexes equally but is diagnosed more often in women by reason of their greater lifetime experience of hemostatic challenge, especially the stress of menstruation during the reproductive years. Genetic and laboratory (in the sense of coagulation factor assay) diagnoses are mutually supportive of accurate diagnosis, the essential prerequisite of treatment planning and genetic counseling. Therefore, the two will be considered together under each diagnostic heading.

Inherited Bleeding Disorders in Women, 1st edition. By CA Lee, RA Kadir and PA Kouides. Published 2009 by Blackwell Publishing, ISBN: 978-1-4051-6915-8.

Hemophilia A

Incidence in females

X-linked hereditary factor VIII deficiency/hemophilia A is due to mutations in the factor VIII gene locus at Xq2.8 (gene symbol *f8*). Thus defined, the incidence of hemophilia A worldwide at birth is about 1 in 5000 males. Since the population contains twice as many X chromosomes in females as males the birth incidence of hemophilia A carriers is by inference 1 in 2500 females. For each affected male there are many more potentially affected carrier females, sometimes up to 10 in a given family.

Laboratory testing

See Chapters 1 and 3.

X inactivation

Female carriers of hemophilia A have one defective and one normal *f8* gene. However, during the late blastocyst stage of female embryogenesis one of each pair of X chromosomes in each cell of the epiblast is randomly inactivated. Consequently, the resulting embryo and the woman into which it eventually develops has a variable proportion of defective and normal *f8* genes contributing to the circulating level of factor VIII. Hence, whereas the general population has factor VIII levels approximately normally distributed around a mean of 100 units/dL (range ± 2 SD 50–150 units/dL), hemophilia A carriers have a distribution of factor VIII levels around a mean of 50 units/dL (range ± 2 SD 10–90 units/dL). Carriers with a factor VIII level of 20 units/dL are not unusual and a few have levels as low 5 units/dL because of skewed X inactivation. These patients are in the range of mild (factor VIII >5 units/dL to <50 units/dL) or moderate (factor VIII >1 units/dL to 5 units/dL) hemophilia A. They are sometimes referred to as "manifesting carriers" since they have a clinical bleeding tendency. About a third of carriers manifest mild or moderate hemophilia A. A rare but well-described situation is where the "non-hemophilic" X chromosome has a major defect, such that only cells in which the "hemophilic" X chromosome is not inactivated can survive development. These women can have severe hemophilia A. There are also a few girls born to carrier mothers whose partner has hemophilia and who are homozygous or doubly heterozygous for hemophilia A.

Combining the family tree with assay data

The first step in diagnosis of any inherited disorder is of course the construction of an accurate family tree or genogram. From this the likelihood of an X-linked recessive disorder will usually be obvious (see Fig. 8.1).

The consultand (Fig. 8.1, marked with an arrow) is the daughter of an obligate carrier of hemophilia A, herself the daughter of an affected male. Her factor VIII activity level was normal at 55 units/dL but about half her von Willebrand factor (VWF) antigen (VWF:Ag) level of 90 units/dL. Subsequent to the consultand III:4 had two affected sons by different partners. The daughter has 50% chance on pedigree to be a carrier. Combining this with her low factor VIII to VWF:Ag

ratio made it highly likely she was a carrier. So it was not a surprise to find that her factor VIII sequence was heterozygous at codon 593 for wild-type arginine and mutant cysteine, thus proving her to be a carrier as this is a known cause of hemophilia A, albeit with a wide range of phenotype from moderate to mild [1].

Genetic diagnosis

After the cloning of the factor VIII gene in 1984, advances followed rapidly in linkage analysis for families segregating hemophilia A. The *f8* gene contains 26 exons (protein-coding segments) separated by 25 introns (non-coding segments that are spliced out during mRNA maturation). The basis of linkage analysis is to use a non-pathogenic normal variation in the gene sequence as a marker to follow a mutated gene through a family. The first intragenic polymorphism in the *f8* gene was described in 1985. This was a single nucleotide change within intron 18 and sufficiently frequent in the Caucasian population that about half of the female population is heterozygous and therefore informative. The first antenatal diagnoses using this polymorphism were reported the following year. Later other polymorphisms were found, including a highly polymorphic dinucleotide repeat in intron 13 that is informative in about 90% of females. However, even with these tools for gene tracking [which became technically easier to perform with the advent of polymerase chain reaction (PCR) technology in the late 1980s], family structure or the absence of an affected male relative often frustrated attempts to identify carriers. Although the first

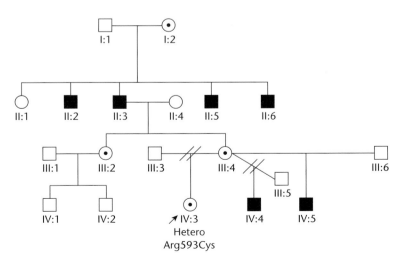

Fig. 8.1 Family tree or genogram, showing an X-linked recessive disorder.

mutations in the *f8* gene were reported in 1986, it was not until the technology for direct automated sequencing became widespread early this century that mutation-specific diagnosis and carrier detection became widely available. The great advantage of this approach is that a specific causative mutation may be found in over 95% of patients with hemophilia A. In carriers the mutation will be heterozygous and it is no longer necessary to have even an index case in a family if a candidate mutation is found in a carrier. Hence, carrier determination by mutation detection succeeds in about 95% of families and is the method of choice. It also allows confident antenatal diagnosis.

Hemophilia A is highly heterogeneous at the mutational level with over 1000 different unique mutations now recorded on the international database (Hamsters http://europium.csc.mrc.ac.uk/WebPages/Main/main. htm). This mutational variation, the most diverse recorded for any human genetic disease, underlies and explains the clinical variation ranging from severe to mild disease in affected males. New mutations continue to be described, with about a third in any series being novel. Since the protein sequence of factor VIII is highly conserved, it is usually obvious which changes are likely to be pathogenic. For a full discussion of factor VIII molecular pathology the interested reader is referred to reviews listed in the references [4, 6, 7]. Although severe gene lesions such as stop codons, deletions, or inversions are consistently associated with severe disease, for individual missense mutations (amino acid substitutions), the clinical factor VIII level can vary quite widely. About half of patients with severe hemophilia A have an inversion involving intron 22 and about 5% have an inversion involving intron 1. Therefore, specific methods for detecting these inversions are usually carried out first in members of kindred segregating severe disease.

From the viewpoint of genetic counseling, the large online database [1] allows inference of the likely range of severity of disease in the offspring of a woman carrying a particular mutation. Also, there is an association of some mutations with the risk of developing inhibitors to factor VIII, which may influence reproductive choices. All these advances follow from direct mutation detection, but there remain about 5% of hemophilia A patients in whom up to now no mutation has been found in the regions of the gene sequenced (exons and flanking sequences). For practical reasons, only about 5% of the gene is sequenced, so it is likely that the remaining mutations lie within the very large intronic regions of the *f8* gene. In these families, linkage analysis can still be used as a last resort.

Sources of difficulty in diagnosis

The laboratory but not the genetic diagnosis of hemophilia A may be confused by the chance co-inheritance of VWD, which lowers the factor VIII level but also usually reduces the VWF:Ag level to a greater extent. Figure 8.2 illustrates such a case, with the family tree giving a clue to the fact that two independent conditions, hemophilia A and VWD, are segregating in the family.

The consultand (Fig. 8.2, arrow) was reviewed for VWD and it was noted that her factor VIII level was consistently lower than her already low VWF:Ag. It was also noticed that two antecedent males in the family had died of bleeding. Since the VWD was mild in the surviving females it was highly unlikely that it could have caused death in a male so affected. Therefore, sequence of her factor VIII gene was undertaken and revealed a mutation causative of moderate or severe hemophilia A in heterozygosity (Arg372Cys). She was pregnant at the time with a male fetus but elected to continue the pregnancy, with a delivery plan reflecting the 50% risk of a severely affected child. Happily the boy was normal. Of note, two other females in the third generation and the consultand's daughter are potential carriers of this mutation and their status remains to be determined.

It should be noted that the now standard approach of using PCR to amplify each exon for sequencing will miss a deletion in a heterozygous female. Hence, if an affected index case is not available, it is technically difficult or impossible to rule out such a possibility when no sequence variation from wild type is found in a putative carrier. Figure 8.3 illustrates this situation.

The consultand IV:2, marked with an arrow, is the first patient to come to recent medical attention in her family and is the person through whom the family tree was ascertained. In this particular family there is no living male relative with a bleeding disorder and the patient herself has a normal factor VIII level. However her VWF level is double the level of her factor VIII. Three males in earlier generations died of bleeding at a young age without the benefit of diagnosis or treatment. Therefore, her prior chances of carriership on pedigree, assuming X-linked inheritance are 1 in 8. The factor VIII to VWF ratio of 0.5

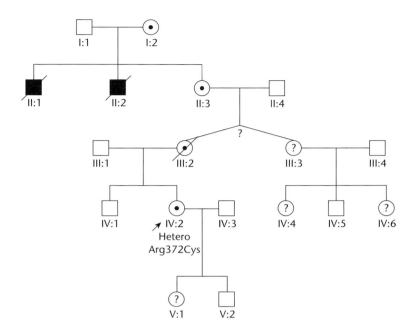

Fig. 8.2 Family tree segregated into two conditions, hemophilia A and von Willebrand disease.

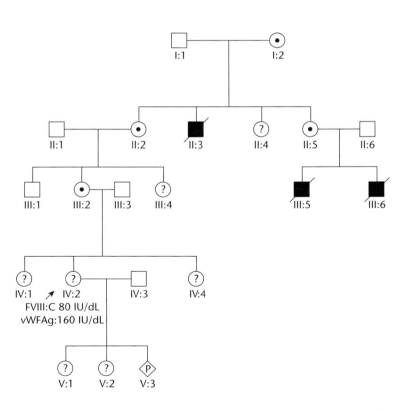

Fig. 8.3 An affected index case is not available.

combined with the family history make it strongly probable that she is a carrier of severe hemophilia A. As she had presented in the third trimester of pregnancy with a male fetus and termination was not an option she and her husband were counseled about the risk of an affected son (approaching 50%) and delivery planned accordingly. Meanwhile her DNA was sent for *f8* gene analysis. The common inversion involving intron 22 was not present but nor was there any other defect found on sequencing. Homozygosity for many polymorphisms suggested the presence of a large deletion. Her male infant proved to be normal, but her two daughters could be carriers and await further investigation.

The Normandy variant of VWD produces a phenocopy of hemophilia in males and females because of mutations in the VWF gene that reduce the binding of factor VIII (see Chapter 4 for specific diagnostic tests). It should be excluded by specific tests where the inheritance pattern is anomalous and/or no mutation can be found in the *f8* gene.

Summary for hemophilia A

The combination of the factor VIII activity assay, other assays to exclude alternative causes of a low factor VIII level, the ratio of factor VIII to VWF:Ag, an accurate family tree, and sequencing of the *f8* gene essential regions or linkage analysis will deliver secure confirmation or exclusion of hemophilia A carriership in over 95% of consultands. A small minority of women at risk of carriership remain of undetermined status pending further advances in our understanding of the genetic causes of hemophilia A.

Hemophilia B

Incidence in females

X-linked hereditary factor IX deficiency/hemophilia B is due to mutations in the factor IX gene locus at Xq2.6 (gene symbol *f9*). The incidence of hemophilia B worldwide at birth is about 1 in 25 000 males. Since the population contains twice as many X chromosomes in females as males the birth incidence of hemophilia B carriers is by inference 1 in 12 500 females. As noted for hemophilia A, for each affected male there are many more potentially affected carrier females. The ratio of patients and carriers with hemophilia A to

hemophilia B is about 5:1 but this can be altered by local founder effects, often in favor of hemophilia B.

Laboratory testing

See Chapters 1 and 3 for details.

X inactivation

Female carriers of hemophilia B have one defective and one normal *f9* gene. All comments made above in relation to hemophilia A apply to hemophilia B, such that carrier women have a variable proportion of defective and normal *f9* genes contributing to their circulating levels of factor IX. Hence, whereas the general population has factor IX levels normally distributed around a mean of 100 units/dL (range ± 2 SD 60–140 units/dL), hemophilia B carriers have a distribution of factor IX levels around a mean of 50 units/dL (range ± 2 SD 10–90 units/dL). Carriers with a factor IX level of 20 units/dL are not unusual because of skewed X inactivation. These patients are in the range of mild hemophilia B (factor IX >5 units/dL to <50 units/dL). Referred to as "manifesting carriers," they have a clinical bleeding tendency. About a third of carriers manifest mild hemophilia B.

Combining the family tree with assay data

From the construction of the family tree it may be clear whether an X-linked recessive bleeding disorder is segregating in the consultand's family. However, this will give no clue whether it is hemophilia A or B. Measuring the consultand's factor IX level may be helpful if low or discrepant from other vitamin K-dependent factor levels. If a surviving male relative is known to have hemophilia B then one may proceed directly to genetic diagnosis looking for a specific mutation if known. However, this is often not the case as illustrated in the family represented in Fig. 8.4.

The consultand, marked with an arrow, is the first patient in her family to come to medical attention in the UK, being a recent immigrant, and is the person through whom the family tree was ascertained. In this particular family there is no living male relative with a bleeding disorder, but the patient herself had a factor IX level at the lower limit of the normal range, with levels of all other vitamin K-dependent factors 95–105 units/dL. An uncle died of bleeding at a young age

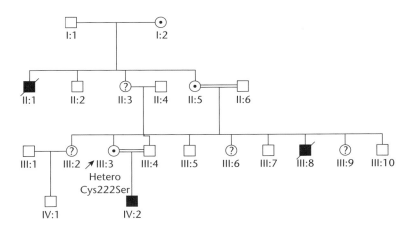

Fig. 8.4 Family where there is no living male relative with a bleeding disorder.

as did her younger brother without the benefit of specific diagnosis or effective treatment in her country of origin. Therefore, her prior chances of carriership on pedigree, assuming X-linked inheritance, are 1 in 2. The factor IX to factor X ratio of 0.5 combined with the family history made it strongly probable that she is a carrier of severe hemophilia B. As she had presented in the second trimester of pregnancy with a male fetus she and her husband were counseled about risk of an affected son (approaching 50%). They elected to continue the pregnancy and delivery was planned accordingly. Meanwhile her DNA was sent for *f9* gene sequencing. A mutation associated with moderately severe hemophilia B was found (Cys222Ser) in heterozygosity. She delivered a boy with severe hemophilia B diagnosed on the cord blood sample. The patient was happy with her decision and with the opportunity that prior diagnosis had provided for preparation and counseling for the eventual outcome.

Genetic diagnosis

After the cloning of the *f9* gene in 1982, linkage analysis for families segregating hemophilia B soon advanced based on many polymorphisms found in the coding and non-coding regions of the gene. The *f9* gene contains eight exons (protein-coding segments) separated by seven introns. The large number of polymorphisms present made it possible to track mutant *f9* genes in most families with a suitable structure and an available index case. However, as with hemophilia A, defects of family structure or the absence of an affected male relative often frustrated attempts to identify carriers. The

first mutation in the *f9* gene causing hemophilia B was reported in 1986. Ingenious approaches to detecting mutations causing hemophilia B were developed that relied on PCR amplification of each exon followed by screening for sequence variation by a variety of methods.

It soon emerged that hemophilia B is highly heterogeneous at the mutational level with 1000 different unique mutations now recorded on an international database [2]. This mutational variation underlies and explains the clinical variation ranging from severe to mild disease in affected males. New mutations continue to be described, but the rate for novel amino acid substitutions is slowing as saturation is reached for all possible variants. Since the protein sequence is highly conserved and the crystallographic structure of factor IX is known, it is usually obvious which changes are pathogenic. For a full discussion of factor IX molecular pathology the interested reader is referred to reviews listed in the references [4–6]. Severe gene lesions such as stop codons and deletions are consistently associated with severe disease and a high risk of inhibitor development.

From the viewpoint of genetic counseling, the large database allows inference of the likely range of severity of disease in the offspring of a woman carrying a particular mutation.

Sources of difficulty in diagnosis

The absence of an affected male is the most likely reason for difficulty in carrier determination, but since nearly all patients with hemophilia B have been found to have mutations on sequencing their essential gene regions, there is good reason to believe that a woman whose factor IX genes are both normal is not a carrier. There are two important caveats to this. Some mutations causing hemophilia B lie well into the promoter region or near the end of the 3′ untranslated region, so full sequencing of those regions as well as the exons and flanking regions is required. Even more important is the point that the now standard approach of using PCR to amplify each exon for sequencing will miss a deletion in a heterozygous female. Hence, if an affected index case is not available, Southern blotting with cDNA probes is required to rule out such a possibility.

Summary for hemophilia B

The combination of factor IX activity assay, other assays to exclude alternative causes of a low factor IX level, an accurate family tree, and sequencing of the *f9* gene essential regions or linkage analysis will deliver secure confirmation or exclusion of hemophilia B carriership in over 95% of consultands. A small minority of women at risk of carriership remain of undetermined status because of the unavailability of an index case and lack of detected sequence variation.

von Willebrand disease

The diagnosis of VWD is a complex and still evolving topic that can only be summarized here. This is due to the highly heterogeneous nature of the disease, the many functional attributes of von Willebrand factor and the correspondingly large number of tests needed to assess them, as well as the variable penetrance of the phenotype, compounded by modifier genes. Furthermore the genetics of VWD in the commonest form has come into question since it has recently become clear that a large proportion of patients with mild disease have no mutation at the VWF locus. Other causes of their phenotype (moderately low levels of VWF activity in the range of 30–50 units/dL) need to be sought [8]. The relationship between phenotype and genotype in VWD is less clear than it is for the X-linked hemophilias.

Incidence in females

The population frequency of VWD is debatable and depends on the diagnostic criteria adopted. At one extreme it was found that about 1% of children in the Veneto region of Italy met the criteria of having VWF:Ag levels below the locally established normal range and a family history of a bleeding tendency.

At the other extreme based on registration data in countries having a national database of hemorrhagic disorders (e.g., the UK and Italy) the ratio of patients with a diagnosis of VWD to those with hemophilia A is near unity, that is, 1 in 10 000. Given that ascertainment is delayed or never reached for milder forms of VWD (the majority of cases) it is likely that the true figure lies between these extremes. In north London with a population catchment of about 5 000 000 there are almost 500 cases registered at the Royal Free Hospital, which is 1 in 1000. As an autosomal disorder this should be equally divided amongst males and females, but is not, because of the ascertainment bias in favor of females with their greater lifetime hemostatic stress than males. Whatever the true incidence specialist hemostasis centers undertaking detailed tests find that the most frequent diagnosis in newly referred children and adults with a history of bleeding is VWD, followed closely by platelet disorders. type 3 severe VWD occurs in outbreed populations at a frequency of about 1 in 1 000 000 with equal sex incidence.

Laboratory diagnosis

See Chapter 4.

Combining the family tree with assay data

Type 3 von Willebrand disease, being recessive, usually occurs in families with consanguinity. All other types of VWD are dominant, except for some of the milder forms of type 1 where there is variable penetrance (but see comment under "Genetic diagnosis" below). Lack of a bleeding history in males in such families does not rule out VWD, for which laboratory confirmation is required. The finding of lower factor VIII activity than VWF:Ag in a female should raise the suspicion of hemophilia A carriership or type N (Normandy) VWD. The factor VIII binding assay is essential to make this distinction. Having VWD does not rule out co-inheritance of *f8* gene mutation. Sometimes it may be necessary to sequence *f8* to rule out this possibility (as in Fig. 8.3).

Genetic diagnosis

The VWF gene is located at chromosome 12p13 (gene symbol *VWF*). It is extremely large with 52 exons separated by 51 introns. Consequently, it is a major undertaking to sequence all its coding and flanking regions. Where this has been done the results are of great interest for understanding the molecular pathology of the disease with its diverse phenotypes. An international database [3] records several hundred different unique mutations found in patients with every subtype of VWD. However, only a few of those found in type 1 disease have been reliably proven to be causative by functional studies. The puzzle in type 1 disease is that only cases with VWF:Ag below 30 units/dL have been found to have a plausible mutation at their *VWF* locus. For type 2 VWD, most subtypes have one of a limited number of repetitive mutations in the relevant functional region of the VWF protein sequence. These have been tested by *in vitro* expression and by modeling on the known crystallographic structures of the relevant domains. Hence molecular diagnosis is becoming relatively secure and rational for type 2 VWD. The dominant effect of these mutations can be understood by considering that VWF is assembled from protomers into very large multimers. Therefore, every multimer will have half its protomers derived from the mutated allele, with a consequent global effect on each assembled multimeric molecule in the circulation.

For type 3 VWD, null mutations have been found scattered across the whole gene including deletions. The fact that these mutations are recessive accords with the concept that a single normal gene output, if not interfered with by the alternative allele's product, is sufficient for hemostasis. Hence heterozygotes are unaffected.

A limited approach to molecular diagnosis that provides useful confirmatory evidence and even potentially an approach to antenatal diagnosis is to sequence only those regions of the gene known to carry most of the mutations in specific type-2 subtypes of VWD. These are exon 28 for types 2A and 2B, exons 27 and 28 for 2M, and exons 18, 19, and 20 for type 2N.

However, each molecular diagnostic laboratory will decide whether to set up such extensive sequencing for perhaps rather limited clinical dividends. This is still largely an area where academic research predominates.

Sources of difficulty in diagnosis

Phenotypic and assay variability together with the large number of specialized tests required combine to make VWD one of the more difficult diagnostic areas, especially for the milder forms and for the rarer variants. For example a diagnosis of type 2B VWD could be missed if ristocetin-induced platelet aggregation is not tested. Multimer analysis, which is crucial for subtyping, is technically demanding and not kit based; therefore, it is not widely available outside specialized centers. Genotyping is highly specialized as well, and is not fully established in its interpretation apart from type 2 variants. The evaluation of mild type 1 VWD has undergone radical reinterpretation since it was discovered that most cases have no mutation at the *VWF* locus. Altogether these factors mean that some diagnostic uncertainty is inevitable at the margins of this disorder. The clinician may need to revise the diagnosis in some cases and review the test results over time with resource to newer tests as these become available. It is desirable to avoid labeling patients with a disease category when they are simply at the lower limit of the normal range for one or other assay.

Summary for von Willebrand disease

VWF is a large and complex molecule with multiple functional domains and diverse functional defects. A correspondingly complex array of diagnostic tools is required for evaluation and diagnosis of its defects. Although the disease was first described by Eric von Willebrand in 1926, understanding of this disorder continues to grow as do the diagnostic categories into which individual patients are placed. Nevertheless VWD is one of the commoner causes of bleeding in women and since the response to available treatments varies according to the subtype it is important to continue to develop expertise in defining the range of variation encountered in practice. Expert clinical and academic laboratories are continuing to expand our knowledge in this field.

Conclusion

The role of the clinical laboratory, working closely with clinicians interested in hemostatic disorders, is central to establishing secure diagnosis. This in turn allows and is essential for rational management of the conditions described above, which all have a major impact on the health of women affected by them. These disorders range in frequency from quite common to extremely rare, so that experience of some of them will only be gained in tertiary referral units. The range of tests required for full evaluation demands specialized dedicated facilities and laboratory workers for their completion. Nevertheless the basic clinical skills of detailed personal and family history taking, combined with widely available screening tests and assays, will guide those who first see such patients in making the referral onward to an expert center where the final diagnosis and recommendations for treatment can be made according to the methods summarized in this chapter.

References

1 Haemophilia A structure test and resource site (Hamsters); http://europium.csc.mrc.ac.uk/WebPages/Main/main.htm/.

2 Haemophilia B mutation database; http://www.kcl.ac.uk/ip/petergreen/haemBdatabase.html/.

3 ISTH SSC VWF Information Home Page; http://www.vwf.group.shef.ac.uk/sequences.html/.

4 Tuddenham EGD, Cooper DN. *The molecular genetics of haemostasis and its inherited disorders. Oxford Monographs on Medical Genetics.* Oxford University Press: Oxford 1994.

5 Lillicrap D. The molecular basis of haemophilia B. *Haemophilia* 1998; **4**: 350–357.

6 Antonarakis SE, Kazazian HH, Tuddenham GD. Molecular etiology of factor VIII deficiency in hemophilia A. *Hum Mutat* 1995; **5**: 1–22

7 Bogdanova N, Markoff A, Eisert R, *et al.* Spectrum of molecular defects and mutation detection rate in patients with severe hemophilia A. *Hum Mutat* 2005; **26**: 249–254

8 Lillicrap D. Von Willebrand disease – phenotype versus genotype: deficiency versus disease. *Thromb Res* 2007; **120** (Suppl 1): S11–16.

9 Antenatal diagnosis

Claudia Chi and Rezan A Kadir

Introduction

Inherited bleeding disorders are lifelong conditions that present with a broad spectrum of bleeding manifestations ranging from easy bruising and epistaxis to potentially debilitating musculoskeletal bleeding and life-threatening intracranial hemorrhages. Despite advances in their treatments, they remain incurable and are commonly associated with significant long-term morbidity. Women with inherited bleeding disorders can pass on the gene defect to their offspring and therefore are at risk of having an affected child depending on the inheritance pattern of the condition. The decision regarding reproduction is fundamentally complex and challenging and further complicated for these women because of their genetic risks. Developments in molecular genetics and technologies have created new opportunities and expanded the reproductive options for these women. The aims of this chapter are to explore the reproductive choices of women with inherited bleeding disorders and to examine their views and attitudes towards reproduction and prenatal diagnosis.

Genetic counseling

Inherited bleeding disorders can profoundly affect the daily life and psychological wellbeing of both the

Inherited Bleeding Disorders in Women, 1st edition. By CA Lee, RA Kadir and PA Kouides. Published 2009 by Blackwell Publishing, ISBN: 978-1-4051-6915-8.

affected individuals and the family. It is essential for women who are known carriers or have the possibility of carrying the disorder to have the opportunity to consider the implications for themselves and their offspring. The aims of genetic counseling are to provide them with sufficient information to make a decision appropriate to their own situation and to support them throughout the process. It should ideally be carried out before conception to allow sufficient time for the individuals to gain a full understanding of the information provided and for the laboratory to perform genetic testing. Furthermore, pre-pregnancy planning prevents the parents from having to make difficult decisions under time pressure during early pregnancy and avoids limitations to their reproductive choices. Genetic counseling should be provided by individuals with good communication skills and a detailed knowledge of the disorder including the molecular genetics, the care and treatment involved in the relevant country and the available reproductive options.

To make an informed decision on reproductive options, it is vital to first establish the carrier status of the prospective parents and their genetic risk of having an affected child. This involves obtaining an accurate and detailed family history as well as carrying out phenotypic and genotypic assessments to ascertain the diagnosis, the coagulation factor level and the mutation within the family. Individuals undergoing genetic testing should have an understanding of the purposes and implications of the test. They should also be aware of its accuracy and limitations. Aspects of carrier testing and genetic diagnosis are covered in Chapters 3 and 8.

For prospective parents, the risk of having an affected child is determined by the inheritance pattern of the condition. Hemophilia A and B are X-linked recessive bleeding disorders caused by a deficiency in coagulation factor VIII (FVIII) and IX (FIX), respectively. Males inherit the condition whereas females are affected as carriers. The incidence of hemophilia A is approximately 1 in 5000 male births and of hemophilia B 1 in 25 000 male births. Given that females have two X chromosomes, the birth incidence of hemophilia carriers by inference would be 1 in 2500 and 1 in 12 500 females, respectively. For each affected male in a particular family, there are potentially many more carrier females. Assuming a normal genotype in the partner, these women have a 1:4 chance of having a child with hemophilia in each pregnancy; there is a 50% chance that a son will be affected and a 50% chance that a daughter will also be a carrier of the condition (Fig. 9.1). Since the severity of hemophilia is fairly consistent among family members, carriers can be informed whether their risk is for severe, moderate, or mild hemophilia, although for some missense mutations the range can span two categories.

von Willebrand disease (VWD) is an autosomal condition that affects both males and females. It is the most common inherited bleeding disorder, with a reported prevalence of approximately 1% in population studies [1, 2]. It displays both dominant and recessive inheritance. Type 1, the commonest (60–80%) and generally the milder form of VWD, is transmitted as an autosomal dominant trait. It is characterized by a partial quantitative deficiency of von Willebrand factor (VWF). Type 2 refers to a qualitative deficiency of VWF and is subdivided into four variants (2A, 2B, 2M, and 2N). Type 2A, 2B, and 2M are mainly inherited in an autosomal dominant pattern, whereas type 2N is inherited recessively. Type 3 also has an autosomal recessive inheritance and is the most severe form of VWD with a virtually complete deficiency of VWF.

Rare bleeding disorders include afibrinogenemia, hypoprothrombinemia, and deficiencies of factor V, combined factors V and VIII, factor VII, factor IX, factor X, and factor XIII. They are inherited as autosomal recessive traits and generally are expressed in homozygotes or compound heterozygotes. Their estimated incidence in the severe (homozygous) form ranges from 1 in 500 000 (factor VII deficiency) to 1 in 2 million (factor II deficiency). However, they are more prevalent in racial groups, communities, or countries, such as Asian communities and some Muslim countries, where consanguineous marriages are common.

Other factors that may influence the reproductive decision-making include the likely clinical phenotype of the disorder, its severity and potential complications, the potential risk of inhibitor development, the expected quality of life of affected children and the possible impact on the family. Thus, these predictors should be provided as part of the genetic counseling. Details on the efficacy, safety and side-effects of current treatment should also be addressed. When discussing these issues, it is important to take into consideration the individual's and the family's previous experience with the condition. The implications of a

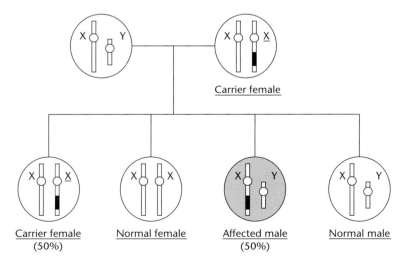

Fig. 9.1 Inheritance of hemophilia (with permission from Peyvandi [190]).

genetic disorder can undoubtedly cause great anxiety and distress; therefore, genetic counseling should not only encompass the technical issues but also the emotional aspects. Adequate support should be provided throughout the whole process.

Reproductive options

The reproductive options for women with inherited bleeding disorders, in general, are:
1 not having children;
2 declining prenatal diagnosis and accepting the outcome of the pregnancy;
3 conceiving naturally and having prenatal diagnosis with the option of termination of affected pregnancy;
4 adoption or fostering;
5 assisted conception with donor gametes;
6 pre-implantation genetic diagnosis.

Women with or carriers of inherited bleeding disorders may choose to abstain from having children in fear of passing the genetic defect to their offspring, especially when adequate treatment and/or the option of prenatal diagnosis is not available. They may choose to use non-biological methods such as adoption or fostering. On the other hand, they may decide to accept any outcome by taking a chance of having an affected child. Over time, reproductive options have been broadened by advances in molecular technology and developments in the techniques for prenatal diagnosis and assisted reproduction. They can choose to have antenatal diagnosis and selective termination of an affected pregnancy or consider assisted conception with the use of donor gametes. There is even the possibility of selecting embryos that are free of the genetic disorder before implantation to prevent the birth of an affected child. In order for the prospective parents to make an informed choice on their reproductive options, it is vital that they are provided with adequate information regarding the availability of these options and the procedures involved, including their accuracy, limitations, and risks. The options of prenatal diagnosis and pre-implantation genetic diagnosis will be further explored in the following sections.

Prenatal diagnosis

Prenatal diagnosis should be undertaken following adequate counseling and in centers with full genetic, hematological, and obstetric expertise. It is generally considered in pregnancies at risk of moderate or severe inherited bleeding disorders and when termination of pregnancy is contemplated if an affected fetus is identified. This is because the techniques for definitive prenatal diagnosis are usually invasive and carry risks to the pregnancy. However, women's attitudes toward prenatal diagnosis and termination of pregnancy differ considerably depending on various personal, social, and cultural factors. They may opt for antenatal diagnosis for other reasons such as psychological preparations in the case of an affected child and planning for place and methods of delivery.

Prenatal diagnostic techniques
Prenatal diagnosis of inherited bleeding disorders entails non-invasive and/or invasive tests. Ultrasound plays an essential role in the antenatal diagnosis of hemophilia as it provides a non-invasive means of determining fetal sex. At present, the definitive prenatal diagnosis of inherited bleeding disorders can only be achieved through invasive procedures such as chorionic villus sampling (CVS), amniocentesis, and fetal cord blood sampling (cordocentesis). These techniques are carried out by skilled operators and are mainly based on obtaining fetal materials for genetic analysis or clotting factor assays.

The identification of the causative mutation or informative markers is a prerequisite for any DNA-based prenatal diagnosis. As this can take up to several weeks, it needs to be done well before considering prenatal diagnosis. Advanced planning and careful coordination between the obstetrician and hematologist as well as the genetic laboratory and the fetal medicine unit are necessary to ensure the successful attainment of accurate results and to minimize the risks of complications.

Furthermore, before embarking on these options, it is important to explain to the women what the procedure involves and the benefits, risks, and limitations of each method. The options of screening for fetal chromosomal and structural abnormalities (e.g., fetal nuchal translucency) and of karyotyping, in the event of invasive testing, should also be discussed and offered, as appropriate, in the pre-test counseling. When planning for invasive testing, apart from the standard precautions for the prevention of rhesus isoimmunization, additional measures, such as prophylactic cover, may be required to minimize the risk of bleeding complications.

(Refer to Chapter 10 for further discussions on the requirement of prophylactic cover.)

Invasive tests Chorionic villus sampling is a prenatal diagnostic test that is currently the method of choice for obtaining fetal materials for the prenatal diagnosis of inherited bleeding disorders. It offers the advantage of attaining an early diagnosis and thus a shorter period of uncertainty than amniocentesis. Early diagnosis is of particular importance when selective termination of an affected pregnancy is being considered, as there may be personal or religious prohibitions on late termination of pregnancy. Furthermore, termination at a later gestation is likely to be more traumatic. CVS is usually performed between 10 and 13 weeks of gestation under direct ultrasound guidance to obtain a sample of chorionic villi (placenta) for genetic analysis. The chorionic villus tissue is a rich source of fetal DNA that can be extracted and used for polymerase chain reaction (PCR)-based testing for fetal sexing first in the case of hemophilia and direct mutation detection or polymorphism linkage analysis. Results are usually available within 48–72 hours of receipt of samples.

Prior to the CVS procedure, an ultrasound assessment is performed to confirm the viability of the pregnancy, the gestation, the number of fetuses and the positions of the fetus and the placenta. CVS can be performed using the percutaneous transabdominal or the transcervical approach (Fig. 9.2). The transabdominal route is performed under local anesthetic. It entails the insertion of the needle through the abdominal and uterine walls under direct ultrasound guidance and obtaining a sample from the placenta either by single or double needle aspiration using syringe suction or a vacuum aspirator. The transcervical route involves the use of a speculum and passing a fine forceps or aspiration cannula through the cervix to obtain a placental sample under ultrasound guidance. The choice of instruments is currently based on the experience and the preference of the operator [3]. However, the transabdominal route is preferable and more widely used because the transcervical route is associated with more vaginal bleeding (10% vs 1.6%) and technically more demanding with a higher rate of multiple insertions (11.2% vs 4.1%) [4].

CVS is associated with an approximately 1–2% risk of pregnancy loss [5]. It is recommended that CVS should not be performed before 10 weeks of gestation because of its association with limb reduction deformities when carried out before this gestation [6, 7]. Sampling failure can occur because of technical difficulties. There is a small (<1%) chance of failing to

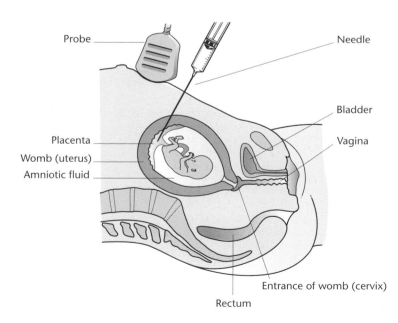

Probe — Needle

Placenta — Bladder

Womb (uterus) — Vagina

Amniotic fluid

Entrance of womb (cervix)

Rectum

Fig. 9.2 Chorionic villus sampling (transabdominal) (with permission from the RCOG patient information leaflet).

obtain a result from the laboratory test. False-negative or -positive results may result from maternal cell contamination or placental mosaicism. There is also a very small (less than 1 in 1000) risk of serious infection from inadvertent puncture of the bowel or from contaminates on the skin or the ultrasound probe/gel. Standard procedures for infection control are recommended to avoid this complication. The risk of injury to the fetus is minimal and is decreased by the use of real-time ultrasound guidance.

Amniocentesis is generally performed between 15 and 18 gestational weeks. It involves the insertion of a fine 20- or 22-gauge needle through the maternal abdominal wall into the amniotic cavity and obtaining a sample of the amniotic fluid through needle aspiration Fig. 9.3. Ultrasound assessment is carried out prior to the procedure to ascertain the positions of the placenta and the fetus. Local anesthetic is usually not required for this procedure. Amniotic fluid contains fetal cells (amniocytes) from which rapid detection of specific chromosomes, including the sex chromosomes in cases of hemophilia, can be achieved by fluorescence *in situ* hybridization (FISH). DNA can also be extracted directly and used for PCR-based testing for linkage analysis or direct mutation detection with results usually available within 48–72 hours. However, there is often insufficient DNA present in the sample for analysis. Therefore, the testing has to be delayed until cultured cells are available which takes approximately 2 weeks. A selection of polymorphic markers unrelated to the gene under investigation should always be included in the analysis of results to ensure that maternal contamination is detected. Full karyotyping is also performed on cultured samples.

It is recommended that amniocentesis be performed under direct ultrasound control with continuous needle tip visualization to reduce the chance of obtaining a "bloody tap" as the presence of blood can interfere with cell culture [2]. This also helps to minimize the risk of fetal trauma, which is rare. The incidence of procedure-related pregnancy loss is approximately 0.5–1% [5, 8]. In some cases, reinsertion of the needle may be required when inadequate amounts of amniotic fluid can be taken in the first attempt. Other complications include a small chance (<1%) of not obtaining a definitive diagnosis due to inconclusive results or culture failure and an even smaller risk (<0.1%) of serious infection caused by skin or ultrasound probe/gel contaminants or by inadvertent puncturing of the bowel.

Amniocentesis has the disadvantage of providing a diagnosis in the second trimester, and thus the option of termination of pregnancy in affected cases at a later gestation. Although amniocentesis can be performed

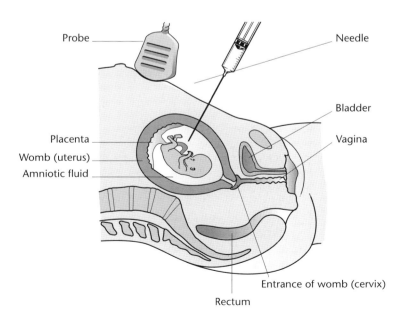

Fig. 9.3 Amniocentesis (with permission from RCOG patient information leaflet).

Probe — Needle

Placenta — Bladder

Womb (uterus) — Vagina

Amniotic fluid

Entrance of womb (cervix)

Rectum

at an earlier gestation (before 14 weeks of gestation), it is not a safe alternative to second trimester amniocentesis or CVS because of the increased risk of miscarriage and fetal talipes [7, 9]. In a large Canadian randomized trial, early (between 11^{+0} and 12^{+6} gestational weeks) amniocentesis was associated with an increased incidence of fetal loss (7.6% vs 5.9%), talipes (1.3% vs 0.1%) and amniotic fluid leakage post procedure (3.5% vs 1.7%) compared with mid-trimester (between 15^{+0} and 16^{+6} gestational weeks) amniocentesis [9]. Furthermore, early amniocentesis was found to be technically more difficult with higher rates of multiple needle insertions and cytogenetic-culture failure [9]. This may be attributed to the presence of two separate membranes (amnion and chorion) until the 15th gestational week. When compared with transabdominal CVS, the rate of spontaneous miscarriage following early amniocentesis was significantly higher (4% vs 2%) [4]. For these reasons, transabdominal CVS is preferable to early amniocentesis for attaining early antenatal diagnosis.

Amniocentesis is also carried out in the third trimester in certain circumstances including late karyotyping and evaluation of infection in preterm labor or rupture of the membrane. The deferment of amniocentesis for prenatal diagnosis until the third trimester has been suggested as a possible option in certain situations (for example, previous fetal loss or in multiple pregnancies where the risk of pregnancy loss following second trimester amniocentesis may be higher [10]) to avoid the risk of miscarriage or severe prematurity associated with second trimester amniocentesis [11–13]. Current data on the risks of late amniocentesis are limited as most of the existing data were obtained prior to the use of continuous ultrasound guidance for amniocentesis. The procedure-related complications then (including rupture of membranes, infections, maternal hemorrhage, uterine vessels injury, fetal injury and fetal hemorrhage) were more common and the failure rates were higher [14]. With the use of continuous ultrasound guidance, the risks of third trimester amniocentesis are considerably less and equally its success rate is much higher [15, 16]. In addition, it does not appear to be associated with a significant risk of requiring emergency delivery [7, 15, 17]. Nonetheless, there is still an approximately 1% risk of procedure-related complications such as preterm delivery, premature rupture of membranes and placental abruption [15, 16]. Complications such

as multiple attempts (>5%) and bloodstained fluid (5–10%) are also more common compared with mid-trimester procedures [7, 15, 16]. Furthermore, there is an approximately 1% chance of failing to obtain a sample and a higher culture failure rate in amniotic fluid samples taken in the third compared with the second trimester (10% vs <1%) [18, 19].

In pregnancies at risk of severe inherited bleeding disorders, prenatal diagnosis by third trimester amniocentesis is a possible option that enables appropriate planning and management of labor and delivery (see Chapter 10) for parents who are unwilling to accept the risk of fetal loss associated with earlier prenatal testing. However, a positive diagnosis could become a psychological burden in advance of delivery. There is also the risk of unexpected delivery before the test or the availability of the test result. Even though third trimester amniocentesis could provide an antenatal diagnosis while obviating the risk of miscarriage associated with first or second trimester testing, its benefits must be carefully weighed against its risks and implications. It also raises several ethical and moral dilemmas that are beyond the scope of this chapter. Currently, there is no evidence to support the routine use of third trimester amniocentesis in this situation.

Cordocentesis, or percutaneous umbilical cord blood sampling, is another invasive diagnostic technique performed after around 18 weeks of gestation. It involves the insertion of a 22-gauge needle under continuous ultrasound guidance through the maternal abdomen and uterine walls and into the umbilical cord to obtain a sample of fetal blood for laboratory analysis. It is performed under aseptic conditions with or without the use of local anesthesia. Similar to other invasive tests, it carries an approximately 1–2% risk of procedure-related fetal loss when performed by an experienced operator [20–25]. Factors that increase this risk include gestational age of less than 20 weeks [26], the indication of the procedure, e.g., fetal anomaly or severe growth restricture [27, 28], maternal obesity, the number of attempts, and the duration of the procedure [29, 30]. There is a risk of cord hematoma or bleeding from the puncture site, which is usually transient but could potentially be significant in the presence of an abnormal coagulation. Fetuses affected with a bleeding disorder are at particular risk of this hemorrhagic complication and this should be taken into consideration when planning for the procedure [31]. Measures should be taken to check for maternal blood contamination, including the assessment of red cell mean corpuscular volume with a channelizer, the Kleihauer–Betke test and/or analysis of molecular markers, as it can lead to inaccurate results. Other potential complications include failure in obtaining a sample, fetal bradycardia that may require urgent delivery, infection, premature rupture of membrane, and premature birth.

Cordocentesis has largely been superseded by CVS and amniocentesis in obtaining fetal material for genetic studies. The last two procedures allow earlier diagnosis, are less technically demanding, and are associated with a lower risk of complications. Nevertheless, cordocentesis still has a role in pregnancies at risk of inherited bleeding disorders where prenatal genetic testing is not possible or available by allowing direct access to fetal blood for the evaluation of coagulation factor levels.

Non-invasive tests Prenatal determination of fetal gender can be achieved non-invasively through ultrasound assessment or the analysis of free fetal DNA (ffDNA) present in the maternal blood. This is valuable in the management of pregnancies at risk of X-linked genetic disorders such as hemophilia. Knowledge of fetal sex enables carriers of hemophilia to avoid invasive diagnostic procedures with its associated risks in pregnancies involving a female fetus. It also allows planning for the management of labor and mode of delivery. Non-invasive means of determining fetal sex will help to relieve anxiety in 50% of the cases where the fetus is female. Furthermore, women who are

reluctant to have invasive prenatal testing due to the risks involved are likely to accept non-invasive testing.

Ultrasound has given accurate assessment of fetal gender in the second trimester for over 20 years, based on ultrasound visualization of the external genitalia [32, 33]. Since the development of the external genitalia is similar in both sexes until 14 weeks' gestation, fetal gender determination by ultrasound was initially limited to the second trimester onwards. It enabled the exclusion of female fetal gender prior to amniocentesis but for early prenatal diagnosis, female pregnancies were subjected to the risks of CVS. Improvements in the resolution of ultrasound have subsequently allowed early identification of fetal gender from as early as 11 weeks' gestation by assessing the direction in which the genital tubercle develops [34, 35]. Fetal gender can be determined by measuring, in a mid-sagittal plane, the angle between the genital tubercle and a line drawn through the lumbosacral vertebrae. The fetal sex is considered to be male if the phallus is directed cranially with an angle to the lumbosacral vertebrae >30° and female if the phallus is directed caudally with an angle <30° [34, 36] (Fig. 9.4). There are two potential limitations to this approach. First, visualization of the genital tubercle is not always possible at the first attempt due to fetal lie, but repeat examination can be arranged. Second, differentiation of the genital tubercle into the male or female phallus only begins at 11 weeks' gestation; therefore, this sign cannot be used prior to this stage [35]. The accuracy of fetal sex determination by ultrasound at 11 weeks' gestation

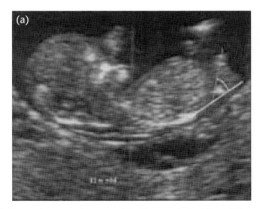 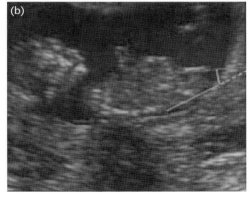

Fig. 9.4 First trimester ultrasound (with permission from Efrat *et al.* [36]). (a) Male fetus with acute angle of the penis shown. (b) Female fetus with converging angle of the clitoris shown.

Table 9.1 Accuracy of first trimester fetal sex determination by ultrasound (with permission from Avent and Chitty [38])

Reference	N	Gestation (weeks)	Technique	Accuracy (when attempted)			Gestation for 100% accuracy			Gender not assigned (%)
				Male (%)	Female (%)	All (%)	Male	Female	All	
Efrat et al. 1999 [36]	157	$11-13^6$	TAS	86.7	98.7	92.4	$13-13^6$	$12-12^6$	$13-13^6$	8.7
Benott 1999 [39]	578	12–13	TVS	98.4	100	98.9	$13-13^6$	$12-12^6$	$13-13^6$	37.7
Mazza et al. 1999 [40]	385	(BPD 18–29)	TAS or TVS	91.5	95.9	93.6	13^0	13^2	13^2	12.5
Whitlow et al. 1999 [34]	447	11–14	TAS 76% TVS 24%	87.8	84.1	85.0	Not achieved			15
Mazza et al. 2004 [41]	2182	(BPD 18–29)	TAS or TVS	88.5	99.1	94.1	13^0	13^4	13^4	9
Hyett et al. 2005 [37]	32	10^5-13^2	TAS	100	100	100	n/a			9.4

BPD, biparietal diameter; TAS, transabdominal ultrasound; TVS, transvaginal ultrasound.

is limited, but it increases with advancing gestation (Table 9.1). Most series were able to attain near 100% accuracy from 13 weeks' gestation [34, 36–41].

Analysis of ffDNA in maternal circulation is an alternative non-invasive means of determining fetal sex. In 1997 Lo et al. [42] discovered the presence of cell ffDNA in maternal plasma and serum by the detection of the Y-chromosome-specific DNA sequence derived from a male fetus. Before this discovery, most investigators focused on utilizing intact fetal cells in the maternal circulation as the source of fetal material for DNA analysis in the development of non-invasive prenatal diagnosis [43–45]. This has proven to be very difficult as there is a very low frequency of fetal cells in maternal blood in the order of 1 in 10^5 to 1 in 10^7 [45, 46]. In contrast, the concentrations of ffDNA in the total maternal plasma DNA are much higher at 3.4% and 6.2% in early and late pregnancies, respectively [47]. Although few reports have suggested the persistence of ffDNA [48, 49], most studies have found rapid clearance from the maternal circulation after delivery [50–54] with a reported mean half-life of 16.3 minutes [55]. Conversely, the persistence of fetal cells in the maternal circulation from previous pregnancies is well recognized as a potential source of false-positive results [56]. For these reasons, ffDNA in mater-

nal plasma has become a much more attractive and accessible source for non-invasive prenatal diagnosis. Advances in molecular technology, particularly the development of quantitative real-time PCR, have allowed several groups to demonstrate a high (96–100%) specificity and sensitivity in the determination of fetal gender from the analysis of ffDNA in maternal circulation (Table 9.2) [37, 47, 57–67]. Although ffDNA has been detected as early as the fourth or fifth week of pregnancy, its concentration is relatively low at this stage and thus can lead to unreliable, mainly false negative, results [59, 61, 65, 67, 68]. However, the amount of ffDNA and consequently the sensitivity of the test increase with gestational age. It is, therefore, possible to utilize this technique to accurately identify fetal gender before 11 weeks' gestation and avoid CVS in pregnancies involving a female fetus. This test is generally performed in a research setting and is beginning to be incorporated into clinical practice in certain units for pregnancies at risk of X-linked disorders. It offers the advantage of eliminating the risk of miscarriage associated with invasive prenatal testing in female pregnancies, but it is also susceptible to exploitation. The potential of its use for non-medical reasons raises several ethical and moral issues that are beyond the scope of this chapter. It is essential

Table 9.2 Accuracy of first trimester fetal male gender determination by real-time polymerase chain reaction analysis of free fetal DNA (modified with permission from Avent and Chitty [38])

Reference	Year	N	Gestation (weeks)	Sensitivity (%)	Specificity (%)
Lo *et al.* [47]	1998	25	11–17	100	100
Costa *et al.* [57]	2001	121	8–14	100	100
Rijnders *et al.* [63]	2001	45	8–17	96	100
Sekizawa *et al.* [58]	2001	302	7–16	97	100
Zhong *et al.* [64]	2001	34	13–17	100	100
Honda *et al.* [59]	2002	81	5–10	100	100
Rijnders *et al.* [61]	2003	13	5–10	100	100
Guibert *et al.* [65]	2003	22	4–9	100	100
Hromadnikova *et al.* [60]	2003	44	10–18	100	100
Rijnders *et al.* [62]	2004	72	11–19	97	100
Cremonesi *et al.* [66]	2004	356	6–40	97	100
Hyett *et al.* [37]	2005	35	7–14	100	100
Birch *et al.* [67]	2005	201	5–41	99	100

that patients are counseled regarding its accuracy, limitations, and the implications of its limitations. Furthermore, it should only be carried out in accredited and experienced laboratories.

Prenatal diagnosis of hemophilia

Prenatal diagnosis of hemophilia was initially restricted to fetal sex determination by amniocentesis in the second trimester. Some carriers utilized this opportunity to interrupt pregnancies involving a male fetus, but most found this unacceptable because in half of these cases the male fetus would have been unaffected. The definitive diagnosis of hemophilia became possible towards the end of the 1970s when techniques were introduced for obtaining pure fetal blood samples under fetoscopic guidance [69] alongside the development of sensitive assays for determining coagulation factor VIII and IX on samples so obtained [70, 71]. Prenatal diagnosis of hemophilia was achieved by means of coagulation or immunoradiometric assays for factor VIII or IX on fetal blood samples obtained during the 18–20th weeks of gestation in male pregnancies identified by ultrasound assessment or amniocentesis [71–73]. Owing to the improvements in ultrasound technology, fetal blood sampling under fetoscopic guidance was later replaced by cordocentesis [74, 75], a direct ultrasound-guided approach which is associated with a lower rate of procedure-related fetal loss (~5–6% vs 1–2%, respectively) [20–25, 76]. However, fetal blood sampling by either approach is limited to the second trimester onwards. As a result, early prenatal diagnosis and termination of pregnancy, if opted for, was still unavailable.

The characterization of the genes for factors VIII and IX [77, 78] together with the development of CVS techniques [79, 80] and PCR technology eventually made first trimester prenatal diagnosis of hemophilia feasible during the 1980s. At first, the genetic diagnosis was achieved indirectly through linkage studies using restriction fragment length polymorphisms [81–90]. This approach has several limitations, including uninformative polymorphisms, unavailability of blood samples from key pedigree members, lack of prior family history, mosaicism, risk of recombination with extragenic markers, plus the sensitive and ethical issue regarding paternity. Subsequently, advances in molecular technology and further knowledge of genes for factors VIII and IX have facilitated the antenatal diagnosis of hemophilia through direct identification of the causative mutation [91–95]. Direct mutation detection circumvents the problems associated with linkage analysis and has become widely available in developed countries following the widespread use of direct automated sequencing technology early this century. It is the most reliable method for prenatal diagnosis and should be used if available. However, in situations where the causative mutation cannot be identified because of the complexity of the genes involved, the heterogeneity of mutations or, in many developing countries, the lack of resources and facilities required, linked polymorphic markers can be utilized to achieve prenatal diagnosis [96, 97]. When both direct and indirect genetic analyses are not available or fail, cordocentesis provides an alternative method of prenatal diagnosis through evaluation of fetal clotting factors [98–100].

More recently, non-invasive first trimester fetal sex determination has been proposed as a new approach in the prenatal diagnosis of hemophilia and other X-linked disorders [37, 49, 101–103]. It allows the avoidance of invasive testing, including CVS, and its associated risks in pregnancies with a female fetus. Carriers who would not consider invasive testing are likely to accept non-invasive tests more readily as the results can also help in the planning of labor and delivery. As discussed earlier, fetal gender can be identified non-invasively and reliably in the first trimester by analysis of ffDNA in maternal blood or by ultrasound assessment of the fetal genital tubercle. The former method has the advantage of providing an earlier (prior to 11 weeks' gestation) and a more reliable result. However, at the introduction of new tests, the use of two independent non-invasive techniques may allow clinicians and patients to have greater confidence in the accuracy of the results [101].

Prenatal diagnosis of von Willebrand disease
Antenatal diagnosis is not usually required or requested in pregnancies at risk of type 1 or 2 VWD because the bleeding tendency is relatively mild. It is mainly applicable to families with type 3 or severe VWD. The procedures and methods available are similar to those developed and used for the prenatal diagnosis of hemophilia. Antenatal diagnosis by direct mutation detection is available in certain diagnostic laboratories for type 2 variants where clusters of mutations have been identified. However, direct mutation detection is not practical in VWD because of the large size of the VWF gene and the heterogeneity of the mutations. The causative mutation is unknown in the majority of cases and, in these cases, linkage studies with RFLP or variable number of tandem repeat (VNTR) sequences may be used for prenatal diagnosis. Cordocentesis followed by factor assays provides an alternative option for prenatal diagnosis when genetic diagnosis is not available [100].

Few cases of prenatal diagnosis of severe VWD have been reported in the literature [31, 104–108]. Hoyer *et al.* [105] excluded severe forms of VWD in a fetus through prenatal evaluation of factor VIII-related antigen and coagulant antigen levels in fetal blood samples obtained under fetoscopic guidance at 19 weeks' gestation. Improvements in the assessment of VWF including von Willebrand antigen (VWF:Ag), ristocetin cofactor activity (VWF:RCo) and the multimeric pattern of VWF allowed Rothschild *et al.* [107] to perform prenatal diagnosis in a woman with type 2A VWD and a severe phenotype. Analysis of VWF levels in fetal blood samples obtained by cordocentesis at 20 weeks revealed an unaffected fetus [107]. In another case report, severe type 3 VWD was diagnosed prenatally by DNA analysis on CVS samples obtained at 12 weeks' gestation [31]. The result was further confirmed by assessment of fetal clotting factors following cordocentesis at 20 weeks' gestation. The latter procedure was complicated by a massive fetomaternal hemorrhage, fetal hypovolemia, and persistent bradycardia. The fetal condition recovered following intracardiac blood transfusion. This illustrates the importance of recognizing that fetuses with a bleeding disorder are at particular risk of hemorrhagic complications from this procedure. Peake *et al.* [108] described the use of a VNTR polymorphic marker within intron 40 of the VWF to track the defective gene for prenatal diagnosis. It enabled the identification of a severely affected fetus through DNA analysis of CVS samples obtained at 10 weeks' gestation and the diagnosis was confirmed by fetal blood sampling at 18 weeks' gestation. Trasi *et al.* [104] also utilized this gene-tracking approach successfully for prenatal diagnosis on two occasions in a family with severe type 3 VWD.

Prenatal diagnosis of rare bleeding disorders
Rare bleeding disorders are generally inherited as recessive traits and are more common among consanguineous marriages. In most cases, they are due to mutations in the genes that encode the relevant clotting factors. Multiple mutations have been described for each rare bleeding disorder and they are often unique for each kindred [109]. In approximately 10% of the cases, no causative mutation has been found [110]. This may be due to defects in the non-coding regions or in genes that encode for the regulators of intracellular transport and post-translational modification of clotting factors. Prenatal diagnosis based on genetic analysis is only feasible if the causative mutation is known or if there are informative genetic markers. There have been a small number of reports

on the prenatal diagnosis of rare bleeding disorders, including factor VII [111–114], factor X [115, 116], and factor XIII deficiencies [117, 118], based on direct mutation detection, linkage analysis or a combination of these methods. Similar to the prenatal diagnosis of hemophilia, cordocentesis can be considered when genetic diagnosis in the fetus is unavailable or unfeasible [100, 119].

Future trends

Pre-implantation genetic diagnosis

Pre-implantation genetic diagnosis (PGD) is an alternative reproductive technique available for couples at risk of having a child with a certain genetic disorder. It is a very early form of prenatal diagnosis, in which embryos created *in vitro* are analyzed for the specific genetic abnormality and only unaffected embryos are transferred to the uterus. This can prevent the birth of an affected child and obviates the need for prenatal diagnosis with selective termination of an affected pregnancy, a procedure that can be very traumatic both emotionally and physically to the parents. PGD is an option for couples who would not consider termination of pregnancy for religious or personal reasons and for those with concurrent infertility.

The first successful clinical application of PGD was in couples at risk of having children with X-linked disorders following the report of sex determination in single cells from the pre-implantation embryo [120, 121]. In these cases, male embryos were discriminated from female embryos by PCR amplification of Y-chromosome sequences and only female embryos were transferred. Since then, PGD has been used for an increasing number of monogenic diseases as well as chromosomal abnormalities. These conditions can be diagnosed provided the causative mutation has been identified, the chromosome that carries the gene can be tracked through linkage studies or the specific chromosomal rearrangement is known [122]. In the latest published data collection from the European Society for Human Reproduction and Embryology [123], PGD cycles were initiated for nearly 60 different monogenic disorders and sexing alone for 36 various X-linked disorders in the calendar year 2003. In this report, the clinical pregnancy rate for monogenic diseases is 20% per oocyte retrieval and 27% per embryo transfer. The corresponding rate for sexing only in X-linked diseases is 22% and 39%, respectively [123].

PGD can only be performed in conjunction with *in vitro* fertilization (IVF) to allow the creation of a number of embryos *in vitro*. This involves ovarian stimulation to enable the maturation of several oocytes followed by oocyte retrieval, IVF using intracytoplasmic sperm injection (ICSI), and embryo culture. A biopsy sample for genetic testing can be obtained at various developmental stages: (a) polar bodies from the oocyte/zygote stage, (b) blastomeres from cleavage stage embryos on day 3, and (c) trophectoderm cells from blastocysts. Each of the methods has its advantages and disadvantages and the choice mainly depends on the clinical situation.

Polar body (PB) biopsy involves the manipulation of oocytes rather than embryos, thus obviating the ethical and safety concerns regarding human embryo biopsy. It is unlikely to have a detrimental effect on subsequent embryonic development since the genetic materials removed are byproducts of oocyte division during meiosis. The genotype of the oocyte can be indirectly derived from the opposite diagnosis of the first polar body. However, the analysis can be complicated by recombination events and allele drop out (ADO) resulting in misdiagnosis or inconclusive results. Consecutive biopsy of the first and second PBs may be required and can help to improve the accuracy of the diagnosis [124, 125]. The main disadvantage of PB analysis is that it can only provide information on the maternal genotype. Autosomal dominant and X-linked disorders that are maternally transmitted can be diagnosed. However, paternal alleles cannot be analyzed and gender determination is not possible using this approach. Furthermore, not all oocytes tested will fertilize and form viable embryos. PB biopsy is not the preferred method in most PGD centers, but it may be useful in detecting aneuploidies since many cases are maternally derived. In countries such as Germany where the legislation bans the selection of pre-implantation embryos, PB analysis is the only possible method to perform PGD [126].

Cleavage stage biopsy is the most widely used technique [123] and is performed on the third day after insemination when the fertilized embryos have usually six to eight cells (Fig. 9.5). At this stage, the cells (blastomeres) are still totipotent and the removal of one or two blastomeres does not appear to have an adverse effect on the *in vitro* development of the embryo [127, 128]. Following genetic testing, embryos are transferred to the uterus on day 4 or

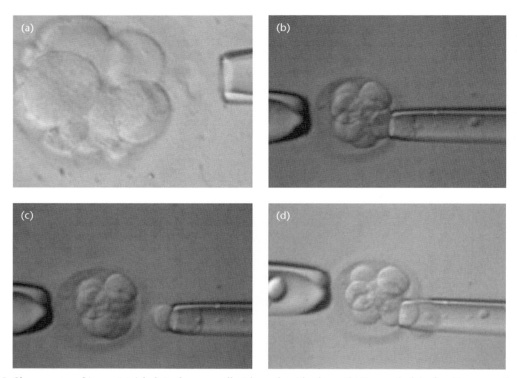

Fig. 9.5 Cleavage-stage biopsy. (a) A hole in the zona pellucida made with a laser. (b) Removal of the first blastomere from the embryo. (c) Deposition of blastomere in the medium. (d) Removal of the second blastomere (with permission from Sermon *et al.* [131]).

5 of development. Cleavage stage biopsy, unlike PB analysis, can provide information on both maternal and paternal alleles. The disadvantages of cleavage stage biopsy include the limited amount of material (often only a single cell) available for analysis, the impact of embryo mosaicism on the risk of misdiagnosis, and the ethical implications of removing a cell that would have contributed to the fetus. Although it has been shown that up to 25% of a human embryo can be removed without disrupting its development, doubt still remains as to whether the biopsy of two versus one cell may have an effect on subsequent embryonic development.

Blastocysts develop 5–6 days after insemination. This is the latest stage for embryo biopsy to enable timely transfer of the embryos back to the uterus for successful implantation. The advantage of biopsy at this stage is that more cells can be obtained for analysis. In addition, it involves the removal of trophectoderm cells that eventually form the placenta

and other extra-embryonic tissue, thereby reducing possible ethical considerations [122]. However, only about 40–50% of the embryos develop to this stage *in vitro*, which limits the application of this biopsy method for PGD [129, 130]. Furthermore, embryos should be transferred before day 5 or 6, thus limiting the time available for diagnosis [131].

PGD is challenging as the diagnosis depends on a single cell. Therefore, strict controls are essential to prevent assay contamination from extraneous DNA sources. This necessitates dedicated equipment and laboratories with filtered air. Testing at the single cell level is also affected by ADO, where one of the two alleles does not amplify during the initial rounds of PCR. Diagnostic assays must therefore be designed and validated to enable the detection of this phenomenon and provide information on the misdiagnosis risk.

Various molecular techniques have been developed and utilized in the genetic testing of biopsy materials. The diagnostic protocols are based on PCR to amplify sufficient DNA from the cells followed by the diagnosis of a specific genetic defect or FISH for the analysis of chromosomes, including sexing. Techniques such as multiplex, fluorescent, and/or real-time PCR and minisequencing are being introduced in an attempt to overcome the inherent difficulties of single cell PCR (including failure of amplification, potential sample contamination, and ADO) due to the limited amount of DNA template and to improve the diagnostic accuracy [131, 132].

Hemophilia is one of the most common indications for PGD (either sexing alone or specific diagnosis) among the X-linked disorders [123], whereas PGD has not yet been applied to other inherited bleeding disorders. Initially PGD in hemophilia only provided diagnosis of fetal sex, but this entails the unnecessary disposal of healthy male embryos and reduces the success rate by decreasing the number of embryos suitable for transfer. More recently, there have been reports of successful mutation-specific PGD of hemophilia [132–134]. Gigarel *et al.* [134] described the use of extragenic linked polymorphic markers for the indirect PGD of hemophilia. Three (one male and two females) embryos identified as unaffected were transferred, resulting in a singleton female pregnancy. Fiorentino *et al.* [132] applied the method known as minisequencing, which identifies the specific mutations without sequencing the entire PCR product, for the PGD of hemophilia A in five cases. Despite the potential of direct mutation detection, an informative intronic single nucleotide polymorphism in IVS 7 was utilized to identify the affected allele. One live birth unaffected by hemophilia was reported. Polymorphic markers are useful when direct detection of mutation is not possible, but they may not be informative and there is also the risk of misdiagnosis because of crossover. Michaelides *et al.* [133] described the first case of PGD based on direct mutation detection in a family with severe hemophilia caused by a single nucleotide substitution mutation in exon 14 of the FVIII gene. This approach resulted in a singleton pregnancy with the birth of a non-carrier female.

PGD is likely to become a realistic option for more couples at risk of having a child affected by hemophilia or other severe inherited bleeding disorders in the near future. Although the reliability and efficiency of PGD are improving with continuous scientific and technological advancement, it remains technically challenging and labor intensive, requiring the close collaboration of a team of specialists. It has raised several ethical and safety issues that still need to be addressed. Further data are required to establish the potential long-term effect of embryo biopsy on children born after the procedure. PGD also has considerable financial implications as it entails the use of IVF in addition to the advance molecular techniques. Apart from being costly, IVF is associated with high levels of stress and anxiety as well as the risks of multiple pregnancies and ovarian hyperstimulation. Unlike IVF for infertility, the number of suitable embryos available for transfer is diminished by excluding affected embryos or those with inconclusive results. In the latest (sixth) European Society of Human Reproduction and Embryology PGD consortium report, there were 2984 PGD cycles resulting in 501 pregnancies and 373 (12.5%) live births [123]. Based on current evid-ence, PGD may be indicated in some individual cases after careful counseling and assessment but should not be regarded as a standard service [135]. It is required by the Human Fertilisation and Embryology Authority (HFEA) for all PGD to be carried out in licensed centers and practice guidelines have been drawn up by the ESHRE PGD Consortium [136].

Sperm sorting

This is an alternative approach for women with X-linked disorders, such as hemophilia, to increase their chance of a female pregnancy by selecting spermatozoa that carry the X chromosome for use in intrauterine insemination (IUI), *in vitro* fertilization (IVF), or ICSI. It can also be utilized as an adjunct to PGD to increase the number of suitable embryos for transfer [137, 138]. The sperm samples are enriched for X- or Y-bearing spermatozoa and the selection process is based on the differences in their dry mass, DNA content, and size. On average, X-bearing spermatozoa have about 2.8% more DNA and are larger and longer [139–141]. However, there are some degrees of variations, and thus overlap, in these characteristics which can make the distinction difficult.

Different sperm-sorting techniques have been developed and they fall broadly into two categories: gradient methods and flow cytometry. Gradient methods typically involve the sperm being put through a dense liquid, such as gradient layers of albumin, and centrifuged to separate the X- and the Y-bearing spermatozoa. The success rate of this technique has been

111

controversial and some laboratory studies have shown that it does not achieve clinically significant enrichment of X- or Y-bearing spermatozoa [142–149]. The flow cytometry method uses a fluorescent dye to stain the X and Y chromosomes of the spermatozoa. Since the X-bearing spermatozoa have about 2.8% more DNA content than Y-bearing spermatozoa, they take up more dye [141]. This allows sperm to be sorted by means of fluorescence detection. The technique (MicroSort, Fairfax, VA) has been shown to be able to sort human spermatozoa to a purity of 80–90% for X spermatozoa and of 60–70% for Y spermatozoa [150]. Fugger [151] reported the use of this sperm-sorting procedure in 332 patients for indications including X-linked disorders or family balancing. The pregnancy rate per cycle was 11.8% (61/518) for IUI and 24.1% (35/145) for IVF/ICSI. The number of pregnancies, with known fetal or birth sex, resulting in the desired sex was 94.4% (37/39) for females and 73% (11/15) for males; 47 pregnancies were ongoing at the time of publication. This technique has raised concerns regarding its safety as the use of chromatin-binding dye and laser energy could potentially cause disruption and damage in the DNA. Although there are no reports to date indicating an increase in birth abnormalities after sorting of human spermatozoa, further data are required, particularly on its long-term effects [152]. This technique is currently only available at two centers in the US and is the subject of an ongoing clinical trial overseen by the US Food and Drug Administration (FDA).

It is important to bear in mind that currently sperm sorting can only increase the chance of, but does not guarantee, a female pregnancy. A misdiagnosis rate of ~10–30% is unlikely to be acceptable to many couples [152], but some may favor the option of IUI with sorted sperm as it is less invasive than PGD and does not involve the disposal of any embryos. Previously, sperm sorting was not regulated in the UK. The Human Fertilisation and Embryology Authority (HFEA), following its public consultation in 1993, recommended that its licensed centers should not use sperm-sorting technique in sex selection [153]. It allowed clinics, subject to license from the HFEA, to select the sex of embryos using PGD only for the avoidance of serious sex-linked disorders [145]. Owing to the developments in sperm sorting techniques, in particular the flow cytometry method, the HFEA has recently produced a review on this topic following a public consultation in 2002–03 [154]. The review concluded that because of the potential risk of harm associated with the manipulation of sperm in the laboratory, all treatment with sorted sperm should be regulated and clinics that provide a sperm sorting service should be brought within the licensing regime [145]. It recommended that centres, subject to licenses from the HFEA, should be permitted to offer treatment using sperm sorted by flow cytometry (whether alone or in combination with PGD) only to patients with clear medical reasons. It also recommended that gradient methods should not be used. At this time, sperm sorting by the gradient method was still available from a few private clinics not under HFEA regulation. However, since the recent implementation of the European Tissues and Cells Directive (EUTD) in July 2007, any center in the UK that processes sperm, including sperm sorting, is now under the HFEA regulation. These clinics are not permitted to sort sperm by the gradient method, and can only use the flow cytometry method if there is a clear medical benefit.

Non-invasive prenatal diagnosis

To date, the definitive prenatal diagnosis of hemophilia or other inherited bleeding disorders can only be achieved by genetic analysis or coagulation assays of fetal samples obtained through invasive procedures. These tests are associated with small but definite risks. Consequently, considerable effort has been made to develop non-invasive prenatal diagnostic techniques that obviate these risks. Fetal cells and, more recently, ffDNA in the maternal circulation represent two potential sources of fetal DNA utilized for this purpose. They both have their advantages and limitations. As mentioned earlier, ffDNA has the attractions of being present at a much higher concentration and having a rapid clearance after delivery. Current advances in real-time quantitative PCR technology have allowed detailed studies of ffDNA in maternal plasma. In addition to the prenatal determination of fetal gender and rhesus blood type, ffDNA has been applied successfully to the prenatal diagnosis of single gene disorders caused by paternally inherited alleles or mutations. Prenatal diagnosis of autosomal dominant diseases such as achondroplasia [155, 156] and myotonic dystrophy [157] has been achieved by the detection of fetal-derived paternally inherited mutations. Whereas in autosomal recessive conditions, for example beta-thalassemia [158–160] and cystic fibrosis [161, 162], prenatal exclusion was inferred by the absence of fetal-derived paternally inherited alleles. It is very difficult to differentiate the maternally inherited allele of the fetus from the background of maternal DNA in the plasma. Therefore, prenatal diagnosis of genetic disorders caused by maternally inherited mutation is at present not possible through the analysis of ffDNA. This limitation could potentially be overcome by the development of an approach based on the use of a universal fetal-specific marker that would then allow detection of fetal-derived maternally inherited DNA in maternal plasma. Single nucleotide polymorphisms and epigenetic markers are two rapidly evolving areas of research that hold promise of a wider application of ffDNA in the field of prenatal diagnosis [163].

In contrast to ffDNA, analysis of intact fetal cells in maternal circulation offers the possibility of diagnosing maternally inherited disorders and aneuploidy. However, the isolation of fetal cells from maternal blood presents a considerable challenge because of their limited numbers. Furthermore, enrichment procedures are required and they are generally very specialized, time-consuming, and technically demanding. Fetal leukocytes can persist for years after delivery [56, 164–166], thus giving rise to inaccurate results in multigravida. Trophoblasts are difficult to enrich because of a lack of specific antibodies [167, 168]. Fetal erythrocytes or nucleated red blood cells (NRBCs) have emerged as the most suitable fetal cell type because they are relatively abundant in early fetal circulation [169], have a short lifespan [170] and express a number of antigens at high levels, which facilitates their enrichment [171, 172]. Nevertheless, the use of NRBCs is still subject to the difficult isolation and enrichment process. Moreover, some NRBCs, even after fetal cell enrichment, are of maternal origin [169, 173–175], hence the origin of each cell must be confirmed when used for prenatal diagnosis. DNA analysis of NRBCs presents a further challenge. Although PCR methods are highly sensitive, single-cell PCR is prone to sources of error, including potential sample contamination, total PCR failure, ADO and preferential amplification of one of the alleles. Continuous efforts are being made in improving current molecular technologies and in developing more sensitive methods of recovering and examining NRBCs. Despite the tremendous challenge, it is not inconceivable that non-invasive prenatal diagnosis of inherited bleeding disorders using ffDNA or fetal cells in maternal circulation may be achieved in the future.

Views and experiences of women in families affected with inherited bleeding disorders towards prenatal diagnosis

Several studies have been conducted on the attitudes of carriers of hemophilia towards prenatal diagnosis and their reproductive behavior. There is a lack of data on these aspects for women with type 3 VWD or rare inherited bleeding disorders because of their rarity. The experiences reported on carriers of hemophilia are likely to reflect those of women with rare bleeding disorders since the developments in their treatment and prenatal diagnosis have followed a similar trend. Nonetheless, further research in these areas is required to confirm this postulation.

Attitudes towards prenatal diagnosis

Women's attitudes towards prenatal diagnosis and termination of pregnancy vary widely between different countries and cultures. Religion is a strong determinant of the individual's decision regarding prenatal diagnosis and termination of pregnancy [176, 177]. For example, Catholic women are less likely to opt for these options than women of other religious belief [178, 179]. Other factors that affect women's views towards prenatal diagnosis include their attitudes towards termination of pregnancy, the severity of the disorder, their experience of the condition within the family, and the nature and availability of the tests involved.

In a survey of 105 carriers of severe or moderate hemophilia in Sweden, those who experienced prenatal diagnosis were significantly more positive towards selective termination of pregnancy than those who did not opt for prenatal diagnosis [180]. This connection is understandable since selective termination is often the primary purpose for prenatal diagnosis. Similarly, in a study of 549 potential and obligate carriers in The Netherlands, one of the main reasons for not choosing prenatal diagnosis was a negative attitude towards termination of pregnancy [181]. In this study, only 11% of women with children had opted for prenatal diagnosis. Most women from affected families objected to prenatal diagnosis because they did not consider

113

hemophilia to be sufficiently serious to justify an abortion [181]. Similar views were expressed among carriers of hemophilia in Scotland, Canada, and the USA [179, 182, 183]. In a review of the obstetric experience of carriers spanning two decades from our centre in the United Kingdom, the uptake of invasive prenatal diagnostic tests remained relatively low at 35% (17/48) and 20% (13/65) over the periods 1985–95 and 1995–2005, respectively [184, 185]. A low (14%) uptake of prenatal diagnosis has also been reported among carriers of severe and moderate hemophilia in Sweden towards the end of the 1990s [180].

Another factor that has been identified as an important determinant of the choice of prenatal diagnosis is the severity of the disorder and the woman's experience of this disorder within the family [180]. Understandably, carriers who have experienced the complications of hemophilia or its treatment were more in favor of prenatal diagnosis than women whose affected children received modern treatment without complications. This appears to apply also to the decision to interrupt an affected pregnancy. In our series [185], carriers who opted to have prenatal diagnosis and eventual termination of affected pregnancy were from families with either severe or moderate hemophilia. None of the carriers of mild hemophilia opted for invasive testing or termination of pregnancy because of hemophilia [185].

Carriers may choose to have prenatal testing without the intention of interrupting an affected pregnancy, but for reasons such as psychological preparations or planning for the management of labor and delivery. In the Swedish study by Tedgard et al. [180], most carriers reported a positive attitude towards prenatal diagnosis itself while expressing a more negative feeling towards termination of pregnancy following prenatal diagnosis, especially among those without previous experience of prenatal diagnosis. Similarly, in a study of 35 mothers of children with hemophilia, 43% would consider prenatal diagnosis, but only 17% would terminate a pregnancy if the fetus was found to be affected [179]. The majority of those interested in prenatal diagnosis only wanted to know if the fetus was affected and did not have the intention of selective termination. In our series, termination of pregnancy was opted for in about 60% of the pregnancies identified to carry an affected male [184, 185]. The majority of pregnancy terminations performed among carriers of hemophilia were for social reasons and not

directly for hemophilia [184]. At the same time, an increasing number of carriers over the two decades (from 52% to 97%) chose to have prenatal fetal sex determination. This could be attributed to the non-invasive nature of the techniques involved but also to an increased awareness of its benefits in optimizing the management of labor and delivery [184, 185].

Timing of the prenatal diagnostic test can also influence the woman's decision on its uptake. Women are more inclined to object to prenatal diagnosis if it is performed at a later stage of gestation. When prenatal diagnosis first became possible through fetoscopic fetal blood sampling in the second trimester, only 3% of all pregnant hemophilia carriers in the USA utilized this option [186]. In the Dutch study by Varekamp et al. [181], 30% of the respondents stated that they would opt for prenatal diagnosis and potential termination in the future if this was done early in pregnancy compared with only 15% if it was only possible in the 18–20th gestational week. Prenatal diagnosis of hemophilia by CVS and gene analysis appears to be generally well accepted by carriers and their partners. In a study involving 29 carriers of hemophilia and 23 of their partners who had experienced first trimester CVS, most women (79%) and all men were positive towards having prenatal diagnosis by CVS in a future pregnancy [187].

A large difference in the attitudes towards prenatal diagnosis and termination of pregnancy for hemophilia has been observed between the developed and the developing countries [188, 189]. The burden of a severe genetic condition is evidently heavy in developing countries where there are limited facilities and resources. The life expectancy and the quality of life of affected individuals are subsequently poorer in these countries. As a result, the prevention of the birth of children with hemophilia is a key objective in these countries [190]. One study compared the views of hemophilic populations in Iran and Italy towards prenatal diagnosis and termination of pregnancy and found the acceptability of termination of pregnancy for hemophilia was four times greater (58% vs 17%) in Iranians than in Italians. This difference could be explained by the higher availability and quality of medical care for hemophiliacs in Italy [188]. Likewise, most families affected by hemophilia in India, where there is poor awareness of the disorder, inadequate diagnostic facilities, and a lack of social support systems, would consider termination of an affected pregnancy [189]. However, despite a high acceptability, the use of prenatal diagnosis is limited by multiple factors such as lack of awareness, financial constraints, inadequate diagnostic facilities and social stigma [191].

The experiences and psychological effects of prenatal diagnosis

Prenatal diagnosis is associated with a considerable amount of anxiety and distress particularly when performed because of a high genetic risk [192–194]. Anxiety arises from the risk of having an affected child with long-term morbidity, having potentially painful and invasive diagnostic tests, having a miscarriage due to these tests, receiving an abnormal result, making the decision whether to continue or have a termination of the pregnancy, and undergoing the process of termination and its complications. The negative psychological effect associated with prenatal diagnosis has been found to be more prominent when prenatal diagnosis is carried out at a more advanced gestation [187, 195–197]. Equally, termination of pregnancy is associated with greater mood disturbances following the procedure when carried out after second compared with first trimester prenatal diagnosis [198]. Among carriers of hemophilia, significantly fewer signs of depressive mood were reported following CVS than fetal blood sampling in the second trimester [187, 199]. Termination of an affected pregnancy was found to be emotionally painful for all carriers despite the gestation, but the negative experience was more profound after second trimester termination [187, 199].

A number of characteristics have been identified among carriers at high risk of having negative psychological reactions in association with a prenatal diagnosis of hemophilia by fetal blood sampling [200]. They include a negative view of oneself in general and of being a carrier, a planned pregnancy, high education, good general knowledge of hemophilia, and a guiding philosophy of life. These women also reported signs of depressive mood significantly more often at follow-up. Although fetal blood sampling has largely been superseded by CVS and amniocentesis for prenatal diagnosis, the results of the study may help to identify women who are likely to have difficulty in coping emotionally with the process of prenatal diagnosis and therefore at particular need for psychological support.

The long-term psychological effects of prenatal diagnosis have been evaluated using a symptom check list questionnaire (SCL-90) [201] among 50 carriers of hemophilia at a median of 5.5 (range 1–17) years since their last prenatal diagnosis [202]. The numbers of carriers who underwent early and late prenatal diagnosis were 29 (58%) and 21 (42%), respectively. Nineteen had termination of pregnancy following prenatal diagnosis. No negative long-term psychological effects were demonstrated among these carriers. They, and particularly those who had late prenatal diagnostic procedures, have a lower tendency for somatization (psychological distress that arises from perceptions of bodily dysfunction) than carriers who did not opt for prenatal diagnosis. The subgroup of carriers with late prenatal diagnosis did however have higher scores on the SCL (symptom checklist) subscales for interpersonal sensitivity, depression, and the general severity index. But this group of carriers appears to have been protected from long-term negative psychological effects by their good sense of coherence and social support. It is reassuring that prenatal diagnosis of hemophilia did not appear to have negative long-term psychological effects. Nevertheless, psychosocial support is recommended and crucial for all couples undergoing prenatal diagnosis and those opting for subsequent termination of affected pregnancy.

Effects on reproduction

The impact of prenatal diagnosis on the incidence of hemophilia had been evaluated in Sweden [203, 204]. The annual incidence of severe and moderate hemophilia was relatively constant prior to the 1980s. It then increased from 0.78/10 000 males in the 1970s to 1.34/10 000 in the 1980s and leveled off at 1.31/10 000 in the 1990s [204]. The increased incidence was thought to be most likely due to the improvements in the treatment of hemophilia, which led to the increased life expectancy and reproductive fitness of affected individuals and subsequently an increased number of carrier daughters. Although prenatal diagnosis did not affect the incidence of hemophilia in the 1970s and 1980s, it appeared to have offset a further increase in the incidence hemophilia in the 1990s. One probable explanation was the introduction of first trimester prenatal diagnosis that resulted in a higher uptake of prenatal diagnosis for hemophilia [204].

In a Swedish study towards the end of the 1990s, carriers of hemophilia have been found, in general, to have the same number of children as other women of similar age [180]. However, many carriers who did not opt for prenatal diagnosis chose not to have further pregnancies after the birth of a hemophilic child. These carriers had significantly fewer children than carriers who had prenatal diagnosis or age-matched non-carriers [180]. In our study, which assessed the reproductive choices of 197 obligate and potential carriers of hemophilia during the same period, 106 (54%) had made a conscious decision not to have children or any more children. Hemophilia was a major factor in this decision for a large proportion of women. The reasons were fear of passing hemophilia on to their child (44%), previous experience with hemophilia in the family/not wanting to cope with another hemophilic child (6%), and the stress of going through prenatal tests when they would not consider termination of pregnancy even if the baby was affected (7%) [205].

It is most likely that with the availability of prenatal diagnosis and improved treatment most carriers are able to have the number of children they wish to have.

Modern treatments in the developed countries have led to decreased morbidity and consequently fewer parents feel obliged to prevent the birth of an affected child. However, at the same time, parents are being presented with more possible options as a result of developments in diagnostic techniques and molecular technology. Many welcome these new opportunities that were previously unavailable, but for others they may add more complications or burden to the decision-making process. This further emphasizes the importance of genetic counseling in helping and supporting prospective parents to come to an often very difficult decision regarding reproduction.

Acknowledgement

We would like to thank Professor Edward Tuddenham and Dr Katerina Michaelides for their useful comments.

References

1 Rodeghiero F, Castaman G, Dini E. Epidemiological investigation of the prevalence of von Willebrand's disease. *Blood* 1987; **69**: 454–459.

2 Werner EJ, Broxson EH, Tucker EL, *et al*. Prevalence of von Willebrand disease in children: a multiethnic study. *J Pediatr* 1993; **123**: 893–898.

3 Alfirevic Z, von Dadelszen P. Instruments for chorionic villus sampling for prenatal diagnosis. *Cochrane Database Syst Rev* 2003; CD000114.

4 Alfirevic Z, Sundberg K, Brigham S. Amniocentesis and chorionic villus sampling for prenatal diagnosis. *Cochrane Database Syst Rev* 2003; CD003252.

5 Mujezinovic F, Alfirevic Z. Procedure-related complications of amniocentesis and chorionic villous sampling: a systematic review. *Obstet Gynecol* 2007; **110**: 687–694.

6 Firth HV, Boyd PA, Chamberlain PF, *et al*. Analysis of limb reduction defects in babies exposed to chorionic villus sampling. *Lancet* 1994; **343**: 1069–1071.

7 RCOG. Amniocentesis and chorionic villus sampling. Guideline No. 8. 2005.

8 Tabor A, Philip J, Madsen M *et al*. Randomised controlled trial of genetic amniocentesis in 4606 low-risk women. *Lancet* 1986; **1**: 1287–1293.

9 The Canadian Early and Mid-trimester Amniocentesis Trial (CEMATGroup). Randomised trial to assess safety and fetal outcome of early and midtrimester amniocentesis. *Lancet* 1998; **351**: 242–247.

10 Yukobowich E, Anteby EY, Cohen SM, *et al*. Risk of fetal loss in twin pregnancies undergoing second trimester amniocentesis (1). *Obstet Gynecol* 2001; **98**: 231–234.

11 Fisk NM, Fordham K, Abramsky L. Elective late fetal karyotyping. *Br J Obstet Gynaecol* 1996; **103**: 468–470.

12 Shalev J, Meizner I, Rabinerson D, *et al*. Elective cytogenetic amniocentesis in the third trimester for pregnancies with high risk factors. *Prenat Diagn* 1999; **19**: 749–752.

13 Rozenberg P. [Third trimester amniocentesis for fetal karyotyping: why so late?]. *Gynecol Obstet Fertil* 2002; **30**: 427–430.

14 Galle PC, Meis PJ. Complications of amniocentesis: a review. *J Reprod Med* 1982; **27**: 149–155.

15 Gordon MC, Narula K, O'Shaughnessy R, Barth WH, Jr. Complications of third-trimester amniocentesis using continuous ultrasound guidance. *Obstet Gynecol* 2002; **99**: 255–259.

16 Stark CM, Smith RS, Lagrandeur RM, *et al*. Need for urgent delivery after third-trimester amniocentesis. *Obstet Gynecol* 2000; **95**: 48–50.

17 Hodor JG, Poggi SH, Spong CY, *et al*. Risk of third-trimester amniocentesis: a case-control study. *Am J Perinatol* 2006; **23**: 177–180.

18 Lam YH, Tang MH, Sin SY, Ghosh A. Clinical significance of amniotic-fluid-cell culture failure. *Prenat Diagn* 1998; **18**: 343–347.

19 O'Donoghue K, Giorgi L, Pontello V, *et al.* Amniocentesis in the third trimester of pregnancy. *Prenat Diagn* 2007; **27**: 1000–1004.

20 Donner C, Rypens F, Paquet V, *et al.* Cordocentesis for rapid karyotype: 421 consecutive cases. *Fetal Diagn Ther* 1995; **10**: 192–199.

21 Buscaglia M, Ghisoni L, Bellotti M, *et al.* Percutaneous umbilical blood sampling: indication changes and procedure loss rate in a nine years' experience. *Fetal Diagn Ther* 1996; **11**: 106–113.

22 Weiner CP, Okamura K. Diagnostic fetal blood sampling-technique related losses. *Fetal Diagn Ther* 1996; **11**: 169–175.

23 Tongsong T, Wanapirak C, Kunavikatikul C, *et al.* Cordocentesis at 16–24 weeks of gestation: experience of 1320 cases. *Prenat Diagn* 2000; **20**: 224–228.

24 Tongsong T, Wanapirak C, Kunavikatikul C, *et al.* Fetal loss rate associated with cordocentesis at midgestation. *Am J Obstet Gynecol* 2001; **184**: 719–723.

25 Liao C, Wei J, Li Q, *et al.* Efficacy and safety of cordocentesis for prenatal diagnosis. *Int J Gynaecol Obstet* 2006; **93**: 13–17.

26 Orlandi F, Damiani G, Jakil C, *et al.* The risks of early cordocentesis (12–21 weeks): analysis of 500 procedures. *Prenat Diagn* 1990; **10**: 425–428.

27 Antsaklis A, Daskalakis G, Papantoniou N, Michalas S. Fetal blood sampling – indication-related losses. *Prenat Diagn* 1998; **18**: 934–940.

28 Maxwell DJ, Johnson P, Hurley P, *et al.* Fetal blood sampling and pregnancy loss in relation to indication. *Br J Obstet Gynaecol* 1991; **98**: 892–897.

29 Daffos F, Forestier F, Capella-Pavlovsky M, *et al.* [Risk factors of fetal blood sampling. The essential risk is its duration]. *Rev Prat* 1994; **44**: 923–926.

30 Duchatel F, Oury JF, Mennesson B, Muray JM. Complications of diagnostic ultrasound-guided percutaneous umbilical blood sampling: analysis of a series of 341 cases and review of the literature. *Eur J Obstet Gynecol Reprod Biol* 1993; **52**: 95–104.

31 Ash KM, Mibashan RS, Nicolaides KH. Diagnosis and treatment of feto-maternal hemorrhage in a fetus with homozygous von Willebrand's disease. *Fetal Ther* 1988; **3**: 189–191.

32 Birnholz JC. Determination of fetal sex. *N Engl J Med* 1983; **309**: 942–944.

33 Elejalde BR, de Elejalde MM, Heitman T. Visualization of the fetal genitalia by ultrasonography: a review of the literature and analysis of its accuracy and ethical implications. *J Ultrasound Med* 1985; **4**: 633–639.

34 Whitlow BJ, Lazanakis MS, Economides DL. The sonographic identification of fetal gender from 11 to 14 weeks of gestation. *Ultrasound Obstet Gynecol* 1999; **13**: 301–304.

35 Mielke G, Kiesel L, Backsch C, Erz W, Gonser M. Fetal sex determination by high resolution ultrasound in early pregnancy. *Eur J Ultrasound* 1998; **7**: 109–114.

36 Efrat Z, Akinfenwa OO, Nicolaides KH. First-trimester determination of fetal gender by ultrasound. *Ultrasound Obstet Gynecol* 1999; **13**: 305–307.

37 Hyett JA, Gardener G, Stojilkovic-Mikic T, *et al.* Reduction in diagnostic and therapeutic interventions by non-invasive determination of fetal sex in early pregnancy. *Prenat Diagn* 2005; **25**: 1111–1116.

38 Avent ND, Chitty LS. Non-invasive diagnosis of fetal sex; utilisation of free fetal DNA in maternal plasma and ultrasound. *Prenat Diagn* 2006; **26**: 598–603.

39 Benott B. Early fetal gender determination. *Ultrasound Obstet Gynecol* 1999; **13**: 299–300.

40 Mazza V, Contu G, Falcinelli C, *et al.* Biometrical threshold of biparietal diameter for certain fetal sex assignment by ultrasound. *Ultrasound Obstet Gynecol* 1999; **13**: 308–311.

41 Mazza V, Di Monte, I, Pati M, *et al.* Sonographic biometrical range of external genitalia differentiation in the first trimester of pregnancy: analysis of 2593 cases. *Prenat Diagn* 2004; **24**: 677–684.

42 Lo YM, Corbetta N, Chamberlain PF, *et al.* Presence of fetal DNA in maternal plasma and serum. *Lancet* 1997; **350**: 485–487.

43 Elias S, Price J, Dockter M, *et al.* First trimester prenatal diagnosis of trisomy 21 in fetal cells from maternal blood. *Lancet* 1992; **340**: 1033.

44 de la Cruz F, Shifrin H, Elias S, *et al.* Prenatal diagnosis by use of fetal cells isolated from maternal blood. *Am J Obstet Gynecol* 1995; **173**: 1354–1355.

45 Hahn S, Sant R, Holzgreve W. Fetal cells in maternal blood: current and future perspectives. *Mol Hum Reprod* 1998; **4**: 515–521.

46 Hamada H, Arinami T, Kubo T, *et al.* Fetal nucleated cells in maternal peripheral blood: frequency and relationship to gestational age. *Hum Genet* 1993; **91**: 427–432.

47 Lo YM, Tein MS, Lau TK, *et al.* Quantitative analysis of fetal DNA in maternal plasma and serum: implications for noninvasive prenatal diagnosis. *Am J Hum Genet* 1998; **62**: 768–775.

48 Invernizzi P, Biondi ML, Battezzati PM, *et al.* Presence of fetal DNA in maternal plasma decades after pregnancy. *Hum Genet* 2002; **110**: 587–591.

49 Santacroce R, Vecchione G, Tomaiyolo M, *et al.* Identification of fetal gender in maternal blood is a helpful tool in the prenatal diagnosis of haemophilia. *Hemophilia* 2006; **12**: 417–422.

50 Lau TW, Leung TN, Chan LY, *et al.* Fetal DNA clearance from maternal plasma is impaired in preeclampsia. *Clin Chem* 2002; **48**: 2141–2146.

51 Rijnders RJ, Christiaens GC, Soussan AA, van der Schoot CE. Cell-free fetal DNA is not present in plasma of nonpregnant mothers. *Clin Chem* 2004; **50**: 679–681.

52 Smid M, Galbiati S, Vassallo A, et al. No evidence of fetal DNA persistence in maternal plasma after pregnancy. *Hum Genet* 2003; **112**: 617–618.

53 Johnson-Hopson CN, Artlett CM. Evidence against the long-term persistence of fetal DNA in maternal plasma after pregnancy. *Hum Genet* 2002; **111**: 575.

54 Benachi A, Steffann J, Gautier E, et al. Fetal DNA in maternal serum: does it persist after pregnancy? *Hum Genet* 2003; **113**: 76–79.

55 Lo YM, Zhang J, Leung TN, et al. Rapid clearance of fetal DNA from maternal plasma. *Am J Hum Genet* 1999; **64**: 218–224.

56 Bianchi DW, Zickwolf GK, Weil GJ, et al. Male fetal progenitor cells persist in maternal blood for as long as 27 years postpartum. *Proc Natl Acad Sci USA* 1996; **93**: 705–708.

57 Costa JM, Benachi A, Gautier E, et al. First-trimester fetal sex determination in maternal serum using real-time PCR. *Prenat Diagn* 2001; **21**: 1070–1074.

58 Sekizawa A, Kondo T, Iwasaki M, et al. Accuracy of fetal gender determination by analysis of DNA in maternal plasma. *Clin Chem* 2001; **47**: 1856–1858.

59 Honda H, Miharu N, Ohashi Y, et al. Fetal gender determination in early pregnancy through qualitative and quantitative analysis of fetal DNA in maternal serum. *Hum Genet* 2002; **110**: 75–79.

60 Hromadnikova I, Houbova B, Hridelova D, et al. Replicate real-time PCR testing of DNA in maternal plasma increases the sensitivity of non-invasive fetal sex determination. *Prenat Diagn* 2003; **23**: 235–238.

61 Rijnders RJ, Van Der Luijt RB, Peters ED, et al. Earliest gestational age for fetal sexing in cell-free maternal plasma. *Prenat Diagn* 2003; **23**: 1042–1044.

62 Rijnders RJ, Christiaens GC, Bossers B, et al. Clinical applications of cell-free fetal DNA from maternal plasma. *Obstet Gynecol* 2004; **103**: 157–164.

63 Rijnders RJ, van der Schoot CE, Bossers B, et al. Fetal sex determination from maternal plasma in pregnancies at risk for congenital adrenal hyperplasia. *Obstet Gynecol* 2001; **98**: 374–378.

64 Zhong XY, Holzgreve W, Hahn S. Risk free simultaneous prenatal identification of fetal Rhesus D status and sex by multiplex real-time PCR using cell free fetal DNA in maternal plasma. *Swiss Med Wkly* 2001; **131**: 70–74.

65 Guibert J, Benachi A, Grebille AG, et al. Kinetics of SRY gene appearance in maternal serum: detection by real time PCR in early pregnancy after assisted reproductive technique. *Hum Reprod* 2003; **18**: 1733–1736.

66 Cremonesi L, Galbiati S, Foglieni B, et al. Feasibility study for a microchip-based approach for noninvasive prenatal diagnosis of genetic diseases. *Ann NY Acad Sci* 2004; **1022**: 105–112.

67 Birch L, English CA, O'Donoghue K, et al. Accurate and robust quantification of circulating fetal and total DNA in maternal plasma from 5 to 41 weeks of gestation. *Clin Chem* 2005; **51**: 312–320.

68 Illanes S, Denbow M, Kailasam C, et al. Early detection of cell-free fetal DNA in maternal plasma. *Early Hum Dev* 2007; **83**: 563–566.

69 Rodeck CH, Campbell S. Sampling pure fetal blood by fetoscopy in second trimester of pregnancy. *BMJ* 1978; **2**: 728–730.

70 Peake IR, Bloom AL, Giddings JC, Ludlam CA. An immunoradiometric assay for procoagulant factor VIII antigen: results in haemophilia, von Willebrand's disease and fetal plasma and serum. *Br J Hematol* 1979; **42**: 269–281.

71 Holmberg L, Gustavii B, Cordesius E, et al. Prenatal diagnosis of hemophilia B by an immunoradiometric assay of factor IX. *Blood* 1980; **56**: 397–401.

72 Firshein SI, Hoyer LW, Lazarchick J, et al. Prenatal diagnosis of classic hemophilia. *N Engl J Med* 1979; **300**: 937–941.

73 Mibashan RS, Rodeck CH, Thumpston JK, et al. Plasma assay of fetal factors VIIIC and IX for prenatal diagnosis of haemophilia. *Lancet* 1979; **1**: 1309–1311.

74 Daffos F, Capella-Pavlovsky M, Forestier F. A new procedure for fetal blood sampling in utero: preliminary results of fifty-three cases. *Am J Obstet Gynecol* 1983; **146**: 985–987.

75 Bang J, Bock JE, Trolle D. Ultrasound-guided fetal intravenous transfusion for severe rhesus haemolytic disease. *BMJ (Clin Res Ed)* 1982; **284**: 373–374.

76 The status of fetoscopy and fetal tissue sampling. The results of the first meeting of the International Fetoscopy Group. *Prenat Diagn* 1984; **4**: 79–81.

77 Gitschier J, Wood WI, Goralka TM, et al. Characterization of the human factor VIII gene. *Nature* 1984; **312**: 326–330.

78 Yoshitake S, Schach BG, Foster DC, et al. Nucleotide sequence of the gene for human factor IX (antihemophilic factor B). *Biochemistry* 1985; **24**: 3736–3750.

79 Ward RH, Modell B, Petrou M, et al. Method of sampling chorionic villi in first trimester of pregnancy under guidance of real time ultrasound. *BMJ (Clin Res Ed)* 1983; **286**: 1542–1544.

80 Smidt-Jensen S, Hahnemann N. Transabdominal fine needle biopsy from chorionic villi in the first trimester. *Prenat Diagn* 1984; **4**: 163–169.

81 Gitschier J, Lawn RM, Rotblat F, *et al.* Antenatal diagnosis and carrier detection of haemophilia A using factor VIII gene probe. *Lancet* 1985; **1**: 1093–1094.

82 Chan V, Tong TM, Chan TP, *et al.* Multiple XbaI polymorphisms for carrier detection and prenatal diagnosis of haemophilia A. *Br J Hematol* 1989; **73**: 497–500.

83 Pecorara M, Casarino L, Mori PG, *et al.* Hemophilia A: carrier detection and prenatal diagnosis by DNA analysis. *Blood* 1987; **70**: 531–535.

84 Sampietro M, Camerino G, Romano M, *et al.* Combined use of DNA probes in first-trimester prenatal diagnosis of hemophilia A. *Thromb Haemost* 1987; **58**: 988–992.

85 Brocker-Vriends AH, Briet E, Kanhai HH, *et al.* First trimester prenatal diagnosis of haemophilia A: two years' experience. *Prenat Diagn* 1988; **8**: 411–421.

86 Chistolini A, Papacchini M, Mazzucconi MG, *et al.* Carrier detection and prenatal diagnosis in haemophilia A and B. *Hematologica* 1990; **75**: 424–428.

87 Sacchi E, Randi AM, Tagliavacca L, *et al.* Carrier detection and prenatal diagnosis of hemophilia A: 5-years experience at a hemophilia center. *Int J Clin Lab Res* 1992; **21**: 310–313.

88 Lavergne JM, Laurian Y, Dudilleux A, *et al.* Carrier detection and prenatal diagnosis in 98 families of haemophilia A by linkage analysis and direct detection of mutations. *Blood Coagul Fibrinolysis* 1991; **2**: 293–301.

89 Van de Water NS, Ockelford PA, Berry EW, Browett PJ. Haemophilia management: the application of DNA analysis for prenatal diagnosis. *N Z Med J* 1991; **104**: 443–446.

90 Caprino D, Acquila M, Mori PG. Carrier detection and prenatal diagnosis of hemophilia B with more advanced techniques. *Ann Hematol* 1993; **67**: 289–293.

91 Acquila M, Bottini F, Valetto A, *et al.* A new strategy for prenatal diagnosis in a sporadic haemophilia B family. *Hemophilia* 2001; **7**: 416–418.

92 Ludwig M, Brackmann HH, Olek K. Prenatal diagnosis of haemophilia B by the use of polymerase chain reaction and direct sequencing. *Klin Wochenschr* 1991; **69**: 196–200.

93 Ljung R, Green P, Sjorin E, *et al.* Antenatal diagnosis of haemophilia B by amplification and electrophoresis of an exon fragment with a short deletion. *Eur J Hematol* 1992; **49**: 215–218.

94 Schwartz M, Cooper DN, Millar DS, *et al.* Prenatal exclusion of haemophilia A and carrier testing by direct detection of a disease lesion. *Prenat Diagn* 1992; **12**: 861–866.

95 Salviato R, Belvini D, Zanotto D, *et al.* Prenatal diagnosis of haemophilia A by using intron 1 inversion detection. *Hemophilia* 2007; **13**: 772–774.

96 Chowdhury MR, Tiwari M, Kabra M, Menon PS. Prenatal diagnosis in hemophilia A using factor VIII gene polymorphism – Indian experience. *Ann Hematol* 2003; **82**: 427–430.

97 Shetty S, Ghosh K, Bhide A, Mohanty D. Carrier detection and prenatal diagnosis in families with haemophilia. *Natl Med J India* 2001; **14**: 81–83.

98 Panigrahi I, Ahmed RP, Kannan M, *et al.* Cord blood analysis for prenatal diagnosis of thalassemia major and hemophilia A. *Indian Pediatr* 2005; **42**: 577–581.

99 Shetty S, Ghosh K, Mohanty D. Prenatal diagnosis in a haemophilia A family by both factor VIII activity and antigen measurements. *J Assoc Physicians India* 2003; **51**: 916–918.

100 Shetty S, Ghosh K. Robustness of factor assays following cordocentesis in the prenatal diagnosis of haemophilia and other bleeding disorders. *Hemophilia* 2007; **13**: 172–177.

101 Chi C, Hyett JA, Finning KM, *et al.* Non-invasive first trimester determination of fetal gender: a new approach for prenatal diagnosis of haemophilia. *Br J Obstet Gynaecol* 2006; **113**: 239–242.

102 Costa JM, Benachi A, Gautier E. New strategy for prenatal diagnosis of X-linked disorders. *N Engl J Med* 2002; **346**: 1502.

103 Mazza V, Falcinelli C, Percesepe A, *et al.* Non-invasive first trimester fetal gender assignment in pregnancies at risk for X-linked recessive diseases. *Prenat Diagn* 2002; **22**: 919–924.

104 Trasi S, Mohanty D, Shetty S, Ghosh K. Prenatal diagnosis of von Willebrand disease in a family. *Natl Med J India* 2005; **18**: 187–188.

105 Hoyer LW, Lindsten J, Blomback M, *et al.* Prenatal evaluation of fetus at risk for severe von Willebrand's disease. *Lancet* 1979; **2**: 191–192.

106 Rodeck CH, Mibashan RS, Peake IR, Bloom AL. Prenatal diagnosis of severe von Willebrand's disease. *Lancet* 1979; **2**: 637–638.

107 Rothschild C, Forestier F, Daffos F, *et al.* Prenatal diagnosis in type IIA von Willebrand disease. *Nouv Rev Fr Hematol* 1990; **32**: 125–127.

108 Peake IR, Bowen D, Bignell P, *et al.* Family studies and prenatal diagnosis in severe von Willebrand disease by polymerase chain reaction amplification of a variable number tandem repeat region of the von Willebrand factor gene. *Blood* 1990; **76**: 555–561.

109 Bolton-Maggs PH, Perry DJ, Chalmers EA, *et al.* The rare coagulation disorders – review with guidelines for management from the United Kingdom Haemophilia Centre Doctors' Organisation. *Haemophilia* 2004; **10**: 593–628.

110 Peyvandi F, Jayandharan G, Chandy M, *et al.* Genetic diagnosis of haemophilia and other inherited bleeding disorders. *Haemophilia* 2006; **12** (Suppl 3): 82–89.

111 Millar DS, Cooper DN, Kakkar VV, *et al.* Prenatal exclusion of severe factor VII deficiency by DNA sequencing. *Lancet* 1992; **339**: 1359.

112 McVey JH, Boswell EJ, Takamiya O, *et al.* Exclusion of the first EGF domain of factor VII by a splice site mutation causes lethal factor VII deficiency. *Blood* 1998; **92**: 920–926.

113 Giansily-Blaizot M, Aguilar-Martinez P, Mazurier C, *et al.* Prenatal diagnosis of severe factor VII deficiency using mutation detection and linkage analysis. *Br J Haematol* 2001; **112**: 251–252.

114 Ariffin H, Millar DS, Cooper DN, *et al.* Prenatal exclusion of severe factor VII deficiency. *J Pediatr Hematol Oncol* 2003; **25**: 418–420.

115 Camire R, Ann DR, Day GA, III, *et al.* Prenatal diagnosis of factor X deficiency using a combination of direct mutation detection and linkage analysis with an intragenic single nucleotide polymorphism. *Prenat Diagn* 2003; **23**: 457–460.

116 Ingerslev J, Herlin T, Sorensen B, *et al.* Severe factor X deficiency in a pair of siblings: clinical presentation, phenotypic and genotypic features, prenatal diagnosis and treatment. *Haemophilia* 2007; **13**: 334–336.

117 Kangsadalampai S, Coggan M, Caglayan SH, *et al.* Application of HUMF13A01 (AAAG)n STR polymorphism to the genetic diagnosis of coagulation factor XIII deficiency. *Thromb Haemost* 1996; **76**: 879–882.

118 Killick CJ, Barton CJ, Aslam S, Standen G. Prenatal diagnosis in factor XIII-A deficiency. *Arch Dis Child Fetal Neonatal Ed* 1999; **80**: F238–F239.

119 Mota L, Ghosh K, Shetty S. Second trimester antenatal diagnosis in rare coagulation factor deficiencies. *J Pediatr Hematol Oncol* 2007; **29**: 137–139.

120 Handyside AH, Pattinson JK, Penketh RJ, *et al.* Biopsy of human preimplantation embryos and sexing by DNA amplification. *Lancet* 1989; **1**: 347–349.

121 Handyside AH, Kontogianni EH, Hardy K, Winston RM. Pregnancies from biopsied human preimplantation embryos sexed by Y-specific DNA amplification. *Nature* 1990; **344**: 768–770.

122 Braude P, Pickering S, Flinter F, Ogilvie CM. Preimplanta-tion genetic diagnosis. *Nat Rev Genet* 2002; **3**: 941953.

123 Sermon KD, Michiels A, Harton G, *et al.* ESHRE PGD Consortium data collection VI: cycles from January to December 2003 with pregnancy follow-up to October 2004. *Hum Reprod* 2007; **22**: 323–336.

124 Verlinsky Y, Rechitsky S, Cieslak J, *et al.* Preimplantation diagnosis of single gene disorders by two-step oocyte genetic analysis using first and second polar body. *Biochem Mol Med* 1997; **62**: 182–187.

125 Strom CM, Ginsberg N, Rechitsky S, *et al.* Three births after preimplantation genetic diagnosis for cystic fibrosis with sequential first and second polar body analysis. *Am J Obstet Gynecol* 1998; **178**: 1298–1306.

126 Tomi D, Griesinger G, Schultze-Mosgau A, *et al.* Polar body diagnosis for hemophilia A using multiplex PCR for linked polymorphic markers. *J Histochem Cytochem* 2005; **53**: 277–280.

127 Hardy K, Martin KL, Leese HJ, *et al.* Human preimplantation development in vitro is not adversely affected by biopsy at the 8-cell stage. *Hum Reprod* 1990; **5**: 708–714.

128 Van de Velde H, De Vos A, Sermon K, *et al.* Embryo implantation after biopsy of one or two cells from cleavage-stage embryos with a view to preimplantation genetic diagnosis. *Prenat Diagn* 2000; **20**: 1030–1037.

129 Jones GM, Trounson AO, Lolatgis N, Wood C. Factors affecting the success of human blastocyst development and pregnancy following in vitro fertilization and embryo transfer. *Fertil Steril* 1998; **70**: 1022–1029.

130 Schoolcraft WB, Gardner DK, Lane M, *et al.* Blastocyst culture and transfer: analysis of results and parameters affecting outcome in two in vitro fertilization programs. *Fertil Steril* 1999; **72**: 604–609.

131 Sermon K, Van Steirteghem A, Liebaers I. Preimplantation genetic diagnosis. *Lancet* 2004; **363**: 1633–1641.

132 Fiorentino F, Magli MC, Podini D, *et al.* The minisequencing method: an alternative strategy for preimplantation genetic diagnosis of single gene disorders. *Mol Hum Reprod* 2003; **9**: 399–410.

133 Michaelides K, Tuddenham EG, Turner C, *et al.* Live birth following the first mutation specific preimplantation genetic diagnosis for haemophilia A. *Thromb Hemost* 2006; **95**: 373–379.

134 Gigarel N, Frydman N, Burlet P, *et al.* Single cell co-amplification of polymorphic markers for the indirect preimplantation genetic diagnosis of hemophilia A, X-linked adrenoleukodystrophy, X-linked hydrocephalus and incontinentia pigmenti loci on Xq28. *Hum Genet* 2004; **114**: 298–305.

135 Department of Health. Preimplantation genetic diagnosis (PGD): guiding principles for commissioners of NHS services. Department of Health: London 2002.

136 Thornhill AR, deDie-Smulders CE, Geraedts JP, *et al.* ESHRE PGD Consortium "Best practice guidelines for clinical preimplantation genetic diagnosis (PGD and preimplantation genetic screening (PGS)". *Hum Reprod* 2005; **20**: 35–48.

137 Levinson G, Keyvanfar K, Wu JC, *et al.* DNA-based X-enriched sperm separation as an adjunct to preimplantation genetic testing for the prevention of X-linked disease. *Hum Reprod* 1995; **10**: 979–982.

138 Fugger EF, Black SH, Keyvanfar K, Schulman JD. Births of normal daughters after MicroSort sperm separation and intrauterine insemination, in-vitro fertilization, or

intracytoplasmic sperm injection. *Hum Reprod* 1998; **13**: 2367–2370.

139 Sumner AT, Robinson JA. A difference in dry mass between the heads of X- and Y-bearing human spermatozoa. *J Reprod Fertil* 1976; **48**: 9–15.

140 Cui KH. Size differences between human X and Y spermatozoa and prefertilization diagnosis. *Mol Hum Reprod* 1997; **3**: 61–67.

141 Johnson LA, Welch GR, Keyvanfar K, *et al.* Gender preselection in humans? Flow cytometric separation of X and Y spermatozoa for the prevention of X-linked diseases. *Hum Reprod* 1993; **8**: 1733–1739.

142 Claassens OE, Oosthuizen CJ, Brusnicky J, *et al.* Fluorescent in situ hybridization evaluation of human Y-bearing spermatozoa separated by albumin density gradients. *Fertil Steril* 1995; **63**: 417–418.

143 Wang HX, Flaherty SP, Swann NJ, Matthews CD. Assessment of the separation of X- and Y-bearing sperm on albumin gradients using double-label fluorescence in situ hybridization. *Fertil Steril* 1994; **61**: 720–726.

144 Flaherty SP, Michalowska J, Swann NJ, *et al.* Albumin gradients do not enrich Y-bearing human spermatozoa. *Hum Reprod* 1997; **12**: 938–942.

145 HFEA. *Sex selection: options for regulation.* HFEA: London, 2003.

146 Lobel SM, Pomponio RJ, Mutter GL. The sex ratio of normal and manipulated human sperm quantitated by the polymerase chain reaction. *Fertil Steril* 1993; **59**: 387–392.

147 Vidal F, Moragas M, Catala V, *et al.* Sephadex filtration and human serum albumin gradients do not select spermatozoa by sex chromosome: a fluorescent in-situ hybridization study. *Hum Reprod* 1993; **8**: 1740–1743.

148 Wang HX, Flaherty SP, Swann NJ, Matthews CD. Discontinuous Percoll gradients enrich X-bearing human spermatozoa: a study using double-label fluorescence in-situ hybridization. *Hum Reprod* 1994; **9**: 1265–1270.

149 Lin SP, Lee RK, Tsai YJ, *et al.* Separating X-bearing human spermatozoa through a discontinuous Percoll density gradient proved to be inefficient by double-label fluorescent in situ hybridization. *J Assist Reprod Genet* 1998; **15**: 565–569.

150 Vidal F, Fugger EF, Blanco J, *et al.* Efficiency of MicroSort flow cytometry for producing sperm populations enriched in X- or Y-chromosome haplotypes: a blind trial assessed by double and triple colour fluorescent in-situ hybridization. *Hum Reprod* 1998; **13**: 308–312.

151 Fugger EF. Clinical experience with flow cytometric separation of human X- and Y-chromosome bearing sperm. *Theriogenology* 1999; **52**: 1435–1440.

152 Bjorndahl L, Barratt CLR. *Sex selection: a survey of laboratory methods and clinical results.* HFEA scientific paper: London, 2002.

153 HFEA. *HFEA sex selection consultation.* HFEA: London, 1993.

154 HFEA. *Sex selection: choice and responsibility in human reproduction.* HFEA consultation: London, 2002.

155 Saito H, Sekizawa A, Morimoto T, *et al.* Prenatal DNA diagnosis of a single-gene disorder from maternal plasma. *Lancet* 2000; **356**: 1170.

156 Li Y, Holzgreve W, Page-Christiaens GC, *et al.* Improved prenatal detection of a fetal point mutation for achondroplasia by the use of size-fractionated circulatory DNA in maternal plasma – case report. *Prenat Diagn* 2004; **24**: 896–898.

157 Amicucci P, Gennarelli M, Novelli G, Dallapiccola B. Prenatal diagnosis of myotonic dystrophy using fetal DNA obtained from maternal plasma. *Clin Chem* 2000; **46**: 301–302.

158 Li Y, Di Naro E, Vitucci A, *et al.* Detection of paternally inherited fetal point mutations for beta-thalassemia using size-fractionated cell-free DNA in maternal plasma. *JAMA* 2005; **293**: 843–849.

159 Chiu RW, Lau TK, Leung TN, *et al.* Prenatal exclusion of beta thalassaemia major by examination of maternal plasma. *Lancet* 2002; **360**: 998–1000.

160 Vrettou C, Traeger-Synodinos J, Tzetis M, *et al.* Rapid screening of multiple beta-globin gene mutations by real-time PCR on the LightCycler: application to carrier screening and prenatal diagnosis of thalassemia syndromes. *Clin Chem* 2003; **49**: 769–776.

161 Nasis O, Thompson S, Hong T, *et al.* Improvement in sensitivity of allele-specific PCR facilitates reliable noninvasive prenatal detection of cystic fibrosis. *Clin Chem* 2004; **50**: 694–701.

162 Gonzalez-Gonzalez MC, Garcia-Hoyos M, Trujillo MJ, *et al.* Prenatal detection of a cystic fibrosis mutation in fetal DNA from maternal plasma. *Prenat Diagn* 2002; **22**: 946–948.

163 Lo YM. Recent developments in fetal nucleic acids in maternal plasma: implications to noninvasive prenatal fetal blood group genotyping. *Transfus Clin Biol* 2006; **13**: 50–52.

164 Schroder J, Tiilikainen A, De la Chapelle A. Fetal leukocytes in the maternal circulation after delivery. I. Cytological aspects. *Transplantation* 1974; **17**: 346–354.

165 Hsieh TT, Pao CC, Hor JJ, Kao SM. Presence of fetal cells in maternal circulation after delivery. *Hum Genet* 1993; **92**: 204–205.

166 Liou JD, Hsieh TT, Pao CC. Presence of cells of fetal origin in maternal circulation of pregnant women. *Ann NY Acad Sci* 1994; **731**: 237–241.

167 Bertero MT, Camaschella C, Serra A, *et al.* Circulating "trophoblast" cells in pregnancy have maternal genetic markers. *Prenat Diagn* 1988; **8**: 585–590.

168 Covone AE, Kozma R, Johnson PM, *et al.* Analysis of peripheral maternal blood samples for the presence of placenta-derived cells using Y-specific probes and McAb H315. *Prenat Diagn* 1988; 8: 591–607.

169 Ganshirt D, Garritsen H, Miny P, Holzgreve W. Fetal cells in maternal circulation throughout gestation. *Lancet* 1994; 343: 1038–1039.

170 Pearson HA. Life-span of the fetal red blood cell. *J Pediatr* 1967; 70: 166–171.

171 Bianchi DW, Flint AF, Pizzimenti MF, *et al.* Isolation of fetal DNA from nucleated erythrocytes in maternal blood. *Proc Natl Acad Sci USA* 1990; 87: 3279–3283.

172 Holzgreve W, Garritsen HS, Ganshirt-Ahlert D. Fetal cells in the maternal circulation. *J Reprod Med* 1992; 37: 410–418.

173 Hamada H, Arinami T, Sohda S, *et al.* Mid-trimester fetal sex determination from maternal peripheral blood by fluorescence in situ hybridization without enrichment of fetal cells. *Prenat Diagn* 1995; 15: 78–81.

174 Slunga-Tallberg A, el Rifai W, Keinanen M, *et al.* Maternal origin of nucleated erythrocytes in peripheral venous blood of pregnant women. *Hum Genet* 1995; 96: 53–57.

175 Slunga-Tallberg A, el Rifai W, Keinanen M, *et al.* Maternal origin of transferrin receptor positive cells in venous blood of pregnant women. *Clin Genet* 1996; 49: 196–199.

176 Kadir RA, Sabin CA, Goldman E, *et al.* Reproductive choices of women in families with haemophilia. *Hemophilia* 2000; 6: 33–40.

177 Beeson D, Golbus MS. Decision making: whether or not to have prenatal diagnosis and abortion for X-linked conditions. *Am J Med Genet* 1985; 20: 107–114.

178 Kadir RA, Sabin CA, Goldman E, *et al.* Reproductive choices of women in families with haemophilia. *Hemophilia* 2000; 6: 33–40.

179 Kraus EM, Brettler DB. Assessment of reproductive risks and intentions by mothers of children with hemophilia. *Am J Med Genet* 1988; 31: 259–267.

180 Tedgard U, Ljung R, McNeil TF. Reproductive choices of haemophilia carriers. *Br J Hematol* 1999; 106: 421–426.

181 Varekamp I, Suurmeijer TP, Brocker-Vriends AH, *et al.* Carrier testing and prenatal diagnosis for hemophilia: experiences and attitudes of 549 potential and obligate carriers. *Am J Med Genet* 1990; 37: 147–154.

182 Markova I, Forbes CD, Inwood M. The consumers' views of genetic counseling of hemophilia. *Am J Med Genet* 1984; 17: 741–752.

183 Francis RB, Jr., Kasper CK. Reproduction in hemophilia. *JAMA* 1983; 250: 3192–3195.

184 Kadir RA, Economides DL, Braithwaite J, *et al.* The obstetric experience of carriers of haemophilia. *Br J Obstet Gynaecol* 1997; 104: 803–810.

185 Chi C, Lee CA, Shiltagh N, *et al.* Pregnancy in carriers of haemophilia. *Hemophilia* 2008; 14: 56–64.

186 Hoyer LW, Carta CA, Golbus MS, *et al.* Prenatal diagnosis of classic hemophilia (hemophilia A by immuno-radiometric assays. *Blood* 1985; 65: 1312–1317.

187 Tedgard U, Ljung R, McNeil TF. How do carriers of hemophilia and their spouses experience prenatal diagnosis by chorionic villus sampling? *Clin Genet* 1999; 55: 26–33.

188 Karimi M, Peyvandi F, Siboni S, *et al.* Comparison of attitudes towards prenatal diagnosis and termination of pregnancy for haemophilia in Iran and Italy. *Hemophilia* 2004; 10: 367–369.

189 Pandey GS, Panigrahi I, Phadke SR, Mittal B. Knowledge and attitudes towards haemophilia: the family side and role of haemophilia societies. *Community Genet* 2003; 6: 120–122.

190 Peyvandi F. Carrier detection and prenatal diagnosis of hemophilia in developing countries. *Semin Thromb Hemost* 2005; 31: 544–554.

191 Ghosh K, Shetty S, Pawar A, Mohanty D. Carrier detection and prenatal diagnosis in haemophilia in India: realities and challenges. *Hemophilia* 2002; 8: 51–55.

192 Sjogren B, Uddenberg N. Prenatal diagnosis for psychological reasons: comparison with other indications, advanced maternal age and known genetic risk. *Prenat Diagn* 1990; 10: 111–120.

193 Evers-Kiebooms G, Swerts A, van den Berge H. Psychological aspects of amniocentesis: anxiety feelings in three different risk groups. *Clin Genet* 1988; 33: 196–206.

194 Robinson J, Tennes K, Robinson A. Amniocentesis: its impact on mothers and infants. A 1-year follow-up study. *Clin Genet* 1975; 8: 97–106.

195 Spencer JW, Cox DN. Emotional responses of pregnant women to chorionic villi sampling or amniocentesis. *Am J Obstet Gynecol* 1987; 157: 1155–1160.

196 Robinson GE, Garner DM, Olmsted MP, *et al.* Anxiety reduction after chorionic villus sampling and genetic amniocentesis. *Am J Obstet Gynecol* 1988; 159: 953–956.

197 Sjogren B, Uddenberg N. Prenatal diagnosis and psychological distress: amniocentesis or chorionic villus biopsy? *Prenat Diagn* 1989; 9: 477–487.

198 Black RB. A 1 and 6 month follow-up of prenatal diagnosis patients who lost pregnancies. *Prenat Diagn* 1989; 9: 795–804.

199 Tedgard, Ljung R, McNeil T, *et al.* How do carriers of hemophilia experience prenatal diagnosis (PND)? Carriers' immediate and later reactions to amniocentesis and fetal

blood sampling. *Acta Paediatr Scand* 1989; **78:** 692–700.

200 Tedgard U, Ljung R, McNeil TF, Tedgard E. Identifying carriers at high risk for negative reactions when performing prenatal diagnosis of haemophilia. *Hemophilia* 1997; **3:** 123–130.

201 Derogatis LR, Lipman RS, Cleary PA. Confirmation of the dimensional structure of the SCL-90. A study in construct validity. *J Clin Psychol* 1977; **33:** 981–989.

202 Tedgard U, Ljung R, McNeil TF. Long-term psychological effects of carrier testing and prenatal diagnosis of haemophilia: comparison with a control group. *Prenat Diagn* 1999; **19:** 411–417.

203 Larsson SA, Nilsson IM, Blomback M. Current status of Swedish haemophiliacs. I. A demographic survey. *Acta Med Scand* 1982; **212:** 195–200.

204 Ljung R, Kling S, Tedgard U. The impact of prenatal diagnosis on the incidence of haemophilia in Sweden. *Hemophilia* 1995; **1:** 190–193.

205 Kadir RA, Sabin CA, Goldman E, *et al*. Reproductive choices of women in families with haemophilia. *Hemophilia* 2000; **6:** 33–40.

10 Obstetric management

Claudia Chi and Rezan A Kadir

Introduction

Childbirth presents an intrinsic hemostatic challenge to women with inherited bleeding disorders who could otherwise remain asymptomatic. Pregnancy in these women requires specialized and individualized management provided by a multidisciplinary team of obstetricians, hematologists, and anesthetists. Advance planning in addition to a good understanding and awareness of the potential maternal and neonatal complications are essential in ensuring an optimal outcome. This chapter will address (a) the hemostatic changes in pregnancy, (b) the antenatal, intrapartum, and postnatal management of women with inherited bleeding disorders, and (c) the hemostatic agents available for treatment during pregnancy. In each section, inherited bleeding disorders are broadly categorized into carriers of hemophilia, von Willebrand disease (VWD) and rare bleeding disorders [afibrinogenemia and deficiencies of prothrombin (factor II, FII), factor V (FV), factor VII (FVII), factor X (FX), factor XI (FXI), factor XIII (FXIII) and combined factor deficiencies]. Specific areas on prenatal diagnosis, obstetric analgesia/anesthesia and neonatal management are covered in further detail in Chapters 9, 11 and 12.

Inherited Bleeding Disorders in Women, 1st edition. By CA Lee, RA Kadir and PA Kouides. Published 2009 by Blackwell Publishing, ISBN: 978-1-4051-6915-8.

Hemostatic changes in pregnancy

Normal pregnancy

Various hemostatic changes occur during normal pregnancy (Table 10.1). They are generally in the direction of hypercoagulability and are considered to be in preparation for the hemostatic challenge of delivery. These physiological alternations include a progressive increase in the levels of coagulation FVII, FVIII, FX, FXII, von Willebrand factor (VWF), and fibrinogen [1–9]. The rise in these coagulation factors, in particular FVIII and VWF, is generally more marked in the third trimester [1, 3, 4]. The increase in FVIII and VWF appear to occur in parallel during the first half of the pregnancy but then diverge because of a greater increase in VWF antigen (VWF:Ag) [3, 10]. The ratio of VWF:Ag to FVIII coagulant (FVIII:C) activity rises from 1.09 at 11–15 weeks to 1.77 at 36–40 weeks' gestation [3]. FII, FV and FIX levels are slightly increased or unchanged during normal pregnancy [3, 4, 11]. Inconsistent changes have also been reported for FXI levels, with different studies demonstrating a slight increase [8], no change [4], or a decrease [1, 12, 13] during pregnancy. The FXIII level decreases overall during pregnancy [14–16]. Despite numerous studies of hemostasis in normal pregnancy, the mechanisms and significance of these changes are still poorly understood.

In women with inherited bleeding disorders similar hemostatic responses to pregnancy are seen, which can lead to normalization of the hemostatic defect in some of these women. However, the response is variable in different inherited bleeding disorders and there are also great interindividual variations in women

Table 10.1 Hemostatic changes during normal pregnancy

Clotting factors	Increase (↑)	No significant change (↔)	Inconsistent (−)
Fibrinogen	↑		
FVII	↑		
FVIII	↑		
FX	↑		
FXII	↑		
VWF	↑		
FII		↔	
FV		↔	
FIX		↔	
FXI			−

F, factor; VWF, von Willebrand factor.

with the same disorder. Furthermore, it is highly likely that women with factor deficiencies do not achieve the same magnitude of rise in the respective factor level during pregnancy as those of women with normal hemostasis [17–20].

Carriers of hemophilia

Both FVIII and VWF levels increase progressively in carriers of hemophilia A during pregnancy, reaching its peak in the third trimester. Consequently, most carriers of hemophilia A have normal (>50 IU/dL) FVIII and VWF levels at term [21, 22]. In contrast, FIX levels do not increase significantly during pregnancy, hence most carriers of hemophilia B with a low baseline (non-pregnant) level will continue to have the hemostatic defect at term [4, 21].

von Willebrand disease

A progressive increase in levels of FVIII:C, VWF:Ag and VWF activity (VWF:AC) is seen during pregnancy in most women with type 1 VWD, with the greatest improvement seen in the third trimester [18, 22–24]. The majority of these women achieve factor levels >50 IU/dL at term. However, lack of improvement in the hemostatic defect has been reported in women with severe type 1 VWD [18, 25] and in women with type 1 VWD due to C1130F mutation [26]. In a series of 24 pregnancies in 13 women with VWD, it was noted that FVIII:C and VWF:Ag rose by a factor of at least 1.5 during pregnancy in most cases [18]. On the

other hand, all women with a baseline VWF:AC of <15 IU/dL had a less marked improvement in VWF:AC and none achieved a third trimester VWF:AC of >50 IU/dL [18]. Similarly, women with type 3 VWD showed little or no increase in their FVIII and VWF levels [23, 27].

In type 2 VWD, FVIII and VWF:Ag levels usually increase during pregnancy, but most studies show minimal or no increase in VWF:AC and a persistently abnormal pattern of multimers, reflecting the increased production of abnormal VWF [18, 22, 28]. This pattern, however, varies between individuals and different subtypes of type 2 VWD. In women with subtype 2A, an increase in FVIII:C with a modest or no response in VWF:Ag and VWF ristocetin cofactor activity (VWF:RCo) have been observed [24, 28]. In women with subtype 2M associated with single (R1205H) and double (R1205H and M740I) mutations, no significant changes in VWF and FVIII levels were observed during pregnancy [29].

In women with subtype 2N (Normandy) VWD, FVIII levels often remain low despite increased FVIII and VWF production during pregnancy due to impaired binding by the abnormal VWF [30–33]. However, correction of low FVIII levels during pregnancy has been described in women homozygous or heterozygous for R854Q mutation [34]. The increase in the FVIII level during pregnancy and after therapy may be dependent on the specific mutation and on the severity of the resulting binding defect [30, 35]. The diagnosis of type 2N VWD during pregnancy could be mistaken for carriership of hemophilia A or it may be masked by

125

an increase in FVIII level to the normal range in milder cases [30, 32]. Accurate diagnosis is important for genetic counseling and appropriate management of pregnancy and delivery, as they differ between women with type 2N VWD and carriers of hemophilia.

In subtype 2B, thrombocytopenia may develop or worsen during pregnancy due to increased production of the abnormal intermediate VWF multimers, which bind to platelets and induce spontaneous platelet aggregation [36, 37]. In some cases, thrombocytopenia developed only during pregnancy, with reversal to normal or minimally reduced platelet count after delivery [36–39]. The platelet count has been reported to fall during pregnancy to a nadir of $10–20 \times 10^9$/L at term [37, 40, 41]. Type 2B VWD should be included in the differential diagnosis of thrombocytopenia during pregnancy, especially in women with a personal or family bleeding history, as it could be misdiagnosed as idiopathic thrombocytopenic purpura, resulting in unnecessary and ineffective therapy [30, 40].

Rare bleeding disorders

Owning to the rarity of these disorders, there are limited data on the hemostatic response to pregnancy in affected women. In general, their hemostatic abnormalities persist throughout pregnancy, especially if the defect is severe. Although pregnancy is associated with an increase in the FX level [8], it often remains low in women with a severe deficiency [42, 43]. Similarly, most studies have found no significant rise in FVII levels during pregnancy in women with homozygous (severe) FVII deficiency [44–47]. On the contrary, a significant rise in FVII levels has been reported among women with heterozygous (mild/moderate) FVII deficiency [48].

Studies on changes in FXI levels during pregnancy in the general obstetric population have yielded controversial results [1, 4, 8]. Similarly, inconsistent changes in FXI levels have been observed in pregnant women with FXI deficiency [23, 49]. Overall, there appears to be no significant increase in FXI levels during pregnancy in these women and most of them are likely to have subnormal factor levels at term [23, 49]. Similarly, prothrombin and FV levels do not alter significantly during normal pregnancy [3, 4, 11]. Therefore, the hemostatic abnormalities in women with prothrombin or FV deficiency are expected to continue throughout pregnancy. Women with FXIII or fibrinogen deficiency,

in general, also have persistent hemostatic defects during pregnancy [50–54].

Antenatal management

Women may be exposed to various hemostatic challenges during pregnancy. They include spontaneous miscarriage and invasive procedures such as prenatal diagnostic tests, termination of pregnancy, and insertion of cervical cerclage. These can be complicated by excessive and prolonged bleeding. In women with inherited bleeding disorders, it is important to assess the relevant clotting factor level and arrange prophylactic cover, if necessary, prior to any invasive procedures and in cases of spontaneous miscarriage to minimize the risk of bleeding complications.

A close and continuing collaboration between obstetricians and hematologists is essential for the management of pregnancy in these women. Ideally, clotting factor levels should be checked at booking, and at 28 and 34 weeks of gestation, especially in those with low pre-pregnancy levels. Having factor levels checked at planned intervals allows their availability in acute situations when factor levels often cannot be assessed easily. Monitoring in the third trimester is of particular importance for appropriate management of labor and delivery, which will be addressed in the next section. Details on prenatal diagnosis can be found in Chapter 9.

Carriers of hemophilia

The risks of miscarriage and bleeding during pregnancy are unknown in carriers of hemophilia. In a review of a total of 172 pregnancies among 65 carriers of hemophilia A and 20 carriers of hemophilia B in the United Kingdom during the periods 1985–95 [21] and 1995–2005 [55], the miscarriage rate was found to be 31% (22/72) and 17% (13/78), respectively. In the remaining pregnancies reviewed over the two decades, no antepartum bleeding (vaginal bleeding after 24 weeks' gestation) was documented in carriers of hemophilia A. Self-limiting mild to moderate antepartum bleeding was reported in three pregnancies among two carriers of hemophilia B. FIX levels were <50 IU/dL when the bleeding occurred. No hemostatic treatment was given and the pregnancies continued to term. During the study periods, a further two carriers of hemophilia B and two carriers of hemophilia A had persistently low (<50 IU/dL) FIX or FVIII levels throughout pregnancy but did not experience antepartum bleeding.

A large concealed subchorionic hematoma diagnosed by ultrasound has been reported in a carrier of hemophilia B at 32 weeks of gestation [56]. Her FIX level had decreased from pre-pregnancy levels of 7–11 to 4 IU/dL with a decreased platelet count of $60 \times 10^9/L$. She was managed conservatively with FIX infusions for 9 days. Subsequent ultrasound showed a significant decrease in the size of the hematoma and a successful pregnancy outcome at term was achieved.

At present there is insufficient evidence to determine whether the risks of miscarriage and bleeding during pregnancy are increased among carriers of hemophilia. It is unknown whether the use of antenatal prophylaxis can prevent these complications in women with low (<50 IU/dL) factor levels. However, they require prophylactic cover for any invasive procedures. As FVIII increases significantly during pregnancy, prophylaxis is not usually required in carriers of hemophilia A during late pregnancy and at delivery. Nevertheless, they may require prophylactic cover for invasive procedures in the first or second trimester since the rise in FVIII levels may only become significant in late gestation. Carriers of hemophilia B with low pre-pregnancy levels usually require hemostatic support for any invasive procedures as FIX levels do not increase significantly during pregnancy. In the UK series [55], recombinant FVIII or FIX was given in 59% (10/17) of the pregnancies to cover invasive prenatal diagnostic procedures because the women's factor levels were <50 IU/dL and no bleeding complication was reported. Desmopressin has also been used safely for this purpose in carriers of hemophilia A (see "Desmopressin") [57].

von Willebrand disease

It is unclear whether VWD is associated with an increased risk of miscarriage. Vaginal bleeding during the first trimester (threatened miscarriage) was reported in 28 (33%) of 84 pregnancies among 31 women with VWD in a UK study [23]. In the general population, first trimester vaginal bleeding has been reported in 7–19% of pregnancies [58–60]. It is possible that women known to have a bleeding disorder present more readily if they experience any bleeding

in pregnancy. In a case–control study, the percentage of pregnancies ending in miscarriage was higher among women with VWD than in controls (15% vs 9%), a difference of borderline statistical significance ($P = 0.05$) [61]. Although higher than controls, a miscarriage rate of 15% is not distinctly different from the rate of 12–13.5% observed in the general population [62–64]. The overall rates of spontaneous miscarriage in affected women in two case series were 21% [23] and 22% [65], respectively. The latter study examined women with VWD who were unresponsive to desmopressin. Interestingly, women classified as type 1 "Other" (because of insufficient data and heterogeneity of the group) had a higher miscarriage rate (31%) than those with types 2 or 3 VWD (11%) [65], suggesting that the bleeding disorder may not contribute to this adverse outcome. In another study including 182 Iranian women with type 3 VWD, the miscarriage rate was not found to be more frequent than in the general population [66]. Caliezi et al. [27] described the use of regular replacement therapy with VWF-containing FVIII concentrate in the first trimester to prevent pregnancy loss in a woman with type 3 VWD who experienced recurrent vaginal bleeding during early pregnancy. Antenatal prophylactic therapy may be considered in cases of severe VWD presenting with recurrent pregnancy loss or the development of a subchorionic hematoma [27, 56]. However, there is currently a lack of evidence in the literature on its efficacy in improving the pregnancy outcome.

Bleeding complications may occur following spontaneous miscarriage or elective termination. In the UK study, excessive bleeding requiring transfusion was reported in 10% of spontaneous miscarriages and elective terminations [23]. Furthermore, 30% of the cases had prolonged, intermittent bleeding after the miscarriage. Several other case reports have also documented bleeding complications during the first few weeks following termination of pregnancy or miscarriage in women with VWD [65, 67–69].

It was generally believed that the risk of antepartum hemorrhage is not increased in women with VWD. However, a recent large case–control study from the USA including 4067 deliveries in women with a diagnosis of VWD found that women with VWD are 10 times more likely to experience antepartum bleeding, but not placental abruption, preterm delivery, fetal growth restriction or stillbirth, than women without VWD [70].

Antenatal management of women with VWD includes regular monitoring of VWF:Ag and VWF:AC together with FVIII:C, particularly prior to any invasive procedures and in the third trimester. The platelet count should also be monitored in women with type 2B VWD as thrombocytopenia may develop or worsen during pregnancy [36]. The extent to which thrombocytopenia contributes to the bleeding risk is unknown but probably depends on its severity [30]. If VWF:AC and/or FVIII:C is less than 50 IU/dL, prophylactic treatment should be given to cover any invasive procedures during the antenatal period as well as labor and delivery [71, 72]. Treatment options include desmopressin, virus-inactivated VWF-containing concentrates and antifibrinolytic agents such as tranexamic acid (see "Hemostatic agents and pregnancy"). Platelet transfusions in addition to replacement therapy with VWF-containing FVIII concentrates may be required in type 2B VWD if the woman develops significant thrombocytopenia [40].

Rare bleeding disorders

Data on the management of pregnancy in affected women is limited and mostly derived from case reports. It is therefore crucial that these women are managed in close collaboration with specialized centers/hematologists to ensure optimal pregnancy outcomes. Although very rare, these autosomal recessive disorders are seen more frequently in communities where consanguineous marriages are common.

Deficiency of FXIII and fibrinogen are two rare inherited bleeding disorders that are strongly associated with pregnacy loss [16]. Both FXIII and fibrinogen play an essential role in placental implantation and the continuation of pregnancy. Several reports have described an increased risk of recurrent miscarriages and placental abruption resulting in fetal loss or premature delivery among women with FXIII [52, 73–79] or fibrinogen [51, 80–82] deficiency. Fortunately, it seems possible to revert these adverse pregnancy outcomes with replacement therapy [51, 54].

FXIII deficiency
In plasma, FXIII circulates as a tetramer composed of two A subunits and two B subunits. The A subunit is the enzymatically active part, whereas the B subunit is a plasma carrier protein [54]. Three subtypes of

FXIII deficiency have been identified according to the presence or absence of the subunits A and B: type I (combined deficiency of both subunits A and B); type II (deficiency of subunit A); and type III (deficiency of subunit B) [83].

In a review of case reports and series in the English literature between 1966 and 1998, 61 women with FXIII deficiency (four type 1, 55 type II, and two type III) were identified [52]. Women with types I and III conceived and delivered normally. However, the majority of women with type II had a history of recurrent miscarriages. There were seven successful pregnancies among women with type II FXIII deficiency and five had received FXIII replacement. Similarly, in a more recent literature review eight successful pregnancies with replacement therapy were reported among six women with FXIII subunit A deficiency [54]. Without substitution therapy, all pregnancies experienced by these women ended in miscarriages. These data suggest that appropriate replacement therapy is critical for pregnancy maintenance in these women. Since pregnancies had been reported to establish spontaneously without replacement therapy [79, 84], it does not seem that FXIIIA is essential for either fertilization or early implantation. However, it is recommended that replacement therapy (to maintain FXIII levels at least >3 IU/dL [50] and, if possible, >10 IU/dL [54]) be commenced as early as possible in pregnancy to prevent bleeding and pregnancy loss. In all severely affected girls, monthly prophylactic infusions of FXIII concentrate are recommended from the time of diagnosis in view of the potentially fatal bleeding complications, including intracranial hemorrhage [50].

Inherited fibrinogen abnormalities
Inherited abnormalities of fibrinogen consist of quantitative (afibrinogenemia and hypofibrinogenemia) and qualitative deficiencies (dysfibrinogenemia). These abnormalities can also coexist as hypodysfibrinogenemia. Afibrinogenemia refers to a total absence of fibrinogen whereas hypofibrinogenemia is a milder form of the disorder with a decreased level of fibrinogen. Both are associated with recurrent miscarriages as well as placental abruption and postpartum hemorrhage [51, 81, 85, 86].

In a total of 20 pregnancies among eight women with afibrinogenemia, there were 12 miscarriages, two perinatal deaths (a stillbirth at 24 weeks and a neonatal death following delivery at 27 weeks' gestation), and six live births between 36 and 40 weeks [51, 80, 81, 87–91]. All successful pregnancies were achieved with fibrinogen replacement therapy throughout pregnancy. Pregnancies were established spontaneously but vaginal bleeding began at around 5 weeks' gestation in cases where fibrinogen infusions were not commenced at 4 weeks' gestation [51, 88]. Based on these observations, it is recommended that regular fibrinogen infusions be commenced as soon as possible in pregnancy to keep the fibrinogen level at least >0.6 g/L (if possible, >1 g/L) [50, 51]. Fibrinogen clearance has been found to increase as the pregnancy progresses [92]. Thus the amount of fibrinogen required to avoid placental abruption also increases with advancing gestation [51]. Similar replacement therapy may be required in women with hypofibrinogenemia, depending on the fibrinogen level, bleeding tendency, and previous obstetric history [93].

Regular monitoring of fibrinogen levels and ultrasound assessment for concealed placental bleeding and fetal growth are also recommended. Aygoren-Pursun et al. [94] reported a woman with congenital afibrinogenemia receiving fibrinogen prophylaxis who developed a subchorionic hematoma in the first trimester. The subchorionic hematoma was identified on ultrasound 1 day after a plasma fibrinogen nadir of 0.29 g/L. This could either suggest the marked fibrinogen deficiency as the cause of the hemorrhage or reflect fibrinogen consumption by the developing hematoma. With subsequent continuous and intensified fibrinogen concentrate replacement, the hematoma resolved over 6 weeks and the woman delivered a healthy infant at term. Paradoxical thrombotic events have also been reported in patients with inherited afibrinogenemia [82, 95, 96]; hence, the risks of bleeding and thrombosis should be balanced during pregnancy.

Dysfibrinogenemia is characterized by abnormal fibrinogen function and has an unpredictable clinical phenotype [50]. It is usually transmitted as an autosomal dominant trait, an exception to the general pattern of rare inherited bleeding disorders as recessive disorders. A database of over 250 patients showed that 53% were asymptomatic, 26% had a tendency to bleed, and 21% had thrombosis, some of whom also had hemorrhage [97]. A study of the Scientific and Standardization Committee of the International Society on Thrombosis and Haemostasis (ISTH) identified 26 cases that fulfilled the criteria of familial dysfibrinogenemia and thrombosis not due to other reasons [98]. The study included 15 women who had at least one pregnancy. A high incidence of spontaneous miscarriages (24/64, 38%) and stillbirth (6/64, 9%) was noted among these women. Placental abruption has also been reported in women with dysfibrinogenemia [99, 100].

The management of pregnancy in women with dysfibrinogenemia needs to be individualized, taking into account the fibrinogen level as well as the patient's personal and family history of bleeding and thrombosis [50]. No specific treatment is required in asymptomatic women unless bleeding occurs or there is a significant bleeding tendency. Women with a personal or family history of thrombosis should be offered antenatal prophylaxis with low-molecular-weight heparin (LMWH) and fibrinogen replacement therapy is given only if bleeding occurs. Conversely, replacement therapy should be considered in women with a personal or family bleeding phenotype, especially if the bleeding tendency is significant or if the patient is undergoing invasive procedures. Thromboprophylaxis with compression stockings and a prophylactic dose of LMWH should also be considered as fibrinogen may precipitate venous thrombosis [50]. There is limited information on the management of women with dysfibrinogenemia who have recurrent miscarriages. The options include the use of prophylactic LMWH and if this fails the use of fibrinogen replacement is considered [50]. Yamanaka et al. [101] described a woman with dysfibrinogenemia who had two first trimester miscarriages and two second trimester fetal losses due to placental abruption. She was treated with fibrinogen replacement to maintain a fibrinogen level of >1 g/L from 8 weeks' gestation in her fifth pregnancy. Although complicated by vaginal bleeding and preterm labor, a live male infant was delivered by an emergency cesarean section at 29 weeks' gestation.

Factor II (prothrombin) deficiency

Prothrombin deficiency is the rarest inherited bleeding disorder with an estimated prevalence of 1:2 million in the general population [102]. It can be classified as hypoprothrombinemia, where there is a parallel decrease in prothrombin antigen and activity levels, or dysprothrombinemia, where prothrombin activity is reduced but antigen level is normal or slightly decreased [103]. The activity level is usually <10 IU/dL in homozygous hypoprothrombinemia and between

40 and 60 IU/dL in heterozygotes. In dysprothrombinemia, the activity levels vary between 1 and 50 IU/dL [103]. Bleeding manifestations may be severe in homozygous but absent in heterozygous hypoprothrombinemia and they are variable in dysprothrombinemia.

There are very limited data on the obstetric complications or management of women with FII deficiency. Catanzarite *et al.* [104] reported eight pregnancies in a woman with congenital hypoprothrombinemia (FII activity <1 IU/dL). All the pregnancies were complicated by first trimester bleeding, four ended in a miscarriage and four progressed to term without replacement therapy. It is difficult to make recommendations on the obstetric management of these women and it is unclear whether routine prophylactic therapy during pregnancy can improve outcome. However, it is imperative to correct the deficiency in the event of serious bleeding or prior to any invasive procedures.

Factor V deficiency
Information on pregnancy management and outcomes in women with FV deficiency is also scarce. In a series of 15 pregnancies in 11 heterozygote women (with FV activity levels about 50 IU/dL) and three pregnancies in two homozygous women (with FV activity levels <5 IU/dL), no bleeding complications in the antenatal period were reported [105]. There did not appear to be an increased incidence of recurrent miscarriages, premature birth, and/or fetal loss in the study [105]. Replacement therapy is required in those with severe deficiency to cover any invasive procedures and delivery [106].

Factor VII deficiency
FVII deficiency is the most common of the rare inherited bleeding disorders. It is associated with a wide spectrum of bleeding symptoms. Furthermore, there is a relatively poor correlation between absolute FVII levels and the bleeding tendency; some individuals with very low FVII levels may have minimal symptoms, whereas others with higher levels have a significant bleeding tendency [50]. In severe (homozygous) FVII deficiency, the FVII levels are usually <10 IU/dL, whereas levels of 40–60 IU/dL are commonly seen in heterozygotes [45, 107]. Despite the poor correlation between FVII level and bleeding risk, it is generally believed that a level between 10 and 20 IU/dL is required to achieve hemostasis for surgery

or invasive procedures, and clinical manifestations do not usually occur unless the FVII level is <10 IU/dL [50, 108].

As previously discussed, a significant rise in FVII level is seen during pregnancy in non-deficient women. This has also been observed in women with mild/moderate forms of FVII deficiency (heterozygotes) [48], but not in women with severe deficiency [44–47]. In a series including 10 pregnancies in four women with mild/moderate FVII no bleeding complications related to delivery were reported, possibly reflecting the protective effect of the pregnancy-induced rise in factor level [48]. However, excessive bleeding was reported after two early pregnancy losses probably due to an inadequate rise in the FVII level in early pregnancy. Consequently, prophylactic cover for invasive procedures or incomplete miscarriage may be required, particularly in women with FVII levels <15–20 IU/dL. Although antepartum bleeding has been reported in two woman with severe deficiency [47, 107], the available data (albeit limited) do not suggest an increased risk of miscarriage or antepartum hemorrhage among women with FVII deficiency.

Factor X deficiency
Although FX deficiency is associated with a variable bleeding tendency, patients with severe deficiency (FX level <1 IU/dL) tend to be the most seriously affected patients with rare coagulation defects [109]. Patients with moderate FX deficiency (FX level 1–5 IU/dL) may bleed only after hemostatic challenge, whereas mildly affected patients (FX level 6–10 IU/dL) may be asymptomatic and may only be identified incidentally during routine screening or family studies [50, 109]. A factor X level of 10–20 IU/dL is generally considered to be sufficient for hemostasis [50, 110].

In a review, 14 pregnancies in nine women with FX deficiency were identified in the literature [111]. Pregnancy-related complications such as antepartum bleeding, retroplacental hematoma [42], preterm delivery [112], and postpartum hemorrhage [113] were reported among these women. Kumar and Mehta [112] described four pregnancies in a woman with severe FX deficiency. The first two pregnancies resulted in the birth of extremely premature babies at 21 and 25 weeks' gestation following preterm labor and both died in the neonatal period. The mother was treated early in pregnancy with regular FX replacement in her subsequent pregnancies and she delivered healthy babies at 34 and 32 weeks' gestation. The authors suggested that the prophylactic factor replacement had led to improved pregnancy outcome. However, several other case reports have described successful term pregnancies in women with severe FX deficiency without antenatal prophylaxis [43, 114, 115]. Nonetheless, these women should be monitored closely for any abnormal bleeding, retroplacental hematoma or premature labor. Replacement therapy should be considered if bleeding occurs or if the patient is undergoing invasive procedures. Women with severe deficiency and a history of adverse pregnancy outcome may benefit from prophylactic replacement therapy during pregnancy [50].

FXI deficiency

FXI deficiency is an autosomally inherited condition. It is particularly common in Ashkenazi Jews with a heterozygote frequency as high as 8% [116]. It has been described in all racial groups, but, in general, the incidence of severe deficiency is very low with an estimated at 1:1 million [117]. Factor XI levels are severely reduced (<15–20 IU/dL) in homozygotes or compound heterozygotes and partially deficient (20–70 IU/dL) in heterozygotes [118–120]. The condition is associated with a variable bleeding tendency and bleeding can occur in homozygous as well as heterozygous individuals. Spontaneous bleeding is rare but hemorrhage can occur at sites prone to fibrinolysis following injury or surgery and women with partial as well as severe deficiency are at risk of excessive uterine bleeding [120, 121]. The bleeding tendency can be inconsistent within an individual and the family. It is also not clearly related to factor levels [119, 121, 122] or the genotype responsible for the condition [123]. This unpredictable nature of factor XI deficiency makes management for pregnancy and delivery difficult; therefore, attempts should be made to identify whether the patient has a clinical bleeding tendency and whether other factors are involved, such as coexistence of VWD and platelet malfunction [124].

Two retrospective case series in the UK including 44 women with FXI deficiency showed that FXI deficiency does not appear to be associated with an increased risk of miscarriage [23, 49]. Severe placental abruption requiring emergency cesarean section was reported in one pregnancy [23]. Both series reported excessive bleeding following miscarriage or termination of pregnancy [23, 49].

In general, women with FXI deficiency who are probable "non-bleeders" undergoing any invasive procedure or presenting with a miscarriage can be managed expectantly with treatment available on standby should bleeding occur. However, in women with a significant bleeding history or a severe deficiency prophylaxis with FXI concentrate or tranexamic acid should be considered. The need for therapy in partially deficient women is guided by the patient's bleeding history, especially in relation to any hemostatic challenges and the nature of the procedure. Management should be individualized and the risks of bleeding balanced against the risks and benefits of treatment.

Combined factor V and factor VIII deficiency

Patients with this rare bleeding disorder have concomitantly low but detectable levels of coagulant activity and antigen of both factors, which are usually between 5 and 20 IU/dL [108]. Since there are no published data on the management of pregnant women with this combined deficiency, the obstetric experience of women with FV deficiency and carriers of hemophilia could probably serve as a useful guide. FV levels in pregnancy do not consistently increase or decrease, whereas FVIII levels rise throughout the pregnancy. Therefore, any possible bleeding, especially at term/during labor and delivery, is likely to be dependent on the FV level. However, it is recommended to monitor both levels antenatally and to maintain FV levels >15–20 U/dL and FVIII levels >50 IU/dL for any invasive procedures [50].

Inherited deficiency of the vitamin K-dependent clotting factors

This disorder has been reported as single case reports in fewer than 20 kindreds worldwide [50]. Plasma defects include low levels of FII, FVII, FIX, and FX ranging from less than 1 to 30 IU/dL [108]. There is one report of a pregnancy in a woman with severe vitamin K-dependent clotting factor deficiency (VKCFD) [125]. Her baseline FII, FVII, FIX, and FX activities were <3 IU/dL. She had been maintained on vitamin K since diagnosis and throughout the pregnancy (15 mg per day orally). The course of her pregnancy was uneventful, but excessive bleeding occurred from the episiotomy site, requiring treatment with fresh-frozen plasma (FFP). These limited data suggest the need to watch for potential bleeding complications. Vitamin K should be continued throughout the pregnancy. Replacement therapy should be considered to cover any invasive procedures.

Intrapartum and postpartum management

General principles for the management of labor and delivery (Table 10.2)

Labor and delivery are critical times for women with inherited bleeding disorders and their affected newborns as they may be exposed to various hemostatic challenges. Delivery at a tertiary obstetric unit with an on-site hemophilia center is not required for all women with inherited bleeding disorders. However, close liaison with the hemophilia center/hematologists throughout the pregnancy is essential and the arrangement for delivery should be made in advance. It is recommended that women with a severe deficiency or carrying an affected/potentially affected fetus deliver at a unit where the necessary expertise in the management of bleeding disorders and resources for laboratory testing and clotting factor treatments are readily available [72].

Women with inherited bleeding disorders are at increased risk of bleeding complications during and after delivery, especially if their factor levels are subnormal. At the beginning of labor, maternal blood samples should be taken for blood group and saved for cross-matching, full blood count, and coagulation screen. Assessment of factor levels may not be possible during labor, thus planning for delivery can be done on the basis of the third trimester levels. Preferably, a management plan is devised during the antenatal period and made available when the woman presents in labor or for a planned delivery. In general, for women with subnormal factor levels, intravenous access should be established and prophylactic treatment given to cover labor and delivery. The suggested hemostatic levels required for labor and delivery in women with inherited bleeding disorders are shown in Table 10.3. However, they can vary depending on the mode of delivery and the individual's bleeding tendency.

When delivery in a tertiary center with an on-site hemophilia center (at a long distance) is deemed necessary, planned induction of labor may be considered to ensure timely arrival of the mother. However, spontaneous labor should be allowed where possible and special consideration should be given when labor is to be induced. Induced labor is likely to be prolonged and associated with the need for instrumental delivery or emergency cesarean section, particularly in primigravida women with unfavorable cervix at the start of induction [126]. In these cases, a multidisciplinary team of obstetrician, hematologist, anesthetist, and neonatologist along with the mother should perform a careful risk assessment. In some circumstances, an elective cesarean section could be considered less traumatic to both the mother and her affected child, although intuitively this carries a greater bleeding risk than a normal spontaneous vaginal delivery.

Table 10.2 General principles in the management of labor and delivery in women with inherited bleeding disorders

• Multidisciplinary approach
• Group and save, full blood count and coagulation screen at the onset of labor. Relevant clotting factor assay for those with low third trimester levels who require treatment
• Prophylactic treatment is recommended when the relevant factor level is below the hemostatic level suggested in Table 10.3. The hemostatic level should be maintained for at least 3 days after vaginal delivery and at least 5 days after cesarean section
• Regional analgesia/anesthesia should only be considered after careful risk assessment and if the factor level and coagulation screen are normal
• Avoid invasive intrapartum fetal monitoring techniques, prolonged labor and traumatic instrumental deliveries if the fetus is at risk
• Active management of third stage
• Obtain cord blood sample for assessment of neonatal coagulation status in neonates at risk of moderate to severe inherited bleeding disorder
• Avoid intramuscular injection in neonates at risk until the coagulation status is known – give oral vitamin K and immunization through intradermal or subcutaneous route

Table 10.3 Suggested hemostatic levels for invasive procedures during pregnancy and for delivery

Inherited bleeding disorder	Clotting factor (activity)	Hemostatic levels suggested (IU/dL)*	Comments
VWD	VWF	50	
Carrier of hemophilia A	FVIII	50	
Carrier of hemophilia B	FIX	50	
Fibrinogen deficiency	Fibrinogen	1.0–1.5†	To maintain >1.0 g/L during pregnancy
FII deficiency	FII	20–30	
FV deficiency	FV	15–25	
FVII deficiency	FVII	10–20	
FX deficiency	FX	10–20	
FXI deficiency	FXI	20–70	
FXIII deficiency	FXIII	20–30	To maintain >3 IU/dL during pregnancy

VWD, von Willebrand disease; VWF, von Willebrand factor; F, factor.
*For general guidance only, personal and family bleeding history must be taken into considerations when deciding the need for prophylaxis. Please refer to text.
†g/L.

Invasive intrapartum monitoring techniques such as fetal scalp electrodes and fetal blood sampling should be avoided in pregnancies where the fetus is at risk of a bleeding disorder because of the potential risk of scalp hemorrhage. There are several case reports of this complication following fetal blood sampling in newborns with coagulopathy [127–129]. Affected fetuses are at risk of serious head bleeding, including cephalohematoma and intracranial hemorrhage, from the process of birth. The safest method of delivery for fetuses at risk is controversial. The available data involve newborns with severe or moderate hemophilia [130, 131], which is the commonest severe inherited bleeding disorder. In a survey of obstetricians in the USA, 57% would "frequently" deliver a known carrier of hemophilia by the vaginal route, whereas 11% preferred cesarean section; 85% and 74% responded that they would rarely use vacuum extraction and forceps delivery, respectively [131]. Ljung *et al.* [130] reviewed 117 children with moderate to severe hemophilia born in Sweden between 1970 and 1990 and found 23 neonatal bleedings associated with delivery. The risk of hemorrhage (all sites) was 10% (9/87) with vaginal delivery, 64% (11/17) with vacuum extraction, and 23% (3/13) with cesarean section. The

risk of head bleeding specifically was 3% (3/87) with vaginal delivery, 64% (11/17) with vacuum extraction, and 15% (2/13) with cesarean section. There have also been reports of head bleeding after elective cesarean section in neonates with severe bleeding disorders [24, 132]. These data, albeit relatively small in sample size, indicate that the risk of serious bleeding during normal vaginal delivery is probably small and that delivery of all fetuses at risk of hemophilia by cesarean section is not expected to eliminate this risk [130]. Therefore, normal vaginal delivery is generally not contraindicated in pregnancies at risk of inherited bleeding disorders. On the other hand, the use of vacuum extraction or forceps, and prolonged labor especially prolonged second stage of labor, should be avoided since they are associated with an increased risk of head bleeding [21, 130].

In a UK study, cephalohematoma was reported in two neonates affected with hemophilia [21]. The first neonate developed a large cephalohematoma after a ventouse delivery requiring blood transfusion. The second neonate was delivered by cesarean section after a 2 hour second stage. In principle, delivery should be achieved by the least traumatic method and early recourse to cesarean section should be considered to minimize the risk of neonatal bleeding complications. Low forceps delivery may be considered less traumatic than cesarean section when the head is deeply engaged in the pelvis and an easy outlet delivery is anticipated. Care should also be taken in minimizing maternal genital and perineal trauma in order to reduce the risk of excessive bleeding at delivery [23, 70, 125].

A cord blood sample should be collected from neonates at risk of moderate or severe inherited bleeding disorders to assess the coagulation status and clotting factor levels. This enables early identification and management of newborns at risk of hemorrhagic complications. If delivery has been traumatic or if there are clinical signs suggestive of head bleeding, a cranial ultrasound should be performed. It is also advisable to consider prophylactic cover in these cases [72]. Intramuscular injections should be avoided in neonates at risk until the coagulation status is known. Vitamin K should be given orally and routine immunizations given intradermally or subcutaneously. Any surgical procedures (e.g., circumcision) should be delayed until the coagulation status of the neonate is known. When assessing the neonatal clotting factor levels, it should be appreciated that these correlate with gestational age and reach adult levels at 6 months of age. Furthermore, the vitamin K-dependent coagulation factors are low at delivery. It is therefore not reliable to diagnose mild forms of inherited bleeding disorders at birth. Further details on the management of newborns with inherited bleeding disorders can be found in Chapter 12.

General principles for postpartum management

Postpartum hemorrhage (PPH) is a major cause of maternal morbidity and mortality. It accounts for an estimated 140 000 maternal deaths each year worldwide and many suffer from the long-lasting and debilitating consequences of the resultant anemia [133]. It is generally classified as primary or secondary PPH. Primary PPH is traditionally defined as a blood loss of more than 500 mL (or 1000 mL for severe PPH) in the first 24 hours after delivery, whereas secondary PPH refers to excessive bleeding occurring between 24 hours and 6 weeks after delivery. They affect approximately 5–8% and 0.8 % of pregnancies, respectively [134, 135]. However, the incidence of PPH varies widely, with much higher rates occurring in developing countries and rural settings. Further-more, the estimation of blood loss following delivery is difficult and commonly underestimated. Although the majority (90%) of the cases are attributed to uterine atony, coagulation disorders are a recognized cause of PPH.

Women with inherited bleeding disorders are at increased risk of both primary and secondary PPH [17]. In most women with inherited bleeding disorders the risk of PPH is often related to the factor levels. For this reason, prophylactic replacement therapy is generally given to cover labor, delivery, and the immediate postpartum period (at least 3 days for vaginal delivery and 5 days for cesarean section) in women with subnormal factor levels [72]. Table 10.3 shows the suggested hemostatic levels required for delivery in women with inherited bleeding disorders. As the pregnancy-induced rise in clotting factors can reverse rapidly after delivery [20], the use of oral tranexamic acid for 3–4 days after vaginal delivery or 7–10 days following cesarean section has been suggested for the prevention of secondary PPH, even among those with normal factor levels at term [72]. Women with inherited bleeding disorders may be at risk for secondary PPH for several weeks postpartum. Combined oral contraceptive pills, if not contraindicated, are also an option for preventing excessive bleeding in the late postpartum period.

Active management of the third stage of labor is associated with a significant reduction in blood loss and the need for blood transfusion compared with expectant management [136], and therefore is recommended in women with inherited bleeding disorders. It entails the administration of prophylactic uterotonics, early cord clamping, and controlled cord traction of the umbilical cord. In the event of an operative delivery, meticulous surgical hemostasis should be practiced to minimize blood loss. Care must also be taken to minimize maternal genital and perineal trauma, as women with inherited bleeding disorders are at particular risk of developing perineal hematoma [22, 23, 70].

Misoprostol, a new and inexpensive prostaglandin E1 analog that can be given orally, sublingually, or rectally, appears to be a promising uterotonic for the prevention of PPH [137]. Its administration can be associated with side-effects, including vomiting, diarrhea, fever, and shivering. A recent pharmacokinetics study has found lower peak levels but a reduction in adverse effects with rectal compared with the

Table 10.4 Obstetric risk factors for postpartum hemorrhage (PPH)*

History of PPH
Previous cesarean section
Obesity
Pre-eclampsia
Placenta previa
Placental abruption
Fibroids
Multiple pregnancies
Macrosomia
Polyhydramnios
Chorioamnionitis
Induced or augmented labor
Prolonged labor
Retained placenta
Operative delivery

*Not exclusive; data from Stones et al. [195] and Sheiner et al. [196].

oral route [138, 139]. In our unit, we recommend the use of misoprostol (600 μg rectally) in adjunct to active management of the third stage in women with inherited bleeding disorders. However, further studies are needed to determine its efficacy and safety in the prevention of PPH in high-risk women and to establish the optimal dose and route of administration.

It is important not to overlook the obstetric risk factors (Table 10.4) and other causes (Table 10.5) of PPH in women with inherited bleeding disorders. In case of hemorrhage, after initial assessment and restoration of circulatory volume, local causes should be excluded and replacement of the deficient clotting factor with monitoring of the factor levels should be

Table 10.5 Causes of postpartum hemorrhage (PPH)

Primary PPH
Uterine atony
Retained placenta
Genital tract laceration/trauma
Coagulation disorders
Secondary PPH
Retained products of conception
Infection
Coagulation disorders

performed. Management of PPH in these women presents a particular challenge, and close collaboration between hematologists, obstetricians, and anesthetists is imperative.

Specific issues for each inherited bleeding disorder

Carriers of hemophilia
Knowledge of fetal sex is very useful for the management of labor in carriers of hemophilia. If the fetus is identified as male, there is a 50% chance of it being affected. If specific prenatal diagnosis has not been performed, it is important to treat the pregnancy as potentially affected and avoid invasive intrapartum monitoring and instrumental deliveries. If the fetus is identified as female, there is a 50% chance of being a carrier like her mother. There are no specific data on the bleeding risks of newborns who are carriers of hemophilia, but they are usually not expected to be at increased risk of bleeding complications. Furthermore, recent data suggest that the process of labor is associated with a significant increase in neonatal factor levels [140]. However, some carriers could have significantly low factor levels due to extreme lyonization [141] and thus be at increased risk of bleeding complications. Therefore, invasive techniques that carry a high risk of head bleeding such as vacuum extraction should preferably be avoided in these cases.

Prophylactic cover for labor and delivery is not normally required in carriers of hemophilia A as their FVIII levels usually normalize at term. However, the individual's hemostatic response to pregnancy can be variable and a significant proportion, particularly those with a severe deficiency, may still have a low factor level (<50 IU/dL) at term [21, 22, 55]. Since FIX levels do not increase significantly during pregnancy, hemostatic support is commonly used for labor and delivery in carriers of hemophilia B.

In a review of 46 pregnancies in 32 carriers of hemophilia, the incidence of primary and secondary PPH were reported as 22% (10/46) and 11% (5/46), respectively, which are significantly higher than that observed in the general obstetric population [21]. A case–control study also found a significantly higher incidence of prolonged bleeding after delivery among carriers of hemophilia A or B (22%) compared with the controls (6%) [142]. In a further study of five carriers of hemophilia B (FIX activity levels <20 IU/dL), four experienced PPH in six of 16 deliveries; PPH was found to be significantly more common among those receiving ≤3 days of FIX replacement [143]. It appears that FVIII or FIX activity has a significant influence on the risk of bleeding among carriers of hemophilia with most of the significant PPH occurring in those with baseline factor levels below 50 IU/dL [21, 142].

Therefore, replacement therapy to cover labor and delivery is recommended in those with factor levels below 50 IU/dL at term or in the third trimester. If treatment is required, it should start at the onset of labor with the aim of raising the factor level above 50 IU/dL. This level should be maintained for at least 3 days after vaginal delivery and at least 5 days after cesarean section [144]. Recombinant products are regarded as the treatment of choice [145]. Desmopressin can also be used in carriers of hemophilia A, but carriers of hemophilia B do not respond to this agent. Since the pregnancy-induced rise in clotting factors (including FVIII but not FIX) falls after delivery, carriers of hemophilia are also at risk of prolonged or intermittent secondary PPH. They should be advised of this potential complication and in cases of heavy lochia, tranexamic acid could be used to reduce blood loss.

von Willebrand disease
Women with VWD are similarly at increased risk of both primary and secondary PPH. In three case series, including 92 deliveries in 51 women with VWD, primary PPH complicated 16–29% of pregnancies whereas secondary PPH complicated 20–29% of pregnancies [18, 22, 23]. In a case–control study, excessive postpartum bleeding was reported in 59% (51/86) of women with VWD compared with 21% (15/76) of the controls [61]. In another case–control study of 81 women with type 1 VWD, PPH was reported in 31% of these women compared with 10% of the control group; and 17% of women with VWD received blood transfusion compared with 3% of the controls [146].

In a recent large case–control study from the USA including 4067 deliveries in women with VWD, affected women were more likely to experience PPH (OR 1.5; 95% CI 1.1–2.0) and had a fivefold increased risk of being transfused (OR 4.7; 95% CI 3.2–7.0) compared with women without VWD [70]. These women were also at risk of perineal hematoma [22, 23, 70]. Consequently, extra care should be taken to minimize maternal genital and perineal trauma in these women.

The risk of PPH could be relatively higher in women with types 2 and 3 VWD since the majority are likely to have a persistent hemostatic defect at term. In a study of Iranian patients with type 3 VWD, 15 of 100 women who had delivered at least one child experienced PPH [66]. Prophylactic treatments were generally given at delivery. This could explain a lower than expected rate of PPH in the study; however, PPH occurred when the treatment was suboptimal in dosage or was given for too short a time period (for 1 day instead of 3–4 days) [66].

Owing to the wide variation in hemostatic response to pregnancy in women with different types of VWD, it is important to assess VWF and FVIII levels in the third trimester to plan appropriate intrapartum and postpartum prophylactic cover. In principle, prophylactic cover with either desmopressin, if responsive, or VWF-containing concentrates is recommended to maintain VWF:AC and/or FVIII:C levels >50 IU/dL during labor and for at least 3 days after vaginal delivery or 5 days if following cesarean section [72]. Prophylactic cover is usually not required in women with type 1 VWD since their FVIII and VWF levels would normally have risen to above 50 IU/dL at term. However, treatment is generally necessary in women with type 3 VWD and in some women with type 2 VWD, particularly if the delivery is by cesarean section or if there is perineal trauma [72].

Pregnancy-induced rises in clotting factors reverse after delivery. The fall in factor levels is variable and can be rapid [18, 20]. There are anecdotal reports of a decrease from 41 to 9 IU/dL over the course of a week [18] and a fall by half in just 6 hours after delivery in another case [20]. The use of prophylactic treatment at delivery may prevent primary PPH, but the risk of secondary PPH may persist for a number of weeks after delivery [27, 28, 65, 147]. The average time of presentation of PPH in women with VWD had been found to be 15.7 ± 5.2 days [148]. This implies the potential need for prophylaxis and/or close observation for up to several weeks postpartum. Tranexamic acid or combined oral contraceptive pills, if not contraindicated, can be used to control this bleeding complication, although replacement therapy may be required in some cases.

Rare bleeding disorders
The general principles of the management of labor and delivery in women with rare bleeding disorders are

similar to those for pregnancies at risk of hemophilia. Owing to limited information available in the literature, recommendations are generally made based on evidence derived from case studies or opinions and experiences of respected authorities [50]. In view of the unpredictable nature of labor and the possibility of requiring an emergency cesarean section, it may be reasonable to maintain hemostatic levels during labor and delivery equivalent to that recommended for major surgery. The inheritance of the rare bleeding disorders is usually autosomal recessive, with the exception of some of the fibrinogen disorders. In families where both parents are either affected or carriers of a rare inherited bleeding disorder, the fetus could potentially be severely affected with the disorder. In these circumstances labor and delivery is managed similarly to carriers of hemophilia with an affected male fetus.

Women with rare bleeding disorders are also at risk of both primary and secondary PPH. In general, if replacement therapy is instituted for intrapartum cover, considerations should be made to maintain the hemostatic level for at least 3–5 days after vaginal delivery or 5–7 days following cesarean section, depending on the severity of the coagulation defect and the bleeding history. The use of oral tranexamic acid for 3–4 days after vaginal delivery or 7–10 days following cesarean section can also be considered in some cases. However, the potential for thrombosis associated with replacement therapy must be carefully evaluated and balanced against the risk of bleeding given the risk of thrombosis as already noted with some of these disorders.

Inherited fibrinogen abnormalities Afibrinogenemia is an autosomal recessive disorder; therefore, if the father is unaffected, the infant at most is heterozygous, in whom atypical hemorrhage is not normally expected [51]. In contrast, hypofibrinogenemia can be inherited as either a dominant or a recessive trait [149] and dysfibrinogenemia is usually transmitted as an autosomal dominant trait. Consequently, it is important to regard the neonate as potentially affected in these cases and avoid invasive monitoring procedures and instrumental deliveries especially if the family phenotype is of bleeding.

Regular fibrinogen infusions are recommended in women with afibrinogenemia from early pregnancy to prevent fetal loss. For labor and delivery, a minimum

fibrinogen level of 1.5 g/L and, if possible, >2.0 g/L has been suggested for the prevention of placental abruption and PPH [51]. The intrapartum management of women with hypofibrinogenemia is dependent on the bleeding tendency, previous obstetric history, and fibrinogen level. Replacement therapy may be required if the fibrinogen level is below 1 g/L and/or if the woman has a significant bleeding history [50].

Similarly, in women with dysfibrinogenemia, intrapartum management is dependent on the fibrinogen level as well as the personal and family history of bleeding and thrombosis. No specific treatment other than close observation is required in asymptomatic women unless bleeding occurs or the family history suggests a high risk of bleeding [50]. In women with a bleeding phenotype, the management options depend on the severity of the personal and family bleeding history. In women with very mild bleeding phenotype, vaginal delivery can be managed conservatively and treatment is only given if bleeding occurs. However, if the bleeding history is significant or if the woman is undergoing cesarean section, prophylactic treatment is recommended to raise the fibrinogen level >1 g/L and maintain the level at >0.5–1 g/L until wound healing has occurred [50].

Women with inherited abnormalities of fibrinogen are at increased risk of PPH. In a literature review (1960–89) on congenital hypofibrinogenemia including 15 women who had a total of 31 pregnancies excluding miscarriages, PPH was the most common obstetric complication occurring in 45% of the pregnancies [85]. Blood transfusion was required in all cases and hysterectomy in two. One patient presented with secondary PPH 1 week after delivery [150].

However, paradoxical thrombotic events have also been reported among patients with hypofibrinogenemia [96] or afibrinogenemia [82, 92, 95] and particularly in women with dysfibrinogenemia [50, 98]. Therefore, a very careful risk assessment of both bleeding and thrombosis is required for women with abnormalities of fibrinogenemia. In asymptomatic women, fibrinogen replacement therapy is only given if bleeding occurs, whereas prophylactic substitution therapy during the immediate postpartum period is considered for those with a significant bleeding tendency. On the other hand, postpartum prophylactic LMWH with compression stockings is recommended for those with a personal or family history of thrombosis or following cesarean section, especially if performed under hemostatic replacement cover [50]. Tranexamic acid should be avoided in women with a personal or family history of thrombosis.

Factor II (prothrombin) deficiency Only a small number of reports are available in the literature on women with FII deficiency. Catanzarite *et al.* [104] described a woman with severe hypoprothrombinemia (FII activity <1 IU/dL) who experienced secondary PPH in one of her four term pregnancies, but no case of PPH was reported in an Iranian series including 14 patients (gender split not specified) [102]. Nevertheless, women with prothrombin deficiency, particularly those with abnormal prothrombin activity levels, should be considered potentially at risk of PPH. Although there are currently very limited published data available on which to base management recommendations, a prothrombin level of >25 IU/dL during labor and delivery has been suggested to minimize bleeding complications [50]. Since there are no specific prothrombin concentrates available, prothrombin complex concentrates are the treatment of choice [145].

FV deficiency In women with heterozygous (partial) deficiency and no history of bleeding, labor and delivery could be managed expectantly [50]. A case series of 15 deliveries among 11 heterozygous women with FV levels of ~50 IU/dL were not accompanied by any bleeding complications. However, women with homozygous (severe) FV deficiency are at increased risk of bleeding complications [105], and substitution therapy with FFP (as no FV concentrate is available) is recommended to raise FV levels to above 15–25 IU/dL [50, 105]. Close monitoring of FV levels is also recommended to ensure that the required hemostatic level has been achieved and further doses may be necessary to maintain these levels during and after delivery.

In a series of 35 Iranian patients (including 10 females) with FV deficiency, postoperative and postpartum bleeding were reported in 43% (15/35) of the patients [151]. A review of 17 deliveries among nine women with FV deficiency found PPH in 13 (76%) of the 17 deliveries [106]. There were two forceps deliveries both complicated with vaginal hematoma [106, 152]. Women with FV deficiency appear to be at increased risk of PPH; therefore, substitution therapy may be required in the postpartum period to maintain FV levels >15 IU/dL [50]. If cesarean section is performed, it is recommended that FV levels are maintained above this level until wound healing is established [50].

Factor VII deficiency The management of affected patients is complicated by the variable bleeding tendency and the poor correlation between FVII level and the bleeding risk [102, 153]. Women with FVII deficiency are at risk of PPH, particularly those with a severe deficiency or a bleeding tendency. A review of 12 published case reports of FVII deficiency in pregnancy found four were complicated by PPH [44]. In a UK series of 14 pregnancies in seven women with mild/moderate FVII deficiency, there were eight full-term deliveries prior to the diagnosis of FVII deficiency and none was associated with bleeding complications. In mild/moderate forms of FVII, there may be a significant rise in FVII level at term and therefore replacement therapy may not be required for labor and delivery [48]. However, this decision should be individualized and must take into account the mother's bleeding tendency, FVII level in the third trimester and the mode of delivery.

Despite case reports of uncomplicated deliveries in women with severe FVII deficiency without replacement therapy [44, 46], prophylactic cover for labor and delivery is generally recommended in women with severe deficiency (FVII level of <10–20 IU/dL at term and/or significant bleeding history), particularly if a cesarean section is performed [44, 47, 107, 154]. Current therapeutic options include recombinant factor VIIa (rVIIa), plasma-derived FVII concentrates, plasma, prothrombin complex concentrates (provided an adequate amount of FVII is present), and antifibrinolytics. However, rVIIa is the treatment of choice [145]. The use of tranexamic acid can also be considered to prevent or control heavy postpartum bleeding in these women.

Factor X deficiency Since FX levels do not increase significantly during pregnancy in women with severe deficiency [42, 43], replacement therapy is required to cover labor and delivery in these women to minimize the risk of bleeding complications. It is also recommended in women with FX deficiency who have a bleeding tendency or a history of adverse outcome in pregnancy [50]. A conservative approach could be adopted in women with mild FX deficiency (FX level >10 IU/dL) and no significant bleeding history. However, the decision for prophylaxis should be individualized, taking into account any bleeding history in relation to previous hemostatic challenges and the mode of delivery [50]. Treatment options include prothrombin complex concentrates or FFP, preferably prothrombin complex concentrates when available because of a lower volume and higher concentration of FX.

The mode of delivery for pregnancy at risk of homozygous severe FX deficiency has been debated. An elective cesarean section has been recommended because of the risk of cranial and/or abdominal hemorrhage in the newborn as a consequence of vaginal delivery [115]. However, there have been case reports of successful neonatal outcomes following normal vaginal deliveries [42, 43]. Furthermore, cesarean section may not completely eliminate the risk of serious bleeding in these neonates and a case of antenatal subdural hemorrhage in a fetus, subsequently found to be homozygous for factor X deficiency, has been reported [155]. With limited data in the literature, elective cesarean section cannot be recommended for all women with FX deficiency and the decision for the mode of delivery needs to be individualized.

PPH has been described in a woman with abnormal FX (FX Friuli variant) [113]. Both her deliveries were complicated with severe PPH requiring several blood transfusions and a hysterectomy in the second delivery. However, no PPH was reported among five other case reports of severe FX deficiency in the literature [42, 43, 114, 115, 156]. This could be explained by the use of peripartum prophylactic cover in these cases. Women with severe FX deficiency or a positive bleeding history are likely to be at increased risk of PPH, thus replacement therapy should be considered for the immediate postpartum period as well as during labor and delivery.

Factor XI deficiency Changes in FXI levels during pregnancy in women with FXI deficiency have been shown to be inconsistent [23, 49] and, in general, no significant rise is observed. Consequently, many will continue to have a subnormal (<70 IU/dL) factor level at term and thus are at risk of excessive bleeding during delivery. In a UK case series including 25 pregnancies in 11 women with FXI deficiency, primary PPH was reported in 16% of the pregnancies and none received prophylactic treatment [23]. In contrast, there was no bleeding complication in five pregnancies where replacement therapy with FXI concentrates or FFP were given to cover labor and delivery. In another retrospective review of a total of 105 pregnancies in 33 women with FXI deficiency, the incidence of PPH was 13% (eight primary and one secondary) and all but one episode occurred in women with a bleeding tendency [49]. A study of 164 pregnancies in 62 women with severe FXI deficiency (FXI levels <17 IU/dL) in Israel showed 69% (43) of the women never experienced postpartum hemorrhage during 93 deliveries (85 vaginal delivery, eight cesarean sections) without any prophylactic cover [123]. The authors argued that prophylactic treatment is not mandatory even for women with severe FXI deficiency, especially for vaginal deliveries [123]. However, excessive bleeding at delivery did occur in 24% (32/132) of vaginal deliveries and 17% (2/12) of cesarean sections not covered by FFP, whereas all six cesarean sections carried out under prophylactic cover were uncomplicated. In this study, the occurrence of excessive bleeding at delivery did not correlate to the abnormal genotype or FXI level [123].

Owing to the unpredictable bleeding tendency in FXI deficiency, the decision for prophylaxis during labor and delivery needs to be individualized and must take into consideration not only the FXI levels but also the personal/family bleeding history and the mode of delivery. Treatment options include tranexamic acid (for milder forms), FXI concentrates, FFP (if FXI concentrates unavailable), and rVIIa. If FFP is used, solvent detergent-treated plasma if available is preferable in terms of reducing the risk of infectious disease transmission. The general recommendation at present is that vaginal delivery can be managed expectantly in women with FXI levels between about 15 and 70 IU/dL and no bleeding history despite hemostatic challenge [50]. For those with FXI levels between 15 and 70 IU/dL and a significant bleeding history or no previous hemostatic challenge, tranexamic acid can be used to provide peripartum cover starting at the onset of labor. FXI concentrates may be required for a cesarean section in these women depending on the bleeding history. However, for women with severe (FXI level <10–20 IU/dL) deficiency, replacement therapy with FXI concentrate is recommended for all modes of delivery. In view of the thrombotic potential of factor XI concentrate [145, 157], the peak level should aim to be 70 IU/dL. As for all blood products there are concerns about the risk of transfusion-transmitted infections. Recombinant factor VIIa is an alternative option that has been used to prevent surgical bleeding in patients with FXI deficiency [158–160]. Its short half-life makes it less suitable for use to cover labor, but it could be used for management of elective cesarean sections. Further studies are needed to assess its use in this situation.

Women with FXI deficiency are also at increased risk of secondary PPH. The incidence of secondary PPH was 24% in a UK case series [23]. Consequently, prophylactic treatment with tranexamic acid should be considered for those with a bleeding phenotype. When given, it should be extended for 3 days postpartum or 5 days following cesarean section. However, the concomitant use of tranexamic acid and FXI concentrates should be avoided because of the potential thrombogenicity of FXI concentrates [157, 161] and attention should be given to simple thromboprophylactic measures, including adequate hydration and early mobilization. LMWH should be considered in women receiving FXI concentrates, in particular if they also have other thrombotic risks factor.

Factor XIII deficiency Since FXIII deficiency is strongly associated with pregnancy loss, regular replacement therapy to maintain FXIII levels >3 IU/dL [50] and, if possible, >10 IU/dL [54] is recommended during pregnancy. This treatment should also be continued during labor and delivery to minimize the risk of bleeding complications. However, higher FXIII levels may be required for delivery [54]. An FXIII level of >20 IU/dL and, if possible, >30 IU/dL during labor/delivery has been suggested to minimize the risk of bleeding complications [54].

Plasma-derived FXIII concentrates is the treatment of choice. They are superior to FFP or cryoprecipitate because they provide reliable and high concentrations of FXIII in minimum volume, have fewer contaminating substances, and are virally inactivated [162]. However, further studies are needed to establish the optimal dose and interval of administration [54].

The incidence of PPH in women with FXIII deficiency is not known. PPH was not reported in most cases of women with type II or FXIII subunit A deficiency in the literature. This is most likely due to the administration of FXIII concentrate throughout the pregnancy and labor that is essential for a successful pregnancy in these women [54]. The long circulating half-life (7–13 days) of FXIII concentrates [163] may also minimize the risk of secondary PPH. In a review

of case reports and series, women with types I and III FXIII deficiency were found to conceive and deliver normally without replacement therapy, but almost uniformly experienced postpartum hemorrhage [52]. Therefore, the use of postpartum prophylaxis should be considered in women with FXIII deficiency.

Combined factor deficiencies Women with subnormal factor levels are likely to be at increased risk of bleeding complications; hence replacement therapy may be required to cover labor and delivery. In one case report of a woman with VKCFD, profuse bleeding from the episiotomy site requiring treatment with FFP was reported [125]. As there are limited data on the management of pregnancy in women with these rare combined factor deficiencies (combined FV and FVIII deficiency and VKCFD), their management is extrapolated from the obstetric experience of women with a single deficiency of the factors involved.

Hemostatic agents and pregnancy

Desmopressin

Desmopressin (1-desamino-8-D-arginine vasopressin) is a synthetic analog of the natural hormone vasopressin. It increases plasma levels of endogenous VWF and FVIII. It is therefore a valuable therapeutic option for the prevention and treatment of bleeding in carriers of hemophilia A and most women with VWD (mainly type 1). It can be administered intravenously, subcutaneously, or as a nasal spray. Intravenous administration (0.3 µg/kg over 20–30 minutes) is preferred for treatment of acute bleeding episodes and before surgery or invasive procedures [164].

Desmopressin increases plasma FVIII and VWF levels, on average, by two- to fivefold, with a peak at 60 minutes after the completion of intravenous infusion and 90–120 minutes after subcutaneous or intranasal application [71]. A trial of desmopressin, preferably as part of the preconceptual assessment, is recommended to establish the individual response and to predict clinical efficacy. When monitoring responses, blood samples should be taken at 1 hour after infusion to check the patient's peak levels and at 4 hours to obtain information on the clearance rate [164]. Further doses may be required at 12 hour intervals to achieve hemostatic levels, but the response should be monitored as there may be a diminished response to successive doses in some patients [71].

There have been some concerns regarding the use of desmopressin during pregnancy because of the potential risks of placental insufficiency due to arterial vasoconstriction and of miscarriage or preterm labor due to an oxytoxic effect [165]. However, in contrast to naturally occurring vasopressin, desmopressin has minimal vasoconstrictive and oxytocic effects, which are consistent with its predominant V2 vasopressin receptor activity, whereas uterine tissue comprises primarily V1 receptors [165]. Nevertheless, there is a risk of maternal and/or neonatal hyponatremia due to the more potent and prolonged antidiuretic effect of desmopressin compared with that of the natural hormone vasopressin [165]. Maternal hyponatremia has been reported in two pregnant women receiving desmopressin, with one developing a grand mal seizure [24]. Therefore, restriction of fluid intake and care in maintaining fluid balance should accompany the use of desmopressin to prevent fluid overload and consequent hyponatremia. Prolonged administration should be avoided in pregnancy and its use in pregnancies complicated with pre-eclampsia is not advisable [71, 72]. Other more common adverse effects of desmopressin include tachycardia, headache, and facial flushing, but they are generally mild.

The efficacy and safety of desmopressin for prophylaxis or treatment of pregnancy-associated bleeding have not been well studied, but evidence of its safety during pregnancy in women with diabetes insipidus using smaller doses is available [166]. In a survey of hematologists from the USA and Canada, 50% and 34% used intravenous and intranasal desmopressin, respectively, for postpartum hemorrhage in women with type 1 VWD and only 31% considered pregnancy as a contraindication [167]. In a series of 27 carriers of hemophilia A and five women with type 1 VWD, desmopressin was given successfully to cover invasive prenatal diagnostic procedures [57]. All women had FVIII levels <50 IU/dL and on average there was a threefold increase in FVIII levels 1 hour after the infusion. No abnormal bleeding occurred and there were no serious side-effects from desmopressin other than mild facial flushing and headache. There are other case reports on the effective use of desmopressin among women with type 1 VWD in providing hemostatic cover or treatment during labor/delivery [18, 26, 29] and in the immediate postpartum

period [26, 28, 29]. In a retrospective case series including 54 women with VWF <50 IU/dL and a bleeding tendency, desmopressin was given during the first trimester in five pregnancies among three women because of vaginal bleeding or insertion of cervical cerclage [168]. It was also administered, as a single dose in intravenous infusion, in 75 deliveries (30 vaginal deliveries and 45 cesarean sections) either at the onset of labor or prior to regional block or general anesthesia. No adverse effects were observed in the mothers or newborns [168] In general, desmopressin is not contraindicated in uncomplicated pregnancy, but it should be used with caution and ideally given after clamping the umbilical cord to avoid the potential risk of neonatal hyponatremia [71]. Desmopressin does not pass into breast milk in significant amounts and therefore is probably safe to the newborn when used in breastfeeding women.

Desmopressin is often effective in patients with type 1 VWD since they have a functionally normal VWF and a releasable store. In contrast, it is of no therapeutic use in patients with type 3 VWD because they lack releasable stores of VWF [169], although there are rare exceptions [170]. In types 2A and 2M VWD, it increases the levels of abnormal VWF, and therefore is not effective in most cases [71]. It is generally contraindicated in type 2B VWD as the release of the abnormal VWF may induce platelet aggregation and thrombocytopenia [164, 171]. In type 2N VWD, it increases FVIII levels, but because of abnormal FVIII binding, the half-life is shortened [172]. Owing to the wide variations in response, it is important for patients with VWD to have a trial of desmopressin to determine whether their response is adequate for hemostasis.

Antifibrinolytic agents

Antifibrinolytic agents such as tranexamic acid and epsilon-aminocaproic acid (EACA) are synthetic fibrinolytic inhibitors that block the lysine binding sites of the plasminogen and plasmin molecules, thereby preventing the binding of plasminogen and plasmin to the fibrin substrate [173, 174]. EACA is approximately seven- to 10-fold less potent than tranexamic acid [175] but is used in the USA as tranexamic acid is not approved by the US Food and Drug Administration. EACA or tranexamic acid can be administered orally, intravenously, or topically. Antifibrinolytic agents have been used for the prevention and treatment of bleeding in patients with various bleeding disorders [176–178]. Since these drugs inhibit fibrinolysis, they carry a potential risk of thrombosis in patients with an underlying prothrombotic state. There have been isolated case reports of cerebral thrombosis [179, 180] and arterial thrombosis [181] in patients receiving tranexamic acid. The hemostatic changes in pregnancy result in a hypercoagulable state. The risk of thrombosis is greater in pregnant women than in non-pregnant women of similar age [182–184]. Delivery by cesarean section further increases the risk of thrombosis [185]. Consequently, pregnant women, especially those delivered by cesarean section, constitute a group at greater risk of the potential thrombotic effect of antifibrinolytic treatment. For these reasons, there have been concerns and reluctance in its use during pregnancy.

However, tranexamic acid has been used successfully to control or prevent bleeding in antepartum hemorrhage, placental abruption, cesarean section, and postpartum hemorrhage in the general obstetric population without apparent maternal or fetal adverse effects [174, 186–189]. In a retrospective review of 256 women treated with tranexamic acid for placental abruption, placenta previa or unspecified antepartum hemorrhage, including 169 women who underwent cesarean section, no thrombogenic effect of tranexamic acid was found [174]. In another 73 cases of placental abruption treated with tranexamic acid and delivered by cesarean section, none was complicated by thrombosis [187]. Similarly there were no thrombotic complications in a Chinese study of 91 women who received tranexamic acid immediately before a cesarean section to reduce perioperative blood loss [188]. Tranexamic acid, alone or as an adjunct to replacement therapy, has also been used effectively in women with inherited bleeding disorders, including carriers of hemophilia and women with VWD or FXI deficiency, to control or prevent excessive bleeding following delivery, miscarriage, or termination of pregnancy [18, 23, 27, 55, 65].

Its use at a dose of 1 g for 6–8 hours starting at the onset of labor and/or for 3–4 days following vaginal delivery and 7–10 days following cesarean section can be considered for the prevention of PPH in women with inherited bleeding disorders. Although its safety during pregnancy and lactation has not been established, current data do not suggest an increased risk

of thrombosis associated with its use in pregnancy [174]. However, as previously noted, its concomitant use with thrombogenic agents such as FXI concentrate should be avoided. It should also be avoided in patients with a history of thromboembolic disease [71]. No evidence of teratogenicity has been found in animal studies [190]. A limited amount of tranexamic acid may be present in breast milk, but an antifibrinolytic effect is unlikely [190]. Side-effects of tranexamic acid include nausea, vomiting, and diarrhea, which may improve with reduced dosage.

Clotting factor replacement

Currently available plasma-derived clotting factor concentrates are treated with virucidal methods which eliminate the risk of transmitting human immunodeficiency virus (HIV) and the hepatitis B and C viruses [191]. However, they have the potential to transmit hepatitis A, parvovirus B19 and any unknown infection [192, 193]. Although parvovirus is not normally a serious infection in non-immunocompromised adults, fetal infection may result in hydrops fetalis and fetal death. It should be noted that solvent detergent plasma, although effective in eliminating lipid-enveloped viruses, does not protect the recipient from non-lipid-enveloped viruses such as parvovirus. Therefore, non-plasma-derived products or treatment options (desmopressin, tranexamic acid, and recombinant products), if available, are generally regarded as the treatment of choice since they carry no or a negligible risk of infection. Cryoprecipitate is not virally inactivated, hence should not be used during pregnancy because of the small risk of transmission of viral or other blood-borne infections, unless other treatment modalities are not available or have failed [194].

Therapeutic options for women with inherited bleeding disorders in pregnancy (Table 10.6)

Carriers of hemophilia
Recombinant FVIII and FIX are the treatments of choice for carriers of hemophilia A and B, respectively. Desmopressin can also be used in carriers of hemophilia A as discussed earlier.

von Willebrand disease
The use of desmopressin should be considered in women with an adequate response.

Table 10.6 Therapeutic options for women with inherited bleeding disorders in pregnancy [145]

Bleeding disorder	Preferred therapeutic option	Other options
VWD	Desmopressin or VWF-containing concentrates	Platelet (type 2B)
Carriers of hemophilia A	Desmopressin or rFVIII	FVIII concentrate
Carriers of hemophilia B	rFIX	FIX concentrate
Fibrinogen abnormalities	Fibrinogen concentrate	SD plasma
FII deficiency	PCC	SD plasma
FV deficiency	SD plasma	SD plasma
FV and FVIII deficiency	SD plasma rVIII	FVIII concentrate
FVII deficiency	rVIIa	FVII concentrate
FX deficiency	PCC	SD plasma
FXI deficiency	FXI concentrates or tranexamic acid	SD plasma
FXIII deficiency	FXIII concentrates	SD plasma
VKCFD	Vitamin K	SD plasma PCC

F, factor; r, recombinant; SD plasma, fresh-frozen plasma virally inactivated using a solvent detergent technique; PCC, prothrombin complex concentrates; VKCFD, hereditary combined deficiency of the vitamin K-dependent clotting factors; VWD, von Willebrand disease.

Virally inactivated VWF-containing FVIII concentrate is the treatment of choice in women with VWD unresponsive to desmopressin or in whom desmopressin is contraindicated [71]. Platelet transfusions may be required in type 2B VWD if the woman has thrombocytopenia and is symptomatic and not responding to infusion therapy with VWF-containing concentrate or she is undergoing surgery [40]. The use of recombinant FVIII or FVIII concentrates to cover labor in a woman with type 2N VWD and low FVIII levels at term has also been described [32].

Rare bleeding disorders
Similar to the treatment of carriers of hemophilia and women with VWD, the therapeutic options for women with rare inherited bleeding disorders consist of replacement of the deficient clotting factor. However, the available therapies and the clinical experience on their use are limited (Table 10.6). They are mostly plasma derived with the exception of rVIIa. FFP is widely available and relatively inexpensive, but it carries the risk of fluid overload when repeated doses are required to maintain the hemostatic factor levels and the risk of viral transmission. Clotting factor concentrates, if available, are the preferred option. If they are unavailable or contraindicated, then virally inactivated plasma can be used.

Hemostatic agents, such as rVIIa, FXI concentrates, VWF-containing concentrates, and prothrombin complex concentrates, carry the risk of thrombotic complications. They should therefore be avoided in patients with a personal or family history of thrombosis. The risk of bleeding must be balanced against the risk of thrombosis. The use of these agents should be accompanied by appropriate thromboprophylactic measures including adequate hydration, early mobilization, compression stockings and, in some cases, LMWH.

References

1 Hellgren M, Blomback M. Studies on blood coagulation and fibrinolysis in pregnancy, during delivery and in the puerperium. I. Normal condition. *Gynecol Obstet Invest* 1981; **12**: 141–154.
2 Beller FK, Ebert C. The coagulation and fibrinolytic enzyme system in pregnancy and in the puerperium. *Eur J Obstet Gynecol Reprod Biol* 1982; **13**: 177–197.
3 Stirling Y, Woolf L, North WR, *et al.* Haemostasis in normal pregnancy. *Thromb Haemost* 1984; **52**: 176–182.
4 Clark P, Brennand J, Conkie JA, *et al.* Activated protein C sensitivity, protein C, protein S and coagulation in

normal pregnancy. *Thromb Haemost* 1998; **79**: 1166–1170.

5 Kjellberg U, Andersson NE, Rosen S, *et al.* APC resistance and other haemostatic variables during pregnancy and puerperium. *Thromb Haemost* 1999; **81**: 527–531.

6 Donohoe S, Quenby S, Mackie I, *et al.* Fluctuations in levels of antiphospholipid antibodies and increased coagulation activation markers in normal and heparin-treated antiphospholipid syndrome pregnancies. *Lupus* 2002; **11**: 11–20.

7 Uchikova EH, Ledjev II. Changes in haemostasis during normal pregnancy. *Eur J Obstet Gynecol Reprod Biol* 2005; **119**: 185–188.

8 Condie RG. A serial study of coagulation factors XII, XI and X in plasma in normal pregnancy and in pregnancy complicated by pre-eclampsia. *Br J Obstet Gynaecol* 1976; **83**: 636–639.

9 Dalaker K. Clotting factor VII during pregnancy, delivery and puerperium. *Br J Obstet Gynaecol* 1986; **93**: 17–21.

10 Bremme KA. Haemostatic changes in pregnancy. *Best Pract Res Clin Haematol* 2003; **16**: 153–168.

11 Nilsson IM, Kullander S. Coagulation and fibrinolytic studies during pregnancy. *Acta Obstet Gynecol Scand* 1967; **46**: 273–285.

12 Phillips LL, Rosano L, Skrodelis V. Changes in factor XI (plasma thromboplastin antecedent) levels during pregnancy. *Am J Obstet Gynecol* 1973; **116**: 1114–1116.

13 Nossel HL, Lanzkowsky P, Levy S, *et al.* A study of coagulation factor levels in women during labour and in their newborn infants. *Thromb Diath Haemorrh* 1966; **16**: 185–197.

14 Coopland A, Alkjaersig N, Fletcher AP. Reduction in plasma factor 13 (fibrin stabilizing factor) concentration during pregnancy. *J Lab Clin Med* 1969; **73**: 144–153.

15 van Wersch JW, Vooijs ME, Ubachs JM. Coagulation factor XIII in pregnant smokers and non-smokers. *Int J Clin Lab Res* 1997; **27**: 68–71.

16 Inbal A, Muszbek L. Coagulation factor deficiencies and pregnancy loss. *Semin Thromb Hemost* 2003; **29**: 171–174.

17 James AH. More than menorrhagia: a review of the obstetric and gynaecological manifestations of von Willebrand disease. *Thromb Res* 2007; **120** (Suppl 1): S17–S20.

18 Ramsahoye BH, Davies SV, Dasani H, Pearson JF. Obstetric management in von Willebrand's disease: a report of 24 pregnancies and a review of the literature. *Haemophilia* 1995; **1**: 140–144.

19 Kouides PA. Obstetric and gynaecological aspects of von Willebrand disease. *Best Pract Res Clin Haematol* 2001; **14**: 381–399.

20 Hanna W, McCarroll D, McDonald T, *et al.* Variant von Willebrand's disease and pregnancy. *Blood* 1981; **58**: 873–879.

21 Kadir RA, Economides DL, Braithwaite J, *et al.* The obstetric experience of carriers of haemophilia. *Br J Obstet Gynaecol* 1997; **104**: 803–810.

22 Greer IA, Lowe GD, Walker JJ, Forbes CD. Haemorrhagic problems in obstetrics and gynaecology in patients with congenital coagulopathies. *Br J Obstet Gynaecol* 1991; **98**: 909–918.

23 Kadir RA, Lee CA, Sabin CA, *et al.* Pregnancy in women with von Willebrand's disease or factor XI deficiency. *Br J Obstet Gynaecol* 1998; **105**: 314–321.

24 Chediak JR, Alban GM, Maxey B. von Willebrand's disease and pregnancy: management during delivery and outcome of offspring. *Am J Obstet Gynecol* 1986; **155**: 618–624.

25 Adashi EY. Lack of improvement in von Willebrand's disease during pregnancy. *N Engl J Med* 1980; **303**: 1178.

26 Castaman G, Eikenboom JC, Contri A, Rodeghiero F. Pregnancy in women with type 1 von Willebrand disease caused by heterozygosity for von Willebrand factor mutation C1130F. *Thromb Haemost* 2000; **84**: 351–352.

27 Caliezi C, Tsakiris DA, Behringer H, *et al.* Two consecutive pregnancies and deliveries in a patient with von Willebrand's disease type 3. *Haemophilia* 1998; **4**: 845–849.

28 Conti M, Mari D, Conti E, *et al.* Pregnancy in women with different types of von Willebrand disease. *Obstet Gynecol* 1986; **68**: 282–285.

29 Castaman G, Federici AB, Bernardi M, *et al.* Factor VIII and von Willebrand factor changes after desmopressin and during pregnancy in type 2M von Willebrand disease Vicenza: a prospective study comparing patients with single (R1205H) and double (R1205H-M740I) defect. *J Thromb Haemost* 2006; **4**: 357–360.

30 Kujovich JL. von Willebrand disease and pregnancy. *J Thromb Haemost* 2005; **3**: 246–253.

31 Watanabe T, Minakami H, Sakata Y. Successful management of pregnancy in a patient with von Willebrand disease Normandy. *Obstet Gynecol* 1997; **89**: 859.

32 Dennis MW, Clough V, Toh CH. Unexpected presentation of type 2N von Willebrand disease in pregnancy. *Haemophilia* 2000; **6**: 696–697.

33 Nishino M, Nishino S, Sugimoto M, *et al.* Changes in factor VIII binding capacity of von Willebrand factor and factor VIII coagulant activity in two patients with type 2N von Willebrand disease after hemostatic treatment and during pregnancy. *Int J Hematol* 1996; **64**: 127–134.

34 Castaman G, Bertoncello K, Bernardi M, Rodeghiero F. Pregnancy and delivery in patients with homozygous or heterozygous R854Q type 2N von Willebrand disease. *J Thromb Haemost* 2005; **3**: 391–392.

35 Federici AB, Mazurier C, Berntorp E, *et al.* Biologic response to desmopressin in patients with severe type 1 and type 2 von Willebrand disease: results of a multicenter European study. *Blood* 2004; **103**: 2032–2038.

36 Rick ME, Williams SB, Sacher RA, McKeown LP. Thrombocytopenia associated with pregnancy in a patient with type IIB von Willebrand's disease. *Blood* 1987; **69**: 786–789.

37 Casonato A, Sartori MT, Bertomoro A, *et al.* Pregnancy-induced worsening of thrombocytopenia in a patient with type IIB von Willebrand's disease. *Blood Coagul Fibrinolysis* 1991; **2**: 33–40.

38 Giles AR, Hoogendoorn H, Benford K. Type IIB von Willebrand's disease presenting as thrombocytopenia during pregnancy. *Br J Haematol* 1987; **67**: 349–353.

39 Ieko M, Sakurama S, Sagawa A, *et al.* Effect of a factor VIII concentrate on type IIB von Willebrand's disease-associated thrombocytopenia presenting during pregnancy in identical twin mothers. *Am J Hematol* 1990; **35**: 26–31.

40 Mathew P, Greist A, Maahs JA, *et al.* Type 2B vWD: the varied clinical manifestations in two kindreds. *Haemophilia* 2003; **9**: 137–144.

41 Burlingame J, McGaraghan A, Kilpatrick S, *et al.* Maternal and fetal outcomes in pregnancies affected by von Willebrand disease type 2. *Am J Obstet Gynecol* 2001; **184**: 229–230.

42 Konje JC, Murphy P, de Chazal R, *et al.* Severe factor X deficiency and successful pregnancy. *Br J Obstet Gynaecol* 1994; **101**: 910–911.

43 Bofill JA, Young RA, Perry KG, Jr. Successful pregnancy in a woman with severe factor X deficiency. *Obstet Gynecol* 1996; **88**: 723.

44 Rizk DE, Castella A, Shaheen H, Deb P. Factor VII deficiency detected in pregnancy: a case report. *Am J Perinatol* 1999; **16**: 223–226.

45 Robertson LE, Wasserstrum N, Banez E, *et al.* Hereditary factor VII deficiency in pregnancy: peripartum treatment with factor VII concentrate. *Am J Hematol* 1992; **40**: 38–41.

46 Braun MW, Triplett DA. Case Report: Factor VII deficiency in an obstetrical patient. *J Indiana State Med Assoc* 1979; **72**: 900–902.

47 Eskandari N, Feldman N, Greenspoon JS. Factor VII deficiency in pregnancy treated with recombinant factor VIIa. *Obstet Gynecol* 2002; **99**: 935–937.

48 Kulkarni AA, Lee CA, Kadir RA. Pregnancy in women with congenital factor VII deficiency. *Haemophilia* 2006; **12**: 413–416.

49 Myers B, Pavord S, Kean L, *et al.* Pregnancy outcome in Factor XI deficiency: incidence of miscarriage, antenatal and postnatal haemorrhage in 33 women with Factor XI deficiency. *Br J Obstet Gynaecol* 2007; **114**: 643–646.

50 Bolton-Maggs PH, Perry DJ, Chalmers EA, *et al.* The rare coagulation disorders – review with guidelines for management from the United Kingdom Haemophilia Centre Doctors' Organisation. *Haemophilia* 2004; **10**: 593–628.

51 Kobayashi T, Kanayama N, Tokunaga N, *et al.* Prenatal and peripartum management of congenital afibrinogenaemia. *Br J Haematol* 2000; **109**: 364–366.

52 Burrows RF, Ray JG, Burrows EA. Bleeding risk and reproductive capacity among patients with factor XIII deficiency: a case presentation and review of the literature. *Obstet Gynecol Surv* 2000; **55**: 103–108.

53 Gilabert J, Reganon E, Vila V, *et al.* Congenital hypofibrinogenemia and pregnancy, obstetric and hematological management. *Gynecol Obstet Invest* 1987; **24**: 271–276.

54 Asahina T, Kobayashi T, Takeuchi K, Kanayama N. Congenital blood coagulation factor XIII deficiency and successful deliveries: a review of the literature. *Obstet Gynecol Surv* 2007; **62**: 255–260.

55 Chi C, Lee CA, Shiltagh N, *et al.* Pregnancy in carriers of haemophilia. *Haemophilia* 2008; **14**: 56–64.

56 Guy GP, Baxi LV, Hurlet-Jensen A, Chao CR. An unusual complication in a gravida with factor IX deficiency: case report with review of the literature. *Obstet Gynecol* 1992; **80**: 502–505.

57 Mannucci PM. Use of desmopressin (DDAVP) during early pregnancy in factor VIII-deficient women. *Blood* 2005; **105**: 3382.

58 Sipila P, Hartikainen-Sorri AL, Oja H, Von Wendt L. Perinatal outcome of pregnancies complicated by vaginal bleeding. *Br J Obstet Gynaecol* 1992; **99**: 959–963.

59 Axelsen SM, Henriksen TB, Hedegaard M, Secher NJ. Characteristics of vaginal bleeding during pregnancy. *Eur J Obstet Gynecol Reprod Biol* 1995; **63**: 131–134.

60 Yang J, Savitz DA, Dole N, *et al.* Predictors of vaginal bleeding during the first two trimesters of pregnancy. *Paediatr Perinat Epidemiol* 2005; **19**: 276–283.

61 Kirtava A, Drews C, Lally C, *et al.* Medical, reproductive and psychosocial experiences of women diagnosed with von Willebrand's disease receiving care in haemophilia treatment centres: a case-control study. *Haemophilia* 2003; **9**: 292–297.

62 Nybo Andersen AM, Wohlfahrt J, Christens P, *et al.* Maternal age and fetal loss: population based register linkage study. *BMJ* 2000; **320**: 1708–1712.

63 Everett C. Incidence and outcome of bleeding before the 20th week of pregnancy: prospective study from general practice. *BMJ* 1997; **315**: 32–34.

64 Blohm F, Friden B, Milsom I. A prospective longitudinal population-based study of clinical miscarriage in an urban Swedish population. *Br J Obstet Gynaecol* 2008; **115**: 176–182.

65 Foster PA. The reproductive health of women with von Willebrand Disease unresponsive to DDAVP: results of an international survey. On behalf of the Subcommittee on von Willebrand Factor of the Scientific and Standardization Committee of the ISTH. *Thromb Haemost* 1995; **74**: 784–790.

66 Lak M, Peyvandi F, Mannucci PM. Clinical manifestations and complications of childbirth and replacement therapy in 385 Iranian patients with type 3 von Willebrand disease. *Br J Haematol* 2000; **111**: 1236–1239.

67 Ito M, Yoshimura K, Toyoda N, Wada H. Pregnancy and delivery in patients with von Willebrand's disease. *J Obstet Gynaecol Res* 1997; **23**: 37–43.

68 Punnonen R, Nyman D, Gronroos M, Wallen O. Von Willebrand's disease and pregnancy. *Acta Obstet Gynecol Scand* 1981; **60**: 507–509.

69 Sorosky J, Klatsky A, Nobert GF, Burchell RC. Von Willebrand's disease complicating second-trimester abortion. *Obstet Gynecol* 1980; **55**: 253–254.

70 James AH, Jamison MG. Bleeding events and other complications during pregnancy and childbirth in women with von Willebrand disease. *J Thromb Haemost* 2007; **5**: 1165–1169.

71 Pasi KJ, Collins PW, Keeling DM, *et al.* Management of von Willebrand disease: a guideline from the UK Haemophilia Centre Doctors' Organization. *Haemophilia* 2004; **10**: 218–231.

72 Lee CA, Chi C, Pavord SR, *et al.* The obstetric and gynaecological management of women with inherited bleeding disorders – review with guidelines produced by a taskforce of UK Haemophilia Centre Doctors' Organization. *Haemophilia* 2006; **12**: 301–336.

73 Fisher S, Rikover M, Naor S. Factor 13 deficiency with severe hemorrhagic diathesis. *Blood* 1966; **28**: 34–39.

74 Boda Z, Pfliegler G, Muszbek L, *et al.* Congenital factor XIII deficiency with multiple benign breast tumours and successful pregnancy with substitutive therapy. A case report. *Haemostasis* 1989; **19**: 348–352.

75 Lak M, Peyvandi F, Ali SA, *et al.* Pattern of symptoms in 93 Iranian patients with severe factor XIII deficiency. *J Thromb Haemost* 2003; **1**: 1852–1853.

76 Padmanabhan LD, Mhaskar R, Mhaskar A, Ross CR. Factor XIII deficiency: a rare cause of repeated abortions. *Singapore Med J* 2004; **45**: 186–187.

77 Inbal A, Kenet G. Pregnancy and surgical procedures in patients with factor XIII deficiency. *Biomed Prog* 2003; **16**: 69–71.

78 Rodeghiero F, Castaman GC, Di Bona E, *et al.* Successful pregnancy in a woman with congenital factor XIII deficiency treated with substitutive therapy. Report of a second case. *Blut* 1987; **55**: 45–48.

79 Kobayashi T, Terao T, Kojima T, *et al.* Congenital factor XIII deficiency with treatment of factor XIII concentrate and normal vaginal delivery. *Gynecol Obstet Invest* 1990; **29**: 235–238.

80 Trehan AK, Fergusson IL. Congenital afibrinogenaemia and successful pregnancy outcome. Case report. *Br J Obstet Gynaecol* 1991; **98**: 722–724.

81 Evron S, Anteby SO, Brzezinsky A, *et al.* Congenital afibrinogenemia and recurrent early abortion: a case report. *Eur J Obstet Gynecol Reprod Biol* 1985; **19**: 307–311.

82 Lak M, Keihani M, Elahi F, *et al.* Bleeding and thrombosis in 55 patients with inherited afibrinogenaemia. *Br J Haematol* 1999; **107**: 204–206.

83 Girolami A, Sartori MT, Simioni P. An updated classification of factor XIII defect. *Br J Haematol* 1991; **77**: 565–566.

84 Asahina T, Kobayashi T, Okada Y, *et al.* Studies on the role of adhesive proteins in maintaining pregnancy. *Horm Res* 1998; **50** (Suppl 2): 37–45.

85 Goodwin TM. Congenital hypofibrinogenemia in pregnancy. *Obstet Gynecol Surv* 1989; **44**: 157–161.

86 Ness PM, Budzynski AZ, Olexa SA, Rodvien R. Congenital hypofibrinogenemia and recurrent placental abruption. *Obstet Gynecol* 1983; **61**: 519–523.

87 Kobayashi T, Asahina T, Maehara K, *et al.* Congenital afibrinogenemia with successful delivery. *Gynecol Obstet Invest* 1996; **42**: 66–69.

88 Inamoto Y, Terao T. First report of case of congenital afibrinogenemia with successful delivery. *Am J Obstet Gynecol* 1985; **153**: 803–804.

89 Grech H, Majumdar G, Lawrie AS, Savidge GF. Pregnancy in congenital afibrinogenaemia: report of a successful case and review of the literature. *Br J Haematol* 1991; **78**: 571–572.

90 Matsuno K, Mori K, Amikawa H. A case of congenital afibrinogenemia with abortion, intracranial hemorrhage and peritonitis. *Jpn J Clin Hematol* 1977; **18**: 1438.

91 Dube B, Agarwal SP, Gupta MM, Chawla SC. Congenital deficiency of fibrinogen in two sisters. A clinical and haematological study. *Acta Haematol* 1970; **43**: 120–127.

92 Roque H, Stephenson C, Lee MJ, *et al.* Pregnancy-related thrombosis in a woman with congenital afibrinogenemia: a report of two successful pregnancies. *Am J Hematol* 2004; **76**: 267–270.

93 Frenkel E, Duksin C, Herman A, Sherman DJ. Congenital hypofibrinogenemia in pregnancy: report of two cases and review of the literature. *Obstet Gynecol Surv* 2004; **59**: 775–779.

94 Aygoren-Pursun E, Martinez Sauger I, Rusicke E, *et al*. Retrochorionic hematoma in congenital afibrinogenemia: resolution with fibrinogen concentrate infusions. *Am J Hematol* 2007; **82**: 317–320.

95 Dupuy E, Soria C, Molho P, *et al*. Embolized ischemic lesions of toes in an afibrinogenemic patient: possible relevance to in vivo circulating thrombin. *Thromb Res* 2001; **102**: 211–219.

96 Chafa O, Chellali T, Sternberg C, *et al*. Severe hypofibrinogenemia associated with bilateral ischemic necrosis of toes and fingers. *Blood Coagul Fibrinolysis* 1995; **6**: 549–552.

97 Hanss M, Biot F. A database for human fibrinogen variants. *Ann N Y Acad Sci* 2001; **936**: 89–90.

98 Haverkate F, Samama M. Familial dysfibrinogenemia and thrombophilia. Report on a study of the SSC Sub-committee on Fibrinogen. *Thromb Haemost* 1995; **73**: 151–161.

99 Takala T, Oksa H, Rasi V, Tuimala R. Dysfibrinogenemia associated with thrombosis and third-trimester fetal loss. A case report. *J Reprod Med* 1991; **36**: 410–412.

100 Edwards RZ, Rijhsinghani A. Dysfibrinogenemia and placental abruption. *Obstet Gynecol* 2000; **95**: 1043.

101 Yamanaka Y, Takeuchi K, Sugimoto M, *et al*. Dysfibrinogenemia during pregnancy treated successfully with fibrinogen. *Acta Obstet Gynecol Scand* 2003; **82**: 972–973.

102 Peyvandi F, Mannucci PM. Rare coagulation disorders. *Thromb Haemost* 1999; **82**: 1207–1214.

103 Girolami A, Scarano L, Saggiorato G, *et al*. Congenital deficiencies and abnormalities of prothrombin. *Blood Coagul Fibrinolysis* 1998; **9**: 557–569.

104 Catanzarite VA, Novotny WF, Cousins LM, Schneider JM. Pregnancies in a patient with congenital absence of prothrombin activity: case report. *Am J Perinatol* 1997; **14**: 135–138.

105 Girolami A, Scandellari R, Lombardi AM, *et al*. Pregnancy and oral contraceptives in factor V deficiency: a study of 22 patients (five homozygotes and 17 heterozygotes) and review of the literature. *Haemophilia* 2005; **11**: 26–30.

106 Noia G, De Carolis S, De Stefano V, *et al*. Factor V deficiency in pregnancy complicated by Rh immunization and placenta previa. A case report and review of the literature. *Acta Obstet Gynecol Scand* 1997; **76**: 890–892.

107 Fadel HE, Krauss JS. Factor VII deficiency and pregnancy. *Obstet Gynecol* 1989; **73**: 453–454.

108 Mannucci PM, Duga S, Peyvandi F. Recessively inherited coagulation disorders. *Blood* 2004; **104**: 1243–1252.

109 Peyvandi F, Mannucci PM, Lak M, *et al*. Congenital factor X deficiency: spectrum of bleeding symptoms in 32 Iranian patients. *Br J Haematol* 1998; **102**: 626–628.

110 Knight RD, Barr CF, Alving BM. Replacement therapy for congenital Factor X deficiency. *Transfusion* 1985; **25**: 78–80.

111 Girolami A, Randi ML, Ruzzon E, *et al*. Pregnancy and oral contraceptives in congenital bleeding disorders of the vitamin K-dependent coagulation factors. *Acta Haematol* 2006; **115**: 58–63.

112 Kumar M, Mehta P. Congenital coagulopathies and pregnancy: report of four pregnancies in a factor X-deficient woman. *Am J Hematol* 1994; **46**: 241–244.

113 Girolami A, Lazzarin M, Scarpa R, Brunetti A. Further studies on the abnormal factor X (factor X Friuli) coagulation disorder: a report of another family. *Blood* 1971; **37**: 534–541.

114 Larrain C. [Congenital blood coagulation factor X deficiency. Successful result of the use prothrombin concentrated complex in the control of ++cesarean section hemorrhage in 2 pregnancies]. *Rev Med Chil* 1994; **122**: 1178–1183.

115 Romagnolo C, Burati S, Ciaffoni S, *et al*. Severe factor X deficiency in pregnancy: case report and review of the literature. *Haemophilia* 2004; **10**: 665–668.

116 Seligsohn U. Factor XI deficiency. *Thromb Haemost* 1993; **70**: 68–71.

117 Peyvandi F, Lak M, Mannucci PM. Factor XI deficiency in Iranians: its clinical manifestations in comparison with those of classic hemophilia. *Haematologica* 2002; **87**: 512–514.

118 Rapaport SI, Proctor RR, Patch MJ, Yettra M. The mode of inheritance of PTA deficiency: evidence for the existence of major PTA deficiency and minor PTA deficiency. *Blood* 1961; **18**: 149–165.

119 Leiba H, Ramot B, Many A. Heredity and coagulation studies in ten families with Factor XI (plasma thromboplastin antecedent) deficiency. *Br J Haematol* 1965; **11**: 654–665.

120 Bolton-Maggs PH, Young Wan-Yin B, McCraw AH, *et al*. Inheritance and bleeding in factor XI deficiency. *Br J Haematol* 1988; **69**: 521–528.

121 Bolton-Maggs PH, Patterson DA, Wensley RT, Tuddenham EG. Definition of the bleeding tendency in factor XI-deficient kindreds – a clinical and laboratory study. *Thromb Haemost* 1995; **73**: 194–202.

122 Ragni MV, Sinha D, Seaman F, *et al*. Comparison of bleeding tendency, factor XI coagulant activity, and factor XI antigen in 25 factor XI-deficient kindreds. *Blood* 1985; **65**: 719–724.

123 Salomon O, Steinberg DM, Tamarin I, *et al*. Plasma replacement therapy during labor is not mandatory for women with severe factor XI deficiency. *Blood Coagul Fibrinolysis* 2005; **16**: 37–41.

124 Bolton-Maggs PH. The management of factor XI deficiency. *Haemophilia* 1998; **4**: 683–688.

125 McMahon MJ, James AH. Combined deficiency of factors II, VII, IX, and X (Borgschulte-Grigsby deficiency) in pregnancy. *Obstet Gynecol* 2001; **97**: 808–809.

126 Rane SM, Guirgis RR, Higgins B, Nicolaides KH. Models for the prediction of successful induction of labor based on pre-induction sonographic measurement of cervical length. *J Matern Fetal Neonatal Med* 2005; **17**: 315–322.

127 Pachydakis A, Belgaumkar P, Sharmah A. Persistent scalp bleeding due to fetal coagulopathy following fetal blood sampling. *Int J Gynaecol Obstet* 2006; **92**: 69–70.

128 Hull MG, Wilson JA. Massive scalp haemorrhage after fetal blood sampling due to haemorrhagic disease. *BMJ* 1972; **4**: 321–322.

129 Reti LL, Adey FD, Brown MF. Excessive bleeding from fetal scalp blood sampling. *Aust N Z J Obstet Gynaecol* 1980; **20**: 55–57.

130 Ljung R, Lindgren AC, Petrini P, Tengborn L. Normal vaginal delivery is to be recommended for haemophilia carrier gravidae. *Acta Paediatr* 1994; **83**: 609–611.

131 Kulkarni R, Lusher JM, Henry RC, Kallen DJ. Current practices regarding newborn intracranial haemorrhage and obstetrical care and mode of delivery of pregnant haemophilia carriers: a survey of obstetricians, neonatologists and haematologists in the United States, on behalf of the National Hemophilia Foundation's Medical and Scientific Advisory Council. *Haemophilia* 1999; **5**: 410–415.

132 Michaud JL, Rivard GE, Chessex P. Intracranial hemorrhage in a newborn with hemophilia following elective cesarean section. *Am J Pediatr Hematol Oncol* 1991; **13**: 473–475.

133 AbouZahr C. Global burden of maternal death and disability. *Br Med Bull* 2003; **67**: 1–11.

134 El Refaey H, Rodeck C. Post-partum haemorrhage: definitions, medical and surgical management. A time for change. *Br Med Bull* 2003; **67**: 205–217.

135 Hoveyda F, MacKenzie IZ. Secondary postpartum haemorrhage: incidence, morbidity and current management. *Br J Obstet Gynaecol* 2001; **108**: 927–930.

136 Prendiville WJ, Elbourne D, McDonald S. Active versus expectant management in the third stage of labour. *Cochrane Database Syst Rev* 2000; CD000007.

137 Gulmezoglu AM, Forna F, Villar J, Hofmeyr GJ. Prostaglandins for preventing postpartum haemorrhage. *Cochrane Database Syst Rev* 2007; CD000494.

138 Khan RU, El Refaey H. Pharmacokinetics and adverse-effect profile of rectally administered misoprostol in the third stage of labor. *Obstet Gynecol* 2003; **101**: 968–974.

139 Hofmeyr GJ, Walraven G, Gulmezoglu AM, *et al.* Misoprostol to treat postpartum haemorrhage: a systematic review. *Br J Obstet Gynaecol* 2005; **112**: 547–553.

140 Kulkarni A, Riddell A, Lee CA, Kadir RA Assessment of factor VIII and von Willebrand factor levels in cord blood. RCOG 6th International Scientific Meeting, 27–30 September 2005, Cairo, Egypt.

141 Lyon MF. Sex chromatin and gene action in the mammalian X-chromosome. *Am J Hum Genet* 1962; **14**: 135–148.

142 Mauser Bunschoten EP, van Houwelingen JC, Sjamsoedin Visser EJ, *et al.* Bleeding symptoms in carriers of hemophilia A and B. *Thromb Haemost* 1988; **59**: 349–352.

143 Yang MY, Ragni MV. Clinical manifestations and management of labor and delivery in women with factor IX deficiency. *Haemophilia* 2004; **10**: 483–490.

144 Walker ID, Walker JJ, Colvin BT, *et al.* Investigation and management of haemorrhagic disorders in pregnancy. Haemostasis and Thrombosis Task Force. *J Clin Pathol* 1994; **47**: 100–108.

145 Keeling D, Tait C, Makris M. Guideline on the selection and use of therapeutic products to treat haemophilia and other hereditary bleeding disorders: a United Kingdom Haemophilia Center Doctors' Organisation (UKHCDO) Guideline approved by the British Committee for standards in Haematology. *Haemophilia* 2008; **14**: 671–684.

146 Kouides PA, Phatak PD, Burkart P, *et al.* Gynaecological and obstetrical morbidity in women with type I von Willebrand disease: results of a patient survey. *Haemophilia* 2000; **6**: 643–648.

147 Lipton RA, Ayromlooi J, Coller BS. Severe von Willebrand's disease during labor and delivery. *JAMA* 1982; **248**: 1355–1357.

148 Roque H, Funai E, Lockwood CJ. von Willebrand disease and pregnancy. *J Matern Fetal Med* 2000; **9**: 257–266.

149 Menache D. Congenital fibrinogen abnormalities. *Ann N Y Acad Sci* 1983; **408**: 121–130.

150 Strickland DM, Galey WT, Hauth JC. Hypofibrinogenemia as a cause of delayed postpartum hemorrhage. *Am J Obstet Gynecol* 1982; **143**: 230–231.

151 Lak M, Sharifian R, Peyvandi F, Mannucci PM. Symptoms of inherited factor V deficiency in 35 Iranian patients. *Br J Haematol* 1998; **103**: 1067–1069.

152 Fajardo LF, Silvert D. Pregnancy and Ac-globulin deficiency; report of a case. *Am J Obstet Gynecol* 1957; **74**: 909–914.

153 Triplett DA, Brandt JT, Batard MA, *et al.* Hereditary factor VII deficiency: heterogeneity defined by combined functional and immunochemical analysis. *Blood* 1985; **66**: 1284–1287.

154 Jimenez-Yuste V, Villar A, Morado M, *et al.* Continuous infusion of recombinant activated factor VII during caesarean section delivery in a patient with congenital factor VII deficiency. *Haemophilia* 2000; **6**: 588–590.

155 de Sousa C, Clark T, Bradshaw A. Antenatally diagnosed subdural haemorrhage in congenital factor X deficiency. *Arch Dis Child* 1988; **63**: 1168–1170.

156 Rezig K, Diar N, Benabidallah D, Audibert J. [Factor X deficiency and pregnancy]. *Ann Fr Anesth Reanim* 2002; **21**: 521–524.

157 Bolton-Maggs PH, Colvin BT, Satchi BT, *et al.* Thrombogenic potential of factor XI concentrate. *Lancet* 1994; **344**: 748–749.

158 O'Connell NM, Riddell AF, Pascoe G, *et al.* Recombinant factor VIIa to prevent surgical bleeding in factor XI deficiency. *Haemophilia* 2008; **14**: 775–781.

159 Lawler P, White B, Pye S, *et al.* Successful use of recombinant factor VIIa in a patient with inhibitor secondary to severe factor XI deficiency. *Haemophilia* 2002; **8**(2): 145–148.

160 Bern MM, Sahud M, Zhukov O, *et al.* Treatment of factor XI inhibitor using recombinant activated factor VIIa. *Haemophilia* 2005; **11**: 20–25.

161 Mannucci PM, Bauer KA, Santagostino E, *et al.* Activation of the coagulation cascade after infusion of a factor XI concentrate in congenitally deficient patients. *Blood* 1994; **84**: 1314–1319.

162 Board PG, Losowsky MS, Miloszewski KJ. Factor XIII: inherited and acquired deficiency. *Blood Rev* 1993; **7**: 229–242.

163 Fukue H, Arai M. Factor XIIIA subunit deficiency. *Jpn J Thromb Hemost* 2001; **12**: 66–73.

164 Mannucci PM. Treatment of von Willebrand's Disease. *N Engl J Med* 2004; **351**: 683–694.

165 Mannucci PM. Desmopressin (DDAVP) in the treatment of bleeding disorders: the first 20 years. *Blood* 1997; **90**: 2515–2521.

166 Ray JG. DDAVP use during pregnancy: an analysis of its safety for mother and child. *Obstet Gynecol Surv* 1998; **53**: 450–455.

167 Cohen AJ, Kessler CM, Ewenstein BM. Management of von Willebrand disease: a survey on current clinical practice from the haemophilia centres of North America. *Haemophilia* 2001; **7**: 235–241.

168 Sanchez-Luceros A, Meschengieser SS, Turdo K, *et al.* Evaluation of the clinical safety of desmopressin during pregnancy in women with a low plasmatic von Willebrand factor level and bleeding history. *Thromb Res* 2007; **120**: 387–390.

169 Ruggeri ZM, Mannucci PM, Lombardi R, *et al.* Multimeric composition of factor VIII/von Willebrand factor following administration of DDAVP: implications for pathophysiology and therapy of von

170 Castaman G, Lattuada A, Mannucci PM, Rodeghiero F. Factor VIII: C increases after desmopressin in a subgroup of patients with autosomal recessive severe von Willebrand disease. *Br J Haematol* 1995; **89**: 147–151.

171 Holmberg L, Nilsson IM, Borge L, *et al.* Platelet aggregation induced by 1-desamino-8-D-arginine vasopressin (DDAVP) in Type IIB von Willebrand's disease. *N Engl J Med* 1983; **309**: 816–821.

172 Mazurier C, Gaucher C, Jorieux S, Goudemand M. Biological effect of desmopressin in eight patients with type 2N ("Normandy") von Willebrand disease. Collaborative Group. *Br J Haematol* 1994; **88**: 849–854.

173 Astedt B. Clinical pharmacology of tranexamic acid. *Scand J Gastroenterol Suppl* 1987; **137**: 22–25.

174 Lindoff C, Rybo G, Astedt B. Treatment with tranexamic acid during pregnancy, and the risk of thrombo-embolic complications. *Thromb Haemost* 1993; **70**: 238–240.

175 Fraser IS, Porte RJ, Kouides PA, Lukes AS. A benefit-risk review of systemic haemostatic agents: part 1: in major surgery. *Drug Safety* 2008; **31**(3): 217–230.

176 Rainsford SG, Jouhar AJ, Hall A. Tranexamic acid in the control of spontaneous bleeding in severe haemophilia. *Thromb Diath Haemorrh* 1973; **30**: 272–279.

177 Forbes CD, Barr RD, Reid G, *et al.* Tranexamic acid in control of haemorrhage after dental extraction in haemophilia and Christmas disease. *BMJ* 1972; **2**: 311–313.

178 Berliner S, Horowitz I, Martinowitz U, *et al.* Dental surgery in patients with severe factor XI deficiency without plasma replacement. *Blood Coagul Fibrinolysis* 1992; **3**: 465–468.

179 Fodstad H, Liliequist B. Spontaneous thrombosis of ruptured intracranial aneurysms during treatment with tranexamic acid (AMCA). Report of three cases. *Acta Neurochir (Wien)* 1979; **49**: 129–144.

180 Rydin E, Lundberg PO. Letter: Tranexamic acid and intracranial thrombosis. *Lancet* 1976; **2**: 49.

181 Davies D, Howell DA. Tranexamic acid and arterial thrombosis. *Lancet* 1977; **1**: 49.

182 Pabinger I, Grafenhofer H. Thrombosis during pregnancy: risk factors, diagnosis and treatment. *Pathophysiol Haemost Thromb* 2002; **32**: 322–324.

183 Prevention of venous thrombosis and pulmonary embolism. *Natl Inst Health Consens Dev Conf Consens Statement* 1986; **6**: 1–8.

184 Rosendaal FR. Risk factors for venous thrombotic disease. *Thromb Haemost* 1999; **82**: 610–619.

185 Greer IA. Thrombosis in pregnancy: maternal and fetal issues. *Lancet* 1999; **353**: 1258–1265.

186 Walzman M, Bonnar J. Effects of tranexamic acid on the coagulation and fibrinolytic systems in pregnancy

complicated by placental bleeding. *Arch Toxicol Suppl* 1982; **5**: 214–220.

187 Svanberg L, Astedt B, Nilsson IM. Abruptio placentae – treatment with the fibrinolytic inhibitor tranexamic acid. *Acta Obstet Gynecol Scand* 1980; **59**: 127–130.

188 Gai MY, Wu LF, Su QF, Tatsumoto K. Clinical observation of blood loss reduced by tranexamic acid during and after caesarian section: a multi-center, randomized trial. *Eur J Obstet Gynecol Reprod Biol* 2004; **112**: 154–157.

189 As AK, Hagen P, Webb JB. Tranexamic acid in the management of postpartum haemorrhage. *Br J Obstet Gynaecol* 1996; **103**: 1250–1251.

190 British Medical Association and the Royal Pharmaceutical Society of Great Britain. *British National Formulary*, 48 edn. London: British Medical Association and the Royal Pharmaceutical Society of Great Britain, 2004.

191 Mannucci PM. The choice of plasma-derived clotting factor concentrates. *Baillieres Clin Haematol* 1996; **9**: 273–290.

192 Azzi A, Ciappi S, Zakvrzewska K, *et al*. Human parvovirus B19 infection in hemophiliacs first infused with two high-purity, virally attenuated factor VIII concentrates. *Am J Hematol* 1992; **39**: 228–230.

193 Mannucci PM, Gdovin S, Gringeri A, *et al*. Transmission of hepatitis A to patients with hemophilia by factor VIII concentrates treated with organic solvent and detergent to inactivate viruses. The Italian Collaborative Group. *Ann Intern Med* 1994; **120**: 1–7.

194 Lusher JM. Clinical guidelines for treating von Willebrand disease patients who are not candidates for DDAVP – a survey of European physicians. *Haemophilia* 1998; 4 Suppl **3**: 11–14.

195 Stones RW, Paterson CM, Saunders NJ. Risk factors for major obstetric haemorrhage. *Eur J Obstet Gynecol Reprod Biol* 1993; **48**: 15–18.

196 Sheiner E, Sarid L, Levy A, *et al*. Obstetric risk factors and outcome of pregnancies complicated with early postpartum hemorrhage: a population-based study. *J Matern Fetal Neonatal Med* 2005; **18**: 149–154.

11 Analgesia and anesthesia for pregnant women with inherited bleeding disorders

Claudia Chi, Adrian England, and Rezan A Kadir

Introduction

Labor, for many women, is one of the most intense and painful life events. Pain in the first stage of labour is caused by uterine contractions and cervical dilation. Painful stimuli from the uterus are transmitted to the posterior nerve roots of the tenth thoracic through to the first lumbar nerves. In the late first stage and second stage of labour, the pain predominantly results from stretching of the pelvic floor, vagina, and perineum. These pain stimuli are transmitted via the pudendal nerve derived from the second to the fourth sacral nerves. Contraction pain is predominantly visceral, hence it is poorly defined and frequently referred, for example, to the lower abdomen and back, whereas delivery pain is somatic and is generally well localized and sharp.

The experience of pain is multifactorial and cannot be accounted for solely by neurophysiological explanation. Pain is defined by the International Association for the Study of Pain as "an unpleasant sensory and emotional experience associated with actual or potential tissue damage, or described in terms of such damage" [1]. Therefore, the experience of pain, including labor pain, is highly individualized and multidimensional. The response to labor pain is modified by physiologic as well as psychosocial and environmental factors. Although satisfaction in childbirth is not dependent on the absence of pain, a woman's birth experience can be influenced by the level of pain experienced and the effectiveness of pain relief provided.

Management of labor pain is an integral part of the care provided for all pregnant women. It entails the provision of appropriate pain relief options with detailed information on their benefits and risks. A wide range of non-pharmacological and pharmacological options is available to assist women in coping with labor pain. The decision to use a particular method is based on the woman's preferences and on her obstetric, fetal, anesthetic, and hemostatic risks.

In women with inherited bleeding disorders, hemostatic risk is of a particular concern. However, this risk is "physiologically" minimized by the pregnancy-induced increase in some coagulation factors or by appropriate prophylactic treatment. A significant rise in levels of factor VIII activity (FVIII:C) and von Willebrand factor antigen (VWF:Ag) and activity (VWF:AC) is observed during pregnancy, particularly in the third trimester [2–4]. Consequently, most carriers of hemophilia A and women with type 1 von Willebrand disease (VWD) have normal clotting factor levels at term. In contrast, levels of factor IX (FIX) and XI (FXI) do not alter significantly during pregnancy [2, 3]; thus, the coagulation defect in carriers of hemophilia B and in women with FXI deficiency usually persist throughout pregnancy. The hemostatic defects in women with platelet function disorders or severe clotting factor deficiencies, such as type 3 VWD, also remain unchanged in pregnancy. Therefore, it is important to assess coagulation during pregnancy, especially during the third trimester, to allow an individualized management plan to be made for each woman. In addition to the assessment of coagulation status and

Inherited Bleeding Disorders in Women, 1st edition. By CA Lee, RA Kadir and PA Kouides. Published 2009 by Blackwell Publishing, ISBN: 978-1-4051-6915-8.

factor levels, considerations of personal and family bleeding history are important in the risk assessment and decision on the need for hemostatic treatments. The hemostatic changes that accompany pregnancy and the selection and use of prophylactic treatments are discussed in Chapter 10. The aim of this chapter is to explore the options of obstetric analgesia and anesthesia specifically for women with inherited bleeding disorders.

Non-pharmacological methods

A wide variety of non-pharmacological methods have been used to help women cope with the pain of childbirth. However, there are very few published scientific studies that have assessed their efficacy and adverse effects. Commonly used techniques include controlled breathing, massage, warm water bath, aromatherapy, acupuncture, acupressure, transcutaneous electrical nerve stimulation (TENS), hypnosis, music, and audio-analgesia. Many women choose non-pharmacological or complementary pain relief methods to avoid invasive or pharmacological measures. They are frequently used at the first instance and in the early stages of labor. A Cochrane systematic review of non-pharmacological methods used by the general obstetric population concluded that acupuncture and hypnosis may help to relieve labor pain, but there is currently insufficient evidence to support the benefits and effectiveness of massage and other complementary therapies [5]. There is a lack of published scientific data on the efficacy or safety of these non-pharmacological methods in women with inherited bleeding disorders. Techniques that involve disruption to maternal tissue such as acupuncture may be considered to be relatively contraindicated because of the potential risk of bleeding or bruising. But non-invasive techniques such as controlled breathing and massage are generally regarded as safe for these women.

Pharmacological methods

Pharmacological methods of controlling pain during labor and delivery have been used for centuries. Techniques commonly used today include Entonox (nitrous oxide premixed with oxygen), opioids, and regional block techniques in the form of epidural or combined spinal–epidural. The use and popularity of these measures evolved concurrently with the changes in social and cultural views towards the pain of childbirth. Over time, various techniques have been developed, some gained popularity while many were discontinued because of significant maternal or neonatal adverse effects. The primary concern when using any pharmacological method in women with inherited bleeding disorders lies mainly in the potential risks of bleeding complications in the mother and the newborn.

Inhalation analgesia

Volatile agents have been used to provide sedation and analgesia during childbirth for over a century and a half. In 1847 James Simpson discovered the effects of chloroform and subsequently introduced anesthesia to obstetric practice. He first used ether to provide analgesia for vaginal delivery [6]. Inhalation labor analgesia became more widely accepted when Queen Victoria received chloroform during the birth of her eighth and ninth children in 1853 and 1857 [7]. Nitrous oxide (as premixed 80% nitrous oxide in air) was first used for pain relief in labor in 1881 [8]. Minnitt [9] later introduced an apparatus allowing self-administration of nitrous oxide in 1934. Since then other volatile agents have also been used, including trichloroethylene, enflurane, isoflurane, and sevoflurane [10–13], but only nitrous oxide is widely used in current obstetric practice. This is likely due to its ease of administration, minimal toxicity, cardiovascular and respiratory effects, its lack of flammability, odor, or effect on uterine contractions, as well as its low cost.

It is delivered premixed as 50% nitrous oxide and 50% oxygen (Entonox). It is self-administered and can be used at any stages of labor depending on the woman's needs and preferences. It has a fast onset of effect of approximately 50 seconds, which is reversed rapidly when inhalation is ceased [14]. Although it is not a potent labor analgesic it can provide substantial pain relief in at least 50% of women when applied properly [15]. Its clearance is predominantly by exhalation rather than metabolism and it does not cause prolonged sedation in the mother or the baby after delivery. Unlike other pharmacological methods of intrapartum pain relief, it does not affect labor physiology or neonatal outcome [16–18] and it does not require additional maternal or fetal monitoring.

Side-effects include nausea, vomiting, dizziness, and a dry mouth, but there are no major side-effects with short-term use. Owing to its non-invasive mode of administration and low incidence of significant side-effects, nitrous oxide is a safe option for women with inherited bleeding disorders.

Opioid analgesia

The use of systemic opioids for labor pain was first documented in ancient Chinese writings [19]. It remains a common option for women today. Meperidine (pethidine) is currently the most frequently used opioid for the relief of labor pain in the United Kingdom. Other opioid drugs that have been assessed include morphine, tramadol, meptazinol, butorphanol, and fentanyl. Opioids provide some pain relief but are associated with maternal sedation, nausea, vomiting, dizziness, and delayed stomach emptying. They can also cause neonatal respiratory depression [20, 21] as they cross the placenta. An opioid antagonist such as naloxone may be required to reverse this effect in the newborn. However, it is often given intramuscularly, which is contraindicated in newborns with an inherited bleeding disorder. Other neonatal adverse effects of opioids include decreased neonatal alertness [22], inhibition of suckling [23–25], a delay in feeding [26, 27], and lower neurobehavioral scores [28]. Opioids can be administered as an intramuscular or intravenous injection or as intravenous patient-controlled analgesia (PCA). In women with uncorrected bleeding disorders, intramuscular injections can cause bleeding or bruising at the site of injection. Intravenous opioid, on the other hand, is more likely to cause severe opioid-related complications such as respiratory depression in both the mother and the newborn baby. Systemic opioids are generally considered unsuitable in women with inherited bleeding disorders because bleeding complications can result from the intramuscular administration of opioid in mothers with an uncorrected coagulation defect and of the antidote in newborns affected by the bleeding disorders.

Remifentanil, a new ultrashort-acting synthetic opioid, has been used recently to provide pain relief in labor [29, 30]. In a UK survey on the use of intravenous opiates given through a PCA device during labor, remifentanil (34.6%) was the most commonly used opioid for live births [31]. It has an effect-site half-life for analgesia of 1.3 minutes [32] and a context-sensitive half-life (the estimated time required for a 50% reduction in blood concentration after stopping an infusion that reached a steady state) of approximately 3 minutes in the general population [33]. It is rapidly hydrolyzed by non-specific tissue and blood esterases to inactive metabolites [34]. Its rapid onset and offset of action can potentially make it an ideal opioid for PCA during labor [35]. Kan et al. [35] first demonstrated its pharmacokinetics in 19 obstetric patients who received intravenous remifentanil during non-urgent cesarean section under epidural anesthesia. The clearance of remifentanil is greater in parturients than in non-obstetric patients. It crosses the placenta readily, but also appears to be rapidly metabolized, redistributed, or both in the fetus [35]. Comparative studies have shown that remifentanil PCA provided better analgesia during labor than inhaled Entonox or meperidine given either intramuscularly or via intravenous PCA apparatus [36–38]. The side-effects are minor and include mild sedation, itching, and nausea [39–41]. In a recent preliminary safety study, no evidence of cardiovascular instability, respiratory depression, cardiotocograph abnormalities requiring intervention in laboring women, or adverse neonatal outcome was found [41]. Remifentanil could be a promising alternate labor analgesic for women with a contraindication for regional analgesia. Few case reports have described the effective use of remifentanil PCA in parturients with coagulopathies where regional block was contraindicated [29, 30, 42]. However, it is currently not licensed for use in obstetric analgesia and further efficacy and safety data are required before its routine use can be recommended [43].

Regional (neuraxial) analgesia and anesthesia

Regional blockade for pain relief in labor, using subarachnoid cocaine, was reported as early as 1900 by Kreis [44]. Caudal extradural (epidural) analgesia for labor was performed in 1909, but the "loss of resistance technique" for cannulation of the extradural space was not developed until 1921 [45]. Ureteric silk catheters and Tuohy's curved bevel needle were developed in the early 1940s [46]. This allows repeated top-ups into the extradural space without the need for recannulation and made continuous extradural analgesia for labor possible. Extradural blockade for pain relief in labor started to gain popularity in the

1950s and its use in obstetrics has steadily increased, particularly in the last 30 years. The use of diluted local anesthetic solutions and the addition of opiates to local anesthetics to augment analgesia while sparing muscle power and proprioception have increased the attractiveness of this technique to control labor pain. Recent data showed that approximately 21% of women in the UK and 58% of women in the USA use this form of pain relief during labor and delivery [47, 48]. However, its use varies greatly between hospitals depending on its availability and the local population. There has also been a remarkable shift from general anesthesia to regional anesthesia for cesarean sections because of its better safety record [49]. The proportion of cesarean sections performed under general anesthesia in the UK has fallen from over 50% in 1989–90 to less than 10% in 2003–4 [47].

Techniques of regional (neuraxial) blockade
Regional block techniques for delivery include epidural, spinal or a combination of the two. Epidural blockade involves the administration of anesthetic drugs into the extradural space, often through a catheter as this allows repeated doses to be administered. Obstetric epidurals are inserted in the lumbar region below the conus medullaris and where the spinal cord has divided to form the filum terminale, usually at the interspace between the second and third or the third and fourth lumbar vertebrae. The intention is to block electrical transmission along the pain fibers running from the uterus and the birth canal as they cross the epidural space. Blockade of the dermatomes supplying the uterus (T10 to L1) is required for labor pain relief, and blockade of sacral nerve roots that supply the vagina and perineum is required for delivery. For a cesarean section the block needs to be intense and spread up from the sacral area, which provides sensation from the bladder, to the level of the fourth thoracic vertebrae to block the sensory fibers from the peritoneum. The volume and concentration of local anesthetic solution can be titrated to achieve an appropriate level of analgesia for each procedure. Recently, there has been a trend to use mixtures of opiates and less concentrated local anesthetics. These provide analgesia while preserving maternal motor function and proprioception [50]. This enables the women to mobilize during labor, an option preferred by many women [51, 52]. In a randomized trial of walking during active labor, 99% of mothers allocated to the ambulatory group stated they would wish to ambulate again during future labor [52].

A spinal block involves the injection of anesthetic drugs into the intrathecal space and is faster to take effect than an epidural. It is not usually used on its own to provide pain relief in labor because of its relatively short duration of effect. However, it is used for cesarean sections and the manual removal of placenta.

A combined spinal epidural (CSE) involves using both a spinal and an epidural for analgesia. It involves the initial administration of an intrathecal dose of local anesthetic/opiate mixture through a spinal needle and at the same time inserting a catheter into the epidural space through a Tuohy needle. This provides the rapid onset of a spinal anesthetic and allows repeated epidural doses to be given through the catheter. It is particularly effective in late labor and for instrumental or cesarean section deliveries as the spinal component provides a faster blockade of the sacral nerve roots than an epidural. Both CSE and epidural have been shown to provide effective pain relief in labor, with no difference in overall maternal satisfaction, mobility, obstetric outcome, and neonatal outcome [53].

Regional analgesia is currently the most effective form of analgesia for pain relief in labor [54] and it does not cause the sedation associated with other forms of analgesia, including opioid-induced neonatal respiratory depression. Regional anesthesia provides an alternative to general anesthesia for cesarean section. It has been shown to allow quicker mobilization, earlier establishment of breast feeding and gastrointestinal function, and better Apgar scores (at 1 and 5 minutes) than general anesthesia [55–57].

Risks and complications of
regional (neuraxial) blockade
Common side-effects of regional block include hypotension, pruritus, and nausea, which are usually mild and often do not require treatment. Hypotension may develop soon after the administration of the local anesthetic agent and occurs secondary to peripheral vasodilation from sympathetic blockade leading to pooling of blood in the venous capacitance vessels, obstruction of venous return from uterine compression, and arteriolar dilation leading to a reduced afterload.

Therefore, it is important to ensure adequate hydration, to monitor blood pressure in women receiving a regional block and to avoid a maternal supine position. Shivering, fever, drowsiness, and urinary retention have also been reported with the use of a regional block [58–60]. Other potential complications of regional block include inadequate or failure of block, inadvertent puncture of a blood vessel ("bloody tap"), and accidental dural puncture. Dural puncture can cause headache (postdural puncture headache), which may be self-limiting, but when it is severe and persistent, an epidural blood patch (insertion of autologous blood into the epidural space) can be performed to improve the symptoms. Serious but rare complications include local anesthetic toxicity, inadvertent high epidural or total spinal block, infection, spinal epidural hematoma, and neurological complications ranging from nerve root damage to spinal cord paralysis. An epidural can also influence the course of labor. A recent Cochrane review of epidural versus non-epidural or no analgesia in labor showed that women randomized to epidural had a longer second stage of labor, an increased need for oxytocin, and a higher rate of instrumental deliveries [54].

Coagulopathy and the risks of neurological complications

In women with inherited bleeding disorders, the greatest concern with the use of regional block is the potential risk of an epidural or spinal hematoma. In the presence of normal coagulation, bleeding from blood vessel injuries sustained during the administration and removal of a regional block is usually self-limiting. In a woman with defective coagulation bleeding is more likely to continue and result in the formation of an epidural hematoma. This can lead to spinal cord compression and permanent neurological damage if not treated promptly. The risk of spinal and epidural hematomas after neuraxial block is rare both in the general population (1 in 150 000–200 000) and in the obstetric population (0.2–3.7 in 100 000) [61–63]. However, this risk is significantly increased in the presence of coagulation abnormalities. In a review by Vandermeulen et al. [63], 42 (69%) of the 61 cases of spinal hematoma related to regional blocks identified in the general population occurred in patients with evidence of hemostatic abnormality, mostly attributable to anticoagulants. Five of these

were pregnant women. In the review by Abramovitz and Beilin [64] looking specifically at spinal/epidural hematoma in obstetric patients, three of the 10 case reports identified were in women with coagulation abnormalities associated with conditions including pre-eclampsia or obstetric cholestasis. For this reason, coagulopathy is regarded as a contraindication to regional block and consequently women with inherited bleeding disorders are often denied this option. Despite correction of the clotting defect, many anesthetists are still hesitant in instituting a regional block because limited data are available on the safety of regional block in these women.

In 13 case reports or series including 35 women with VWD, 19 with heterozygote FXI deficiency and seven carriers of hemophilia [2, 3, 65–75], no complications from regional blockade were reported (Table 11.1). In most cases, women with mild VWD or carriers of hemophilia A did not require prophylactic cover, whereas those with moderate or severe VWD received VWF-containing FVIII concentrate [2, 3, 65–69, 73, 75]. Dhar et al. [72] reported a case of regional block in a woman with hemophilia A (FVIII:C <1%). This condition is very rare in females as hemophilia is an X-linked disorder and such a low FVIII:C level is likely to be the result of extreme lyonization or first cousin marriage. She was maintained throughout pregnancy on recombinant FVIII concentrate (rFVIII) and her FVIII:C was 101 IU/dL prior to epidural insertion. Most of the women with FXI deficiency (17/19) reported in the literature did not receive prophylactic cover [3, 70, 74]; of these, 15 received regional anesthesia prior to diagnosis of their FXI deficiency [70, 74]. David et al. [70] reported two women (FXI levels 26 and 39 IU/dL, respectively) who received fresh-frozen plasma, which corrected the isolated prolonged activated partial thromboplastin time prior to regional block. One of these women had a positive personal and family bleeding history.

In a recent retrospective review of obstetric analgesia and anesthesia in women with inherited bleeding disorders who delivered at the Royal Free Hospital, London, the use of a regional block was described in a further 36 pregnancies [76]. Prophylactic cover was given in 11 pregnancies due to subnormal clotting factor levels at term, whereas the coagulation defect had normalized in the remaining 25 pregnancies. Complications included one case of hypotension

Table 11.1 Case reports and series on the use of regional block in women with inherited bleeding disorders during labor and delivery (from Chi *et al.* [76])

Author and year	Bleeding disorder and number of women	Prophylactic treatment
Cohen *et al.* 1989 [65]	VWD (1)	No
Milaskiewicz *et al.* 1990 [66]	VWD type 1 (1)	No
Kadir *et al.* 1997 [2]	Carrier of hemophilia (6)	No
Kadir *et al.* 1998 [3]	VWD (8) and FXI deficiency (2)	In one moderate VWD (VWF containing concentrate)
Caliezi *et al.* 1998 [67]	VWD type 3 (1)	Yes (FVIII concentrate)
Jones *et al.* 1999 [68]	VWD type 2A (1)	Yes (FVIII concentrate)
Cohen and Zada 2001 [69]	VWD (1)	Yes (FVIII concentrate)
David *et al.* 2002 [70]	FXI deficiency (3)	In two cases (FFP)
Perez-Barrero *et al.* 2003 [71]	VWD type 1(1)	Yes (DDAVP)
Dhar *et al.* 2003 [72]	Hemophilia A	Yes (rFVIII)
Varughese and Cohen 2007 [73]	VWD type 1 (14), type 2A (1)	No
Myers *et al.* 2007 [74]	FXI deficiency (14)	No
Marrache *et al.* 2007 [75]	VWD type 1 (6)	No

VWD, von Willebrand disease; VWF, von Willebrand factor; FVIII, factor VIII; FXI, factor XI; DDAVP, desmopressin; rFVIII, recombinant factor VIII, FFP, fresh-frozen plasma.

following regional anesthesia, which was corrected by fluid replacement, one case of inadequate analgesia due to unilateral block, and one case of inadequate anesthesia requiring conversion to general anesthesia during a cesarean section. Dural puncture was suspected in one woman and was treated conservatively. A bloody tap was noted in two cases with no further complications; both women had normal clotting screen and factor levels at term. No long-term complications from the regional block were reported. [76]

Guidance for the use of regional (neuraxial) block in women with inherited bleeding disorders

The findings from these case reports and series support the idea that it is safe to site a regional block in women with inherited bleeding disorders provided the coagulation defect has returned to normal during pregnancy or has been corrected with prophylactic treatment. Therefore, the option of regional block techniques should not be denied in all women with inherited bleeding disorders.

At the same time, it is important not to overlook the potential risks of regional block techniques, especially in women with severe or unpredictable disorders where hemostasis cannot be guaranteed. The use of a regional block may be contraindicated in these circumstances.

Table 11.2 presents the prerequisites for the use of a regional block in women with inherited bleeding disorders. The decision on its use should be planned on a case by case basis during the antenatal period. The mother should be counseled on the risks and benefits of regional block and its alternatives. Assessment of the coagulation status during pregnancy and planning for the need and availability of prophylaxis are essential. These can be based on factor levels meas-ured in the third trimester, as it can often be difficult to assess clotting factor levels during labor. The management of these women requires collaboration between hematologists, anesthetists, and obstetricians and the management plan should be documented clearly and be readily

Table 11.2 Conditions for the use of regional block in women with inherited bleeding disorders during labor and delivery

Multidisciplinary management involving hematologists, anesthetists, obstetricians, and the mother
Detailed counseling on the benefits and risks of regional block and its alternatives
Informed consent of the patient
Careful assessment of coagulation status including assessment of clotting factor during the third trimester, and personal and family bleeding history
Availability of therapeutic products and adequate response to treatment
Plan of management made antenatally, clearly documented, and readily available to professionals attending the women in labor
Normalization of coagulation defect either because of pregnancy itself or by prophylactic treatment
Meticulous technical skills in the administration of regional block by experienced anesthetist
Awareness and surveillance for symptoms and signs of potential complications

available to professionals attending the women in labor.

Prophylactic treatment is generally required if the measured coagulation defect does not return to normal during pregnancy. However, considerations must also be given to personal and family bleeding history, especially for disorders with an unpredictable bleeding tendency such as FVII and FXI deficiency. Women with mild VWD and carriers of hemophilia A usually do not require prophylaxis during labor because of a pregnancy-induced rise in FVIII and VWF levels. However, carriers of hemophilia B and women with FXI deficiency or other rare bleeding disorders are likely to require prophylactic treatment because their bleeding defects usually persist during pregnancy. The administration of a regional block requires the correction of the coagulation defect. This includes a normal coagulation screen, a platelet count of $>80 \times 10^9$/L [77], and individual clotting factor activities measured in the normal range or above the suggested hemostatic level for each inherited bleeding disorder (see Table 10.3) [78]. Tranexamic acid cover may be sufficient in some women with borderline clotting factor levels and no personal or family bleeding history. Women with low clotting factor levels or a significant bleeding history require prophylactic treatment with clotting factor replacement. Recombinant clotting factors, when available, are the treatment of choice in pregnant women [78]. For women with rare bleeding disorders, therapeutic options are usually plasma derived with the exception of recombinant factor VIIa, which is recommended for the treatment of FVII

deficiency [79, 80]. For further details on the selection of therapeutic products refer to Chapter 10.

A single-shot spinal anesthesia may be a more suitable and safer option in some situations, such as an uncomplicated elective cesarean section, as it removes the potential risk of vessel damage from an epidural catheter [64, 81–82]. Signs and symptoms of spinal hematoma are variable and they include acute onset of back (radicular) pain, bladder dysfunction, as well as sensory and motor deficits [83]. Regular assessment of neurological function is recommended to enable early recognition of potential complications. The use of low concentrations of local anesthetic augmented with opiates is preferred in order that the onset of abnormal neurologic signs is not masked. Any suspicions of a spinal epidural hematoma should trigger prompt assessment with magnetic resonance imaging for early diagnosis. If an epidural hematoma is discovered, immediate surgical decompression should be performed because an adverse neurological outcome is directly related to the time interval from hematoma formation to surgical decompression. The likelihood of a good recovery was found to be greatest in patients who had less than 8 hours' delay from the onset of neurological symptoms to surgery [63]. It is also important to consider the risk of bleeding during removal of the epidural catheter as the pregnancy-induced rise in factor levels may quickly reverse after delivery [84]. Vandermeulen *et al.* [63] found that almost 50% of spinal hematomas associated with epidural catheter use occurred at the time of removal. Therefore, assessment of the coagulation status and continuation of prophylaxis, if indicated, are equally important for the removal of the epidural catheter.

Other regional block techniques

Paracervical block

This can be used to relieve pain during the first stage of labor and involves the injection of local anesthetic into the cervix. Repeated administration may be required because of its relatively short duration of effect. Although it is easy to perform, concerns over its safety to the fetus and the availability of other effective alternatives have diminished its popularity significantly. Many studies have reported its association with fetal bradycardia and acidosis [85–87]. The cause of these effects is uncertain, but the proposed theories include vasoconstriction of the uterine vessels, leading to a reduction in uterine perfusion and fetal hypoxia or a direct toxic effect via placental transfer of local anesthetic [88]. For these reasons, it should be avoided if there is potential fetal compromise.

Pudendal block

This is primarily used to relieve pain during the second stage of labor. This technique involves the injection of local anesthetic solution into the bilateral pudendal nerves in the pelvis, either through a transvaginal or, less commonly, through a transperineal approach. It can provide pain relief for normal delivery, instrumental deliveries, and episiotomy. The potential complications include systemic toxicity as a result of intravascular administration, maternal hematoma, and infection [89–91].

In women with inherited bleeding disorders, paracervical and pudendal blocks are not advisable if the clotting defects have not been corrected. Perineal infiltration with local anesthetic agents is sometimes performed for certain procedures, such as episiotomy repair, but should be carried out with caution because of the risk of bleeding complications. However, if the mother's clotting defect has been corrected, she may be offered these options depending on other maternal and fetal risks.

General anesthesia

When a cesarean section is required for delivery, usually a regional or general anesthesia is administered. In the last few decades, the number of cesarean sections performed in the UK has risen, but anesthetic mortality related to pregnancy has fallen. Obstetric anesthesia for cesarean section in the UK is considerably safer than in the 1960s, when the majority of cesarean sections were performed under general anesthesia [92]. Between 1970 and 1972, there were 37 anesthetic-related maternal deaths, but regional blocks were performed in only two [93]. Between 2000 and 2002, there were six anesthetic-related deaths, all of which were associated with the use of general anesthesia [92]. General anesthesia in the obstetric population is associated with a higher incidence of difficult and failed intubation. Aspiration of the gastric contents is also more likely to occur because of slower gastric emptying in pregnancy. These complications have been identified as the predominant cause of maternal mortality related to anesthesia. The reduction in anesthetic-related maternal mortality over the last few decades is probably due to increased awareness of the important anesthetic issues, better organization of obstetric services, and a change from the widespread use of general anesthesia to the safer regional blockade as the technique of choice for cesarean sections.

Although regional techniques are the preferred method for anesthesia for cesarean sections, there are circumstances when general anesthesia is indicated. They include emergency procedures for which there is not enough time to establish regional blockade, inadequate or failed regional anesthesia, and an uncorrected maternal bleeding diathesis that renders an epidural contraindicated.

Postoperative pain relief is also an issue following general anesthesia because the analgesic benefits of an epidural are not available and non-steroidal drugs are contraindicated in women with bleeding disorders as they interfere with platelet function. A regime containing regular paracetamol and codeine can be given to reduce the postoperative pain. Opiate drugs can be administered intravenously through a PCA device and this is a suitable option for women with inherited bleeding disorders in whom intramuscular injections are contraindicated and postoperative ileus can make absorption via the oral route unreliable.

Conclusion

Management of obstetric analgesia and anesthesia in women with inherited bleeding disorders requires careful planning and risk assessments. Non-pharmacological and non-invasive methods of pain relief are usually not contraindicated in women with inherited bleeding disorders. The use of inhalation analgesia (Entonox) is considered safe in these women, but intramuscular opioids should be avoided in women with uncorrected coagulopathy because of the risk of bleeding and bruising in the mother. Remifentanil PCA presents a promising alternative labor analgesic, but further efficacy and safety data are required before its use can be recommended. It is possible to offer women with inherited bleeding disorders the option of regional block techniques, provided their coagulation defects have been corrected either because of a spontaneous rise in the level of the deficient clotting factor during pregnancy or because of prophylactic treatment. Regional techniques are contraindicated in women with uncorrected coagulopathy because of the increased risk of bleeding complications and subsequent neurological sequelae. The use of a regional block in women with inherited bleeding disorders must be preceded by thorough discussions on its risks and benefits, detailed assessment of coagulation status, and careful planning for any prophylactic treatment required. Close collaboration between hematologists, anesthetists, and obstetricians is crucial for ensuring optimal outcomes.

References

1 Mersky H. Pain terms: a list with definitions and a note on usage. Recommended by the International Association for the Study of Pain (IASP) Subcommittee on Taxonomy. *Pain* 1979; **6**: 249–252.

2 Kadir RA, Economides DL, Braithwaite J, *et al*. The obstetric experience of carriers of haemophilia. *Br J Obstet Gynaecol* 1997; **104**: 803–810.

3 Kadir RA, Lee CA, Sabin CA, *et al*. Pregnancy in women with von Willebrand's disease or factor XI deficiency. *Br J Obstet Gynaecol* 1998; **105**: 314–321.

4 Greer IA, Lowe GDO, Walker JJ, Forbes CD. Haemorrhagic problems in obstetrics and gynaecology in patients with congenital coagulopathies. *Br J Obstet Gynaecol* 1991; **98**: 909–918.

5 Smith CA, Collins CT, Cyna AM, Crowther CA. Complementary and alternative therapies for pain management in labour. *Cochrane Database Syst Rev* 2006; **4**: CD003521.

6 Rae S, Wildsmith J. So just who was James "Young" Simpson? *Br J Anaesth* 1997; **79**: 271–273.

7 Secher O. Chloroform to a Royal family. In: Atkinson RS and Boulton TB, eds. *The history of anaesthesia*. London: Royal Society of Medicine Services, 1987; 242–256.

8 Klikowitsch S. Uber das Stickstoffoxydul als Anaesthetikum bei Geburten. *Arch Gynaekologir* 1881; **18**: 81–108.

9 Minnitt R. Self-administered anaesthesia in childbirth. *BMJ* 1934; **1**: 501–503.

10 McGuiness C, Rosen M. Enflurane as an analgesia in labour. *Anaesthesia* 1984; **39**: 24–26.

11 Wee MY, Hasan MA, Thomas TA. Isoflurane in labour. *Anaesthesia* 1993; **48**: 369–372.

12 Yeo ST, Holdcroft A, Yentis SM, Stewart A. Analgesia with sevoflurane during labour. i. Determination of the optimum concentration. *Br J Anaesth* 2007; **98**: 105–109.

13 Yeo ST, Holdcrof A, Yentis SM, *et al*. Analgesia with sevoflurane during labour. ii. Sevoflurane compared with Entonox for labour analgesia. *Br J Anaesth* 2007; **98**: 110–115.

14 Rosen MA. Nitrous oxide for relief of labour pain: a systematic review. *Am J Obstet Gynecol* 2002; **186**: S110–126.

15 Rosen M. Recent advances in pain relief in childbirth: inhalation and systematic analgesia. *Br J Anaesth* 1971; **43**: 837–848.

16 McAneny T, Doughty A. Self-administered nitrous-oxide/oxygen analgesia in obstetrics. *Anaesthesia* 1963; **18**: 488–497.

17 Committee MRC. Reports to the Medical Research Council of the Committee on Nitrous Oxide and Oxygen Analgesia in Midwifery. Clinical trials of different concentrations of oxygen and nitrous oxide for obstetric analgesia. *BMJ* 1970; **1**: 709–713.

18 Stefani S, Hughes S, Shnider SM, *et al*. Neonatal neurobehavioral effects of inhalation analgesia for vaginal delivery. *Anesthesiology* 1982; **56**: 351–355.

19 Harmer M, Rosen M. Parenteral opioids. In: Van Zundert A, Ostenheimer GW, eds. *Pain relief and anaesthesia in obstetrics*. Edinburgh: Churchill Livingstone; 1996; 365–372.

20 Wiener PC, Hogg MI, Rosen M. Neonatal respiration, feeding and neurobehavioural state. Effects of intrapartum bupivacaine, pethidine and pethidine reversed by naloxone. *Anaesthesia* 1979; **34**: 996–1004.

21 Shnider SM, Moya F. Effects of meperidine on the newborn infant. *Am J Obstet Gynecol* 1964; **89**: 1009–1015.

22 Belsey EM, Rosenblatt DB, Lieberman BA, *et al*. The influence of maternal analgesia on neonatal behaviour. I. Pethidine. *Br J Obstet Gynaecol* 1981; **88**: 398–406.

23 Kron RE, Stein M, Goddard KE. Newborn sucking behavior affected by obstetric sedation. *Pediatrics* 1966; **37**: 1012–1016.

24 Righard L, Alade MO. Effect of delivery room routines on success of first breast-feed. *Lancet* 1990; **336**: 1105–1107.

25 Nissen E, Lilja G, Matthiesen AS, *et al.* Effects of maternal pethidine on infants' developing breast feeding behaviour. *Acta Paediatr* 1995; **84**: 140–145.

26 Matthews MK. The relationship between maternal labour analgesia and delay in the initiation of breastfeeding in healthy neonates in the early neonatal period. *Midwifery* 1989; **5**: 3–10.

27 Crowell MK, Hill PD, Humenick SS. Relationship between obstetric analgesia and time of effective breast feeding. *J Nurse Midwifery* 1994; **39**: 150–156.

28 Hodgkinson R, Bhatt M, Wang CN. Double-blind comparison of the neurobehaviour of neonates following the administration of different doses of meperidine to the mother. *Can Anaesth Soc J* 1978; **25**: 405–411.

29 Jones R, Pegrum A, Stacey RGW. Patient-controlled analgesia using remifentanil in the parturient with thrombocytopenia. *Anaesthesia* 1999; **54**: 461–465.

30 Thurlow JA, Waterhouse P. Patient-controlled analgesia in labour using remifentanil in two parturients with platelet abnormalities. *Br J Anaesth* 2000; **84**: 411–413.

31 Saravanakumar K, Garstang JS, Hasan K. Intravenous patient-controlled analgesia for labour: a survey of UK practice. *Int J Obstet Anesth* 2007; **16**: 221–225.

32 Glass PS, Hardman D, Kamiyama Y, *et al.* Preliminary pharmacokinetics and pharmacodynamics of an ultra-short-acting opioid: remifentanil (GI87084B). *Anesth Analg* 1993; **77**: 1031–1040.

33 Kapila A, Glass PS, Jacobs JR, *et al.* Measured context-sensitive half-times of remifentanil and alfentanil. *Anesthesiology* 1995; **83**: 968–975.

34 Egan TD. Remifentanil pharmacokinetics and pharmacodynamics. A preliminary appraisal. *Clin Pharmacokinet* 1995; **29**: 80–94.

35 Kan RE, Hughes SC, Rosen MA, *et al.* Intravenous remifentanil: placental transfer, maternal and neonatal effects. *Anesthesiology* 1998; **88**: 1467–1471.

36 Volmanen P, Akural E, Raudaskoski T, *et al.* Comparison of remifentanil and nitrous oxide in labour analgesia. *Acta Anaesthesiol Scand* 2005; **49**: 453–458.

37 Thurlow JA, Laxton CH, Dick A, *et al.* Remifentanil by patient-controlled analgesia compared with intramuscular meperidine for pain relief in labour. *Br J Anaesth* 2002; **88**: 374–378.

38 Blair JM, Dobson GT, Hill DA, *et al.* Patient controlled analgesia for labour: a comparison of remifentanil with pethidine. *Anaesthesia* 2005; **60**: 22–27.

39 Blair JM, Hill DA, Fee JP. Patient-controlled analgesia for labour using remifentanil: a feasibility study. *Br J Anaesth* 2001; **87**: 415–420.

40 Volmanen P, Akural EI, Raudaskoski T, Alahuhta S. Remifentanil in obstetric analgesia: a dose-finding study. *Anesth Analg* 2002; **94**: 913–917.

41 Volikas I, Butwick A, Wilkinson C, *et al.* Maternal and neonatal side-effects of remifentanil patient-controlled analgesia in labour. *Br J Anaesth* 2005; **95**: 504–509.

42 Novoa L, Navarro EM, Vieito AM, *et al.* [Obstetric analgesia and anesthesia with remifentanyl in a patient with von Willebrand disease]. *Rev Esp Anestesiol Reanim* 2003; **50**: 242–244.

43 Volmanen P, Alahuhta S. Will remifentanil be a labour analgesic? *Int J Obstet Anesth* 2004; **13**: 1–4.

44 Kreis O. Über medullarnarkose bei gebärenden. *Centralbl Gyn* 1900; **28**: 724–729.

45 Sicard JA, Forestier J. Methode radiographique d'exploration de la cavite epidurale par le lipiodol. *Rev Neurol (Paris)* 1921; **37**: 1264–1266.

46 Tuohy EB. Continuous spinal anaesthesia: a new method utilizing a ureteral catheter. *Surg Clin North Am* 1945; **25**: 834–840.

47 Department of Health. *Statistical bulletin – NHS maternity statistics, England: 2003–2004*. London: Department of Health, 2005.

48 Declerq E, Sakala C, Corry M, *et al.* *Listening to mothers: report of the first national survey of women's childbearing experiences*. New York: Maternity Center Association/Harris Interactive, 2002.

49 Stamer UM, Grond S, Schneck H, Wulf H. Surveys on the use of regional anaesthesia in obstetrics. *Curr Opin Anaesthesiol* 1999; **12**: 565–571.

50 Comparative Obstetric Mobile Epidural trial (COMET) Study Group UK. Effect of low dose mobile versus traditional epidural techniques on mode of delivery: a randomised control trial. *Lancet* 2001; **358**: 19–23.

51 Murphy JD, Henderson K, Bowden MI, *et al.* Bupivacaine versus bupivacaine plus fentanyl for epidural analgesia: effect on maternal satisfaction. *BMJ* 1991; **302**: 564–567.

52 Bloom SL, McIntyre DD, Kelly MA, *et al.* Lack of effect of walking on labor and delivery. *N Engl J Med* 1998; **339**: 76–79.

53 Simmons SW, Cyna AM, Dennis AT, Hughes D. Combined spinal-epidural versus epidural analgesia in labour. *Cochrane Database Syst Rev* 2007; **3**: CD003401.

54 Anim-Somuah M, Smyth R, Howell C. Epidural versus non-epidural or no analgesia in labour. *Cochrane Database Syst Rev* 2005; **4**: CD000331.

55 Juul J, Lie B, Friberg Nielsen S. Epidural analgesia vs. general anesthesia for cesarean section. *Acta Obstet Gynecol Scand* 1998; **67**: 203–206.

56 Lie B, Juul J. Effect of epidural vs. general anesthesia on breastfeeding. *Acta Obstet Gynecol Scand* 1988; **67**: 207–209.

57 Evans CM, Murphy JF, Gray OP, Rosen M. Epidural versus general anaesthesia for elective caesarean section. Effect on Apgar score and acid-base status of the newborn. *Anaesthesia* 1989; **44**: 778–782.

58 Buggy D, Gardiner J. The space blanket and shivering during extradural analgesia in labour. *Acta Anaesthesiol Scand* 1995; **39**: 551–553.

59 Eberle RL, Norris MC. Labour analgesia. A risk-benefit analysis. *Drug Safety* 1996; **14** (4): 239–251.

60 Liang CC, Wong SY, Tsay PT, *et al*. The effect of epidural analgesia on postpartum urinary retention in women who deliver vaginally. *Int J Obstet Anesth* 2002; **11**: 164–169.

61 Crawford JS. Some maternal complications of epidural analgesia for labour. *Anaesthesia* 1985; **40**: 1219–1225.

62 Scott DB, Hibbard BM. Serious non-fatal complications associated with extradural block in obstetric practice. *Br J Anaesth* 1990; **64**: 537–541.

63 Vandermeulen EP, Van Aken H, Vermylen J. Anticoagulants and spinal-epidural anesthesia. *Anesth Analg* 1994; **79**: 1165–1177.

64 Abramovitz S, Beilin Y. Thrombocytopenia, low molecular weight heparin, and obstetric anesthesia. *Anesthesiol Clin North Am* 2003; **21**: 99–109.

65 Cohen S, Daitch JS, Amar D, Goldiner PL. Epidural analgesia for labor and delivery in a patient with von Willebrand's disease. *Reg Anesth* 1989; **14**: 95–97.

66 Milaskiewicz RM, Holdcroft A, Letsky E. Epidural anaesthesia and von Willebrand's disease. *Anaesthesia* 1990; **45**: 462–464.

67 Caliezi C, Tsakiris DA, Behringer H, *et al*. Two consecutive pregnancies and deliveries in a patient with von Willebrand's disease type 3. *Haemophilia* 1998; **4**: 845–849.

68 Jones BP, Bell EA, Maroof M. Epidural labor analgesia in a parturient with von Willebrand's disease type IIA and severe preeclampsia. *Anesthesiology* 1999; **90**: 1219–1220.

69 Cohen S, Zada Y. Neuroaxial block for von Willebrand's disease. *Anaesthesia* 2001; **56**: 397.

70 David AL, Paterson-Brown S, Letsky EA. Factor XI deficiency presenting in pregnancy: diagnosis and management. *Br J Obstet Gynaecol* 2002; **109**: 840–843.

71 Perez-Barrero P, Gil L, Martinez C, *et al*. [Treatment with desmopressin before epidural anesthesia in a patient with type I von Willebrand disease]. *Rev Esp Anestesiol Reanim* 2003; **50**: 526–529.

72 Dhar P, Abramovitz S, DiMichele D, *et al*. Management of pregnancy in a patient with severe haemophilia A. *Br J Anaesth* 2003; **91**: 432–435.

73 Varughese J, Cohen AJ. Experience with epidural anaesthesia in pregnant women with von Willebrand disease. *Haemophilia* 2007; **13**: 730–733.

74 Myers B, Pavord S, Kean L, *et al*. Pregnancy outcomes in Factor XI deficiency: incidence of miscarriage, antenatal and postnatal haemorrhage in 33 women with Factor XI deficiency. *Br J Obstet Gynaecol* 2007; **114**: 643–646.

75 Marrache D, Mercier FJ, Boyer-Neumann C, *et al*. Epidural analgesia for parturients with type 1 von Willebrand disease. *Int J Obstet Anesth* 2007; **16**: 231–235.

76 Chi C, Lee CA, England A, *et al*. Intrapartum pain relief in women with inherited bleeding disorders [Abstract]. *Haemophilia* 2006; **12** (Suppl 2): 146.

77 British Committee for Standards in Haematology. Guidelines for the investigation and management of idiopathic thrombocytopenic purpura in adults, children and in pregnancy. *Br J Haematol* 2003; **120**: 574–596.

78 Lee CA, Chi C, Pavord SR, *et al*. The obstetric and gynaecological management of women with inherited bleeding disorders – review with guidelines produced by a taskforce of UK Haemophilia Centre Doctors' Organization. *Haemophilia* 2006; **12**: 301–336.

79 United Kingdom Haemophilia Centre Doctors' Organisation. Guidelines on the selection and use of therapeutic products to treat haemophilia and other hereditary bleeding disorders. *Haemophilia* 2003; **9**: 1–23.

80 Bolton-Maggs PH, Perry DJ, Chalmers EA, *et al*. The rare coagulation disorders – review with guidelines for management from the United Kingdom Haemophilia Centre Doctors' Organisation. *Haemophilia* 2004; **10**: 593–628.

81 Haljamae H. Thromboprophylaxis, coagulation disorders, and regional anaesthesia. *Acta Anaesthesiol Scand* 1996; **40**: 1024–1040.

82 Verniquet AJW. Vessel puncture with epidural catheters. Experience in obstetric patients. *Anaesthesia* 1980; **35**: 660–662.

83 Wulf H. Epidural anaesthesia and spinal haematoma. *Can J Anaesth* 1996; **43**: 1260–1271.

84 Hanna W, McCarroll D, McDonald T, *et al*. Variant von Willebrand's disease and pregnancy. *Blood* 1981; **58**: 873–879.

85 Nyirjesy I, Hawks BL, Herbert JE, *et al*. Hazards of the use of parcervical block anesthesia in obstetrics. *Am J Obstet Gynecol* 1963; **15**: 231–235.

86 Teramo K, Widholm O. Studies of the effect of anaesthetics on foetus. I. The effect of paracervical block with mepivacaine upon fetal acid-base values. *Acta Obstet Gynecol Scand* 1967; **46** (Suppl 2): 1–39.

87 Gordon HR. Fetal bradycardia after paracervical block: correlation with fetal and maternal blood levels of local anesthetic (mepivacaine). *N Engl J Med* 1968; **279**: 910–914.

88 Thiery M, Vroman S. Fetal bradycardia after paracervical block analgesia in labor. *Acta Anaesthesiol Belg* 1973; **24**: 288–292.

89 Svancarek W, Chirino O, Schaefer G Jr, Blythe JG. Retropsoas and subgluteal abscesses following paracervical and pudendal anesthesia. *JAMA* 1977; **237**: 892–894.

90 Bozynski ME, Rubarth LB, Patel JA. Lidocaine toxicity after maternal pudendal anesthesia in a term infant with fetal distress. *Am J Perinatol* 1987; **4**: 164–166.

91 Kurzel RB, Au AH, Rooholamini SA. Retroperitoneal hematoma as a complication of pudendal block – diagnosis made by computed tomography. *West J Med* 1996; **164**: 523–525.

92 Why Mothers Die. *Report on confidential enquiries into maternal deaths in the United Kingdom 2002–2004.* London: RCOG Press; 2004.

93 Department of Health and Social Security. *Report on health and social subjects, no. 11. Report on confidential enquiries into maternal deaths in England and Wales 1970–1972.* London: HMSO, 1975.

12 The newborn

H Marijke van den Berg and Rochelle Winikoff

Introduction

Bleeding problems in the newborn can have severe consequences. The newborn is in a very vulnerable state and has to survive the serious effects that delivery and early neonatal life have on hemostasis. Therefore it is very important to have knowledge and understanding about specific haemostatic issues in newborns that have an effect on this situation.

Bleeding problems in the newborn can be divided into inherited bleeding disorders, physiologic aberrations of hemostasis, and acquired hemostasic abnormalities such as vitamin K deficiency or septicemia. All of these factors will affect hemostasis and can lead to an increased bleeding tendency in the newborn.

The most common inherited coagulation disorders are hemophilia A and hemophilia B. Hemophilia in the newborn presents a number of challenges in terms of both diagnosis and management unique to this age group [1]. In the presence of a family history of hemophilia, optimal management requires close cooperation between specialists in obstetrics, hematology, and neonatology, each of whom has an important role to play in ensuring a safe outcome for these infants. More problematic is where a family history is absent or has not been adequately elucidated, in which case the diagnosis of hemophilia in the neonate will not be suspected. Diagnostic difficulties may then arise because of failure to recognize the presence of abnormal bleeding, which is often different from that typically observed in older children with hemophilia. In addition, diagnostic investigations are complicated by physiological differences in the neonatal hemostatic system [2, 3].

Although major bleeding directly after birth is relatively uncommon in severe hemophilia, the incidence of intracranial hemorrhage is higher during the first few days of life than at any other stage in childhood. Hemophilia is an inherited disease which is X linked [4]. This means that all daughters of a father with hemophilia will be obligate carriers of hemophilia and none of his sons will be affected with hemophilia. However, from the maternal side, the mode of transmission may seem less clear (unless a mother already has a hemophilic child), since women who are carriers of hemophilia are not always diagnosed as carriers either because they are relatively asymptomatic or because they have minor hemorrhagic symptoms. In these cases, the possibility of hemophilia in a male offspring may not be suspected antenatally. In asymptomatic female carriers 30% of hemophilic mutations are reported to be *de novo*. Moreover, in large prospective studies of newborns with severe hemophilia, it has been observed that >50% of the boys with severe hemophilia did not have a positive family history for hemophilia [5, 6]. This means that hemophilic boys born in these situations have no special care during delivery and the diagnosis is made later in their life. This puts them at risk of serious hemorrhagic complications at the time of delivery, such as intracranial hemorrhage and its associated morbidity. It may also lead to a distressing

Inherited Bleeding Disorders in Women, 1st edition. By CA Lee, RA Kadir and PA Kouides. Published 2009 by Blackwell Publishing, ISBN: 978-1-4051-6915-8.

period in which the parents are suspected of child abuse because of unusual bleeding such as ecchymoses and hemarthroses [7]. In some contemporary reports suspected physical child abuse has affected up to 30% of the newly diagnosed cases of children with severe hemophilia. For the families this is very difficult and leads to mistrusting the care givers even after an appropriate diagnosis is finally made [7].

It is important that physicians are aware that a congenital bleeding disorder should be suspected in every child with an increased hemorrhagic diathesis even when there is a negative family history. Also, in a child for whom the parents are suspected of child abuse, appropriate laboratory tests to exclude a bleeding disorder should be part of the investigations.

Apart from the recognition of congenital bleeding disorders, other acquired disorders may have an impact and can cause an increased bleeding tendency. More knowledge therefore about special disease status and their relationship to a bleeding tendency is important.

Hemostasis is a dynamic and evolving mechanism that is age dependent and begins *in utero*. Recent studies have provided age-dependent reference values that delineate age-dependent features of hemostasis and facilitate the evaluation of infants with hemostatic disorders. The reference values of hemostatic parameters in newborns are very different from those of older children and adults. The prevalence of thromboembolic and hemorrhagic complications is much lower in newborns than in adults. This is true also for sick neonates in whom additional risk factors are necessary for thromboembolic events. However, hemorrhagic complications are common in sick newborns and are often due to vitamin K deficiency and asphyxia [8]. In fact, serious hemorrhagic problems in the first week of life are more frequently due to acquired pathologic disorders. Thus special attention is needed when children with severe inherited bleeding disorders encounter other complications during delivery or shortly after birth.

The evaluation of the laboratory values in a newborn can be a challenge, since the physiological levels of many coagulation proteins are low, and this makes it difficult to establish the diagnosis of an inherited or an acquired disorder. However, severe congenital deficiencies such as hemophilia A can be correctly diagnosed immediately after birth. Milder diagnoses can often be suspected but need to be confirmed some months later.

In this chapter bleeding complications in the neonatal period will be discussed, including hemostatic laboratory differences between preterm and term newborns; the diagnosis of inherited bleeding disorders in the newborn; and the prevention and treatment of bleeding in the newborn.

Hemostatic parameters in the newborn

Platelets

The number of platelets in the preterm and newborn is similar to that in adults, between 150 and 450×10^9/L.

Platelet adhesion is thought to be similar to adults; however, few data are available regarding platelet aggregation in the newborn. Functional assays in neonates are difficult to perform because of the large quantities of blood needed and because of difficulties in venipuncture where impaired blood flow may activate coagulation proteins and platelets. There is also strong evidence that platelets are activated during delivery. It is speculated that thermal changes, hypoxia, acidosis, and adrenergic stimulation may play a role in the increase of thromboxane B2, β-thromboglobulin and platelet factor 4 in the neonate found immediately after birth.

Coagulation factors

Establishing reference values for coagulation factors in newborns is difficult because frequent blood samples and micro-techniques are required to determine the coagulation proteins. Ethically, this is difficult to justify in healthy children and therefore reference values are often obtained from sick newborns. A bleeding diathesis in the newborn is most commonly caused by acquired vitamin K deficiency and therefore the factors II, VII, IX and X are the most studied coagulation factors in this age group [8].

Tables 12.1 and 12.2 [2, 3] give the reference values in preterm and term healthy infants during the first 6 months of their life. Most coagulation proteins will increase to adult levels during the first 6 months of life. Factor VIII is already normal at delivery, which means that a child with hemophilia A can be diagnosed directly after birth. For factor IX the level is lower than normal and will increase to normal levels at 6 months.

Table 12.1 Reference values for coagulation tests in the healthy full-term infant during the first 6 months of life (This research was originally published in *Blood*. Andrew *et al.* [2] © American Society of Hematology)

Tests	Day 1 (*n*)	Day 5 (*n*)	Day 30 (*n*)	Day 90 (*n*)	Day 180 (*n*)	Adult (*n*)
PT (s)	13.0 ± 1.43 (61)*	12.4 ± 1.46 (77)*†	11.8 ± 1.25 (67)*†	11.9 ± 1.15 (62)*	12.3 ± 0.79 (47)*	12.4 ± 0.78 (29)
APTT (s)	42.9 ± 5.80 (61)	42.6 ± 8.63 (76)	40.4 ± 7.42 (67)	37.1 ± 6.52 (62)*	35.5 ± 3.71 (47)*	33.5 ± 3.44 (29)
TCT (s)	23.5 ± 2.38 (58)*	23.1 ± 3.07 (64)†	24.3 ± 2.44 (63)*	26.1 ± 2.32 (62)*	26.5 ± 2.86 (41)*	26.0 ± 2.66 (19)
Fibrinogen (g/L)	2.83 ± 0.58 (61)*	3.12 ± 0.75 (77)*	2.70 ± 0.54 (67)*	2.43 ± 0.68 (60)*†	2.51 ± 0.68 (47)*†	2.78 ± 0.61 (29)
FII (U/mL)	0.48 ± 0.11 (61)	0.63 ± 0.15 (76)	0.68 ± 0.17 (67)	0.75 ± 0.15 (62)	0.88 ± 0.14 (47)	1.08 ± 0.19 (29)
FV (U/mL)	0.72 ± 0.18 (61)	0.96 ± 0.26 (76)	0.98 ± 0.18 (67)	0.90 ± 0.21 (62)	0.91 ± 0.18 (47)	1.06 ± 0.22 (28)
FVII (U/mL)	0.66 ± 0.19 (60)	0.89 ± 0.27 (75)	0.90 ± 0.24 (67)	0.91 ± 0.26 (62)	0.87 ± 0.20 (47)	1.05 ± 0.19 (29)
FVIII (U/mL)	1.00 ± 0.39 (60)*†	0.88 ± 0.33 (75)*†	0.91 ± 0.33 (67)*†	0.79 ± 0.23 (62)*†	0.73 ± 0.18 (47)†	0.99 ± 0.25 (29)
VWF (U/mL)	1.53 ± 0.67 (40)†	1.40 ± 0.57 (43)†	1.28 ± 0.59 (40)†	1.18 ± 0.44 (40)†	1.07 ± 0.45 (46)†	0.92 ± 0.33 (29)†
FIX (U/mL)	0.53 ± 0.19 (59)	0.53 ± 0.19 (75)	0.51 ± 0.15 (67)	0.67 ± 0.23 (62)	0.86 ± 0.25 (47)	1.09 ± 0.27 (29)
FX (U/mL)	0.40 ± 0.14 (60)	0.49 ± 0.16 (76)	0.59 ± 0.14 (67)	0.71 ± 0.18 (62)	0.78 ± 0.20 (47)	1.08 ± 0.23 (29)
FXI (U/mL)	0.38 ± 0.14 (60)	0.55 ± 0.16 (74)	0.53 ± 0.13 (67)	0.69 ± 0.14 (62)	0.86 ± 0.24 (47)	0.97 ± 0.15 (29)
FXII (U/mL)	0.53 ± 0.20 (60)	0.47 ± 0.18 (75)	0.49 ± 0.16 (67)	0.67 ± 0.21 (62)	0.77 ± 0.19 (47)	1.08 ± 0.28 (29)
PK (U/mL)	0.37 ± 0.16 (45)†	0.48 ± 0.14 (51)	0.57 ± 0.17 (48)	0.73 ± 0.16 (46)	0.86 ± 0.15 (43)	1.12 ± 0.25 (29)
HMW-K (U/mL)	0.54 ± 0.24 (47)	0.74 ± 0.28 (63)	0.77 ± 0.22 (50)*	0.82 ± 0.32 (46)*	0.82 ± 0.23 (48)*	0.92 ± 0.22 (29)
FXIIIa (IU/mL)	0.79 ± 0.26 (44)	0.94 ± 0.25 (49)*	0.93 ± 0.27 (44)*	1.04 ± 0.34 (44)*	1.04 ± 0.29 (41)*	1.05 ± 0.25 (29)
FXIIIb (IU/mL)	0.76 ± 0.23 (44)	1.06 ± 0.37 (47)*	1.11 ± 0.36 (45)*	1.16 ± 0.34 (44)*	1.10 ± 0.30 (41)*	0.97 ± 0.20 (29)
Plasminogen (CTA, U/mL)	1.95 ± 0.35 (44)	2.17 ± 0.38 (60)	1.98 ± 0.36 (52)	2.48 ± 0.37 (44)	3.01 ± 0.40 (47)	3.36 ± 0.44 (29)

All factors except fibrinogen and plasminogen are expressed as units per milliliter where pooled plasma contains 1.0 U/mL. Plasminogen units are those recommended by the Committee of Thrombolytic Agents (CTS). All values are expressed as mean ± 1 SD.

*Values do not differ significantly from the adult values.

†These measurements are skewed because of a disproportionate number of high values. The lower limit that excludes the lower 2.5th percentile of the population has been given in the respective figures. The lower limit for factor VIII was 0.50 U/mL at all time points for the infant.

Table 12.2 Reference values for coagulation tests in healthy premature infants during the first 6 months of life (This research was originally published in *Blood*. Andrew *et al.* [15] © American Society of Hematology)

Tests	Day 1 (n)		Day 5 (n)		Day 30 (n)		Day 90 (n)		Day 180 (n)		Adult (n)	
	M	B	M	B	M	B	M	B	M	B	M	B
PT (s)	13.0	(10.6–16.2)*	12.5	(10.0–15.3)*†	11.8	(10–13.6)*	12.3	(10.0–14.6)*	12.5	(10.0–15.0)*	12.4	(10.8–13.9)
APTT (s)	53.6	(27.5–79.4)‡	50.5	(26.9–74.1)‡	44.7	(26.9–62.5)	39.5	(28.3–50.70)	37.5	(21.7–53.3)*	33.5	(26.6–40.3)
TCT (s)	24.8	(18.2–30.4)*	24.1	(18.8–29.4)*	24.4	(18.8–29.9)*	25.1	(19.4–30.80)*	25.2	(18.9–31.5)*	26.0	(18.7–30.3)
Fibrinogen (g/L)	2.43	(1.5–3.73)*†‡	2.80	(1.6–4.18)*†‡	2.54	(1.50–4.14)*†	2.46	(1.50–3.52)*†	2.28	(1.5–3.60)†	2.78	(1.58–4.00)
FII (U/mL)	0.45	(0.20–0.77)†	0.57	(0.28–0.85)‡	0.57	(0.36–0.95)†‡	0.68	(0.30–1.06)	0.87	(0.51–1.23)	1.08	(0.70–1.48)
FV (U/mL)	0.88	(0.41–1.44)*†‡	1.00	(0.48–1.54)	1.02	(0.481.56)	0.99	(0.59–1.39)	1.02	(0.58–1.46)	1.06	(0.62–1.50)
FVII (U/mL)	0.67	(0.21–1.13)	0.84	(0.30–1.38)	0.83	(0.21–1.45)	0.87	(0.31–1.43)	0.99	(0.47–1.51)*	1.05	(0.67–1.43)
FVIII (U/mL)	1.11	(0.50–2.13)*†	1.15	(0.53–2.05)*†‡	1.11	(0.50–1.89)*†‡	1.06	(0.58–1.88)*†‡	0.99	(0.50–1.87)*†‡	0.99	(0.50–1.49)
VWF (U/mL)	1.36	(0.78–2.10)†	1.33	(0.72–2.19)†	1.36	(0.68–2.16)†	0.12	(0.75–1.84)*†	0.98	(0.54–1.58)*†	0.92	(0.50–1.53)
FIX (U/mL)	0.35	(0.19–0.65)†‡	0.42	(0.14–0.74)†‡	0.44	(0.13–0.80)†	0.59	(0.25–0.93)	0.81	(0.50–1.20)†	1.09	(0.55–1.63)
FX (U/mL)	0.41	(0.11–0.71)	0.51	(0.18–0.83)	0.55	(0.20–0.82)	0.67	(0.35–0.89)	0.77	(0.35–1.19)	1.05	(0.70–1.52)
FXI (U/mL)	0.30	(0.08–0.52)†‡	0.41	(0.13–0.69)‡	0.43	(0.15–0.71)‡	0.59	(0.25–0.93)‡	0.78	(0.46–1.10)	0.97	(0.67–1.27)
FXII (U/mL)	0.38	(0.10–0.66)‡	0.39	(0.00–0.69)‡	0.43	(0.11–0.75)	0.61	(0.15–1.07)	0.82	(0.22–1.42)	1.08	(0.52–1.64)
PK (U/mL)	0.33	(0.09–0.57)	0.45	(0.26–0.76)†	0.59	(0.31–0.87)	0.78	(0.37–1.21)	0.78	(0.40–1.16)	1.12	(0.62–1.62)
HMW-K (U/mL)	0.49	(0.09–0.89)	0.62	(0.24–1.00)‡	0.64	(0.16–1.12)‡	0.78	(0.32–1.24)	0.83	(0.41–1.25)*	0.92	(0.50–1.38)
FXIIIa (IU/mL)	0.70	(0.32–1.08)	1.01	(0.67–1.45)*	0.99	(0.51–1.47)*	1.13	(0.71–1.55)*	1.13	(0.85–1.61)*	1.05	(0.55–1.55)
FXIIIb (IU/mL)	0.81	(0.35–1.27)	1.10	(0.68–1.58)*	1.07	(0.57–1.57)*	1.21	(0.75–1.67)	1.15	(0.67–1.63)	0.97	(0.57–1.37)
Plasminogen (CTA, U/mL)	1.70	(1.12–2.48)†‡	1.91	(1.21–2.61)‡	1.81	(1.09–2.53)	2.38	(1.68–3.18)	2.75	(1.68–3.59)‡	3.36	(2.48–4.24)

All factors except fibrinogen and plasminogen are expressed as units per milliliter where pooled plasma contains 1.0 U/mL. Plasminogen units are those recommended by the Committee of Thrombolytic Agents (CTS). All values are given as a mean (M) followed by lower and upper boundary encompassing 95% of the population (B). Between 40 and 96 samples were assayed for each value for newborns.

*Values indistinguishable from those of adults.

†Measurements are skewed because of a disproportionate number of high values. The lower limit that excludes the lower 2.5th percentile of the population has been given (B).

‡Values different from those of full-term infants.

More recently, normal coagulation factor ranges have been published for neonates and children (Table 12.3) [9]. The results reconfirm the age-dependent hemostatic changes and illustrate that the absolute values of reference ranges for coagulation assay in neonates vary with analyzer and reagent systems and in some instances also vary significantly from the results previously reported. This finding confirms the need for laboratories to develop age-related reference ranges specific to their own testing systems.

Inherited bleeding disorders

Hemophilia

Inherited coagulation disorders are rare and the most well characterized inherited bleeding disorder is

Table 12.3 Coagulation factor reference values for neonates and children compared with results from Andrew *et al.* [2] (with permission from Monagle *et al.* [9])

Coagulation factors (%)	Age						
	Day 1	Day 3	1 month–1 year	1–5 years	6–10 years	11–16 years	Adults
II	54* (41–69) n=23 (13F/10M)	62* (50–73) n=22 (11F/11M)	90* (62–103) n=22 (7F/15M)	89* (70–109) n=67 (26F/41M)	89* (67–110) n=64 (23F/41M)	90* (61–107) n=23 (6F/17M)	110 (78–138) n=44
II Andrew et al.	48† (37–59)	63† (48–78)	88† (60–116)	94† (71–116)	88 (67–107)	83† (61–104)	108 (70–146)
V	81* (64–103) n=22 (13F/9M)	122 (92–154) n=22 (11F/11M)	113 (94–141) n=20 (6F/14M)	97* (67–127) n=75 (26F/41M)	99* (56–141) n=64 (23F/41M)	89* (67–141) n=20 (5F/15M)	118 (78–152) n=44
V Andrew et al.	72† (54–90)	99† (70–120)	91† (55–127)	103 (79–127)	90† (63–116)	77† (55–99)	106 (62–150)
VII	70* (52–88) n=22 (12F/10M)	86* (67–107) n=22 (11F/11M)	128 (83–160) n=20 (6F/14M)	111* (72–150) n=66 (25F/41M)	113* (70–154) n=64 (23F/41M)	118 (69–200) n=22 (6F/16M)	129 (61–199) n=44
VII Andrew et al.	66† (47–85)	89† (62–116)	87† (47–127)	82† (55–116)	85 (52–120)	83† (58–115)	105 (67–143)
VIII	182 (105–329) n=20 (9F/11M)	159 (83–274) n=25 (12F/13M)	94* (54–145) n=21 (6F/15M)	110* (36–185) n=45 (26F/19M)	117* (52–182) n=52 (20F/32M)	120* (59–200) n=24 (6F/18M)	160 (52–290) n=44
VIII Andrew et al.	100 (61–139)	88 (55–121)	73† (50–109)	90 (59–142)	95 (58–132)	92 (53–131)	99 (50–149)
IX	48* (35–56) n=24 (11F/13M)	72* (44–97) n=23 (11F/12M)	71* (43–121) n=21 (5F/16M)	85* (44–127) n=44 (25F/19M)	96* (48–145) n=51 (19F/32M)	111* (64–216) n=25 (6F/19M)	130 (59–254) n=44
IX Andrew et al.	53† (34–72)	53† (34–72)	86† (36–136)	73† (47–104)	75† (63–89)	82† (59–122)	109 (55–163)

Table 12.3 (Con't)

Coagulation factors (%)	Age						
	Day 1	Day 3	1 month–1 year	1–5 years	6–10 years	11–16 years	Adults
X	55* (46–67) n=22 (12F/10M)	60* (46–75) n=22 (11F/11M)	95* (77–122) n=21 (6F/15M)	98* (72–125) n=66 (25F/41M)	97* (68–125) n=49 (20F/29M)	91* (53–122) n=24 (7F/17M)	124 (96–171) n=44
X *Andrew et al.*	40† (26–54)	49† (34–64)	78† (38–118)	88† (58–116)	75† (55–101)	79† (50–117)	106 (70–152)
XI	30* (7–41) n=20 (10F/10M)	57* (24–79) n=22 (11F/11M)	89* (62–125) n=22 (6F/16M)	113 (65–162) n=41 (24F/17M)	113 (65–162) n=50 (18F/32M)	111 (65–139) n=24 (5F/19M)	112 (67–196) n=44
XI *Andrew et al.*	38† (24–52)	55† (39–71)	86† (49–134)	97 (56–150)	86 (52–120)	74 (50–97)	97 (67–127)
XII	58* (43–80) n=20 (9F/11M)	53* (14–80) n=21 (11F/10M)	79* (20–135) n=21 (7F/14M)	85* (36–135) n=39 (20F/19M)	81* (26–137) n=45 (17F/28M)	75* (14–117) n=22 (7F/15M)	115 (35–207) n=44
XII *Andrew et al.*	53† (33–73)	47† (29–65)	77† (39–115)	93 (64–129)	92 (60–140)	81† (34–137)	108 (52–164)

Andrew *et al.* results shown for day 3 are actually day 5 results. M = males, F = females.
For each assay the first row shows the mean and boundaries including 95% of the population. The second row shows the number of individual samples and the ratio of males to females for each group.
* Denotes values that are significantly different from adult values ($P < 0.05$).
† Denotes values that are significantly different from adult values for Andrew *et al.* data.

hemophilia. It occurs in 1:10 000 males and the incidence appears to be the same in all ethnicities [4]. However, the reported prevalence of hemophilia patients in countries is variable, reflecting physician awareness, laboratory expertise and socioeconomic context. In countries that are less developed, it is mostly only patients with severe hemophilia who are diagnosed. Because of a lack of treatment in these countries, most of these patients will die before they reach reproductive age. In contrast, in countries where modern hemophilia treatment is available, patients have a normal life expectancy and also will procreate. Moreover, when a patient with mild hemophilia is diagnosed, active counseling of the family members will ultimately lead to more cases being diagnosed. Individuals with mild hemophilia are often unaware of their diagnosis because symptoms or signs of an increased bleeding tendency are rare.

In Western European countries and also in the USA and Canada, a cohort of patients with hemophilia will include the following diagnoses: severe hemophilia in approximately 40%, moderate hemophilia in 20%, and mild hemophilia in 40–50%.

This is very different for countries such as India where genetic counseling is very sensitive. In these countries, both the patients and the female carriers have to live with the burden of a serious disease for which they cannot afford treatment. However, when a newborn is diagnosed with hemophilia, the mother and other relatives should be offered active counseling both to inform them about the risk of giving birth to a child with the disease and to inform carriers that they can transmit the gene to their daughters who will be carriers and to their sons who may be hemophiliacs.

von Willebrand disease

See also Chapter 4.

von Willebrand disease (VWD) is an inherited bleeding disorder that affects both the function of platelets and the coagulation proteins. Patients with VWD will also have a decreased factor VIII:C level because VWF is the carrier protein for FVIII.

The clinical picture of VWD in the neonatal period is mostly less pronounced than for severe haemophilia. However, patients with type 3 VWD suffer from very low FVIII and VWF. These children have an increased risk for intracranial hemorrhage (ICH) and will also demonstrate hematomas and muscle bleeding after a traumatic delivery. This means that, for these children, collaboration between the hematologist, and obstetrician-gynecologist is as important as it is for severe hemophilia. Also in the first 10 days after delivery, physicians should be aware that bleeding can still occur. After the immediate neonatal period, symptoms of subcutaneous bleeding, especially in the mouth, and hematomas will develop after very minor trauma and these symptoms should lead the physician to suspect VWD.

Inherited platelet disorders

Platelet disorders are uncommon, the most well known are Glanzmann disease and Bernard–Soulier. A review of diagnosis and clinical management of these disorders has been published [11]. Bruising and extended bleeding after minor trauma and venipuncture may be the first symptoms. When the number of platelets is above 50×10^9/L and hemophilia and related disorders are excluded, a disorder of platelets should be suspected.

For adequate laboratory diagnosis it is necessary to obtain a sufficient number of platelets for aggregation studies. This is difficult to perform in young children, and therefore studies in affected family members can be extremely helpful in establishing a diagnosis.

Rare bleeding disorders

See also Chapter 5.

Other rare inherited bleeding disorders include fibrinogen, factor II, factor V, factor VII, factor X, factor XI and factor XIII deficiencies. The clinical picture of these deficiencies is different from hemophilia. The bleeding pattern is variable and there seems to be less correlation between the severity of the disease and the factor level. However, clinical data should be interpreted carefully. Especially since ICH is a frequently occurring event in the neonatal period, children may die undiagnosed of their inherited bleeding disorder. This means that there is a predilection for children with milder disorders to end up in clinical series. Special attention should be paid to the potential for selection bias since it may affect interpretation of published results in clinical trials. For this reason, as well as for reasons related to difficulties posed by diagnosis and treatment, it is extremely important that carriers are diagnosed and followed in specialized centers. This will also allow for improved data on childbirth and bleeding problems.

The bleeding diagnosed in patients with factor XIII deficiencies is umbilical cord and central nervous system bleeding. Also it was reported that they had more problems in wound healing.

Laboratory diagnosis

Laboratory diagnosis of inherited bleeding disorders in the newborn is challenging. Difficulties in diagnosis relate both to limitations in blood drawing in the neonate as well as to developmental aspects of neonatal homeostasis. Knowledge of the specific bleeding disorder in the parents is likely to be very informative. Babies felt to be at risk should be managed as if they were affected, and appropriate precautions and interventions taken regardless of the laboratory hemostasis profile. Difficult venipuncture in a small baby may give misleading laboratory coagulation results, especially for platelet function, and repeat samples may be required when there is evidence of hemolysis or clotting in the tube. Care should be taken to use a 21-gauge needle (in the neonates a 22- or 23-gauge needle may be required) whenever possible with minimal stasis to avoid abnormal activation. Underfilling of the trisodium citrate blood collection tube is a common occurrence and should be avoided. Specimens from cord blood are of great value in neonates known to be at risk of an inherited bleeding disorder and should be planned prior to delivery. Although cord blood can be an important source for diagnostic material in neonates, some factors have to be considered. In 50% of newborns with

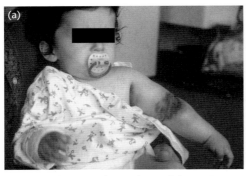
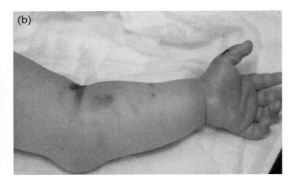

Fig. 12.1 Clinical picture of severe hemophilia. (a) Large muscle and subcutaneous bleed after venous puncture for laboratory tests. (b) Large muscle and subcutaneous bleed with compartment syndrome.

severe hemophilia the diagnosis is not suspected and cord blood is not available for diagnosis. Furthermore, delivery mostly takes place outside office hours and plasma must be frozen directly for tests of hemostasis.

In the neonate there is immaturity of the hepatic gamma-carboxylation steps of vitamin K-dependent coagulation factor production, factors II, VII, IX, and X as well as vitamin K deficiency and thus the exclusion of congenital factor deficiencies is difficult. Disseminated intravascular coagulation (DIC) and liver disease, although uncommon, may complicate the hemostatic picture. Mean values of factor V, XI, and XII are lower than adult values and vary with age [7]. Prematurity further complicates interpretation of these values. Furthermore, difficulties in establishing normal values in neonates makes interpretation of measured values difficult, especially against the usual adult normal ranges. To this end, guidelines have been developed as well as reference ranges for the neonate.

Genetic tests are seldom helpful at birth since clinical decisions and interventions especially in the bleeding child may be urgent and depend heavily on accurate laboratory assessment.

Factor assays are required in all babies at risk of a bleeding disorder or in cases of unexpected bleeding and before surgical procedures such as circumcision. Intramuscular injections and venipunctures must be avoided until a bleeding disorder is excluded. Hepatitis B immunizations should be given intradermally, vitamin K orally [12] and compression should be carried out on all blood puncture sites (Fig. 12.1).

Hemophilia A and B

Factor VIII attains adult levels at birth. A history of a known mother carrier or a family history of hemophilia is very helpful. The cord blood of newborn boys of women known to be carriers should be tested. The activated partial thromboplastin time (APTT) is typically prolonged in hemophilic boys, although borderline normal results are also possible in milder deficiencies and thus specific factor level measures are required. The levels should be measured within 2 hours for accurate results. Accurate and quick diagnostic levels in the offspring of female carriers allows for early management of newborns at risk.

Factor IX levels, in contrast, are low at birth and appropriate age-adjusted normal ranges [7] are essential if a factor deficiency is suspected. It is also important to rule out vitamin K deficiency, and a trial of vitamin K may be appropriate. Liver disease and disseminated intravascular coagulation (DIC) must be excluded as well in newborns who bleed unexpectedly.

Any newborn with unexpected bleeding from puncture sites, surgical interventions, such as circumcision, or easy bruising or bleeding from organs should be suspected of having hemophilia and measurements of coagulation factor VIII and factor IX levels should be made.

von Willebrand disease

Antenatal diagnosis is rarely performed in women with von Willebrand disease (VWD), except for babies at risk of type 3 VWD, hence expectant management is the rule. In newborns at risk for VWD, levels of VWF:Ag, RCoF:Ag and FVIII:C should be measured in cord blood. Normal values may be sufficient to exclude severe forms of VWD in at-risk cases but milder forms may be missed because of increases in these levels induced by the stress of labor [13]. Levels of VWF reach adult levels by 6 months. Type 2b VWD should also be suspected in newborns with a family history and a low platelet count, which may decrease further after stress.

Platelet function disorders

Neonatal testing is not routinely done for the offspring of women with mild, qualitative, or functional platelet defects since neonatal bleeding, even in the most severe Glanzmann and Bernard–Soulier disorders, is unusual. Testing the parents of neonates is particularly important in neonates suspected of inheriting an autosomal recessive type of platelet dysfunction problem such as Glanzmann thrombocytopenia or Bernard–Soulier. The neonate is not at risk of inheriting the full functional platelet defect unless the father is also a heterozygous carrier. It is important to have the paternal carrier status investigated using flow cytometry and the results known prior to delivery. Heterozygote carriers of Bernard–Soulier may on occasion be symptomatic. Maternal antiplatelet antibody status is imperative prior to delivery as well, since fetuses of either disorder are at risk of alloimmune thrombocytopenia and potentially related ICH. Moderate to severe thrombocytopenia in the order of 30×10^9 may be seen occasionally in newborns with Bernard–Soulier and large platelets may be seen on the peripheral blood smear. The platelet count and morphology is typically normal in individuals with Glanzmann disease. In cases where diagnosis is imperative due to genetic transmission or clinical bleeding, flow cytometry should be performed on the neonatal blood and platelet function tests should be carried out in specialized centers. Patients with Glanzmann disease will have a decrease in the number of glycoproteins on their membranes. Absent aggregation to ristocetin is diagnostic of Bernard–Soulier syndrome, whereas isolated aggregation to ristocetin is characteristic of Glanzmann disease.

Neonates at risk of inheriting autosomal dominant platelet function disorders are at risk of bleeding, and the platelet count and function may be measured to triage infants at birth [10].

Acquired deficiency of the vitamin K-dependent coagulation factors and vitamin K deficiency bleeding in infancy

Factors II, VII, IX, and X are vitamin K-dependent coagulation proteins and are typically decreased in the newborn. These reduced levels have been attributed to liver immaturity and can be expected to attain normal adult levels in normal children. Severe deficiencies of these factors because of deficiency in vitamin K may lead to a hemorrhagic diathesis in the newborn called vitamin K deficiency bleeding (VKDB) in infancy. Typically, the international normalized ratio (INR) is prolonged together with a normal fibrinogen and platelet count. Bleeding may be in any form, including ICH, and is preventable and rapidly corrected by the administration of vitamin K. Prolonged jaundice and failure to thrive are predisposing conditions for VKDB. Malabsorption of vitamin K and poor oral intake are other causes of secondary vitamin K deficiency. Vitamin K replacement in the newborn should be instituted to prevent this bleeding.

Since clotting factors may be low because of vitamin K deficiency, it is difficult to diagnose congenital deficiencies of these factors in neonates except for severe deficiencies. All neonates at risk should have factor levels measured on cord blood and should be retested both after a vitamin K challenge and when older. Parental testing for congenital coagulation factor deficiencies prior to pregnancy is useful to identify neonates potentially at risk and to orient coagulation screening at birth. Neonates born to individuals from consanguineous parents are at high risk of severe bleeding diatheses in double heterozygous or homozygous forms.

Rare coagulation factor deficiencies in the newborn

Fibrinogen, coagulation factors II, V, VII, X, XI, XIII. See also Chapter 5.

Inherited disorders of fibrinogen, a hypofibrinogenemia and dysfibrinogenemia, are uncommon disorders with a higher incidence in children of consanguineous parents. The mode of inheritance of dysfibrinogenemia may be autosomal dominant and the clinical phenotype is variable, ranging from asymptomatic to hemorrhagic or thrombotic. Neonates at risk for afibrinogenemia because of consanguineous parents should have levels measured. Typically the prothrombin time (PT) and

171

APTT are prolonged but on occasion can be normal. Thrombin time is a more sensitive test to diagnose dysfibrinogenemia. Dysfibrinogenemia in a neonate should be assumed if the mother is affected and appropriate precautions taken, especially since dysfibrinogenemia is particularly difficult to diagnose in the neonate because of physiologic or acquired dysfibrinogenemia, especially in premature babies. Dysfibrinogenemia with a bleeding phenotype is serious in the neonate and appropriate precautions should be taken to avoid bleeding.

Factor II deficiency is the rarest inherited bleeding disorder and is inherited in an autosomal recessive manner [11]. Newborn bleeding is unusual. The PT and APTT may both be prolonged. Factor II levels may be measured in at-risk neonates but levels must be interpreted in light of age-corrected reference values [7].

Factor V deficiency is an autosomal recessive condition and severe disease is rare except in consanguineous parents. The PT and APTT may be prolonged. Factor V levels should be measured in at-risk babies since ICH is reported in severe cases [11]. Levels increase during the first month of life and so levels should be repeated to exclude mild deficiency.

FVII deficiency is the most common of the rare bleeding disorders and is inherited in an autosomal recessive manner. There is a relatively poor correlation between factor VII deficiency and bleeding. The PT is usually prolonged. This disorder is difficult to diagnose in the newborn owing to low physiologic levels in the newborn. When factor levels are low, screening the parents may be helpful to establish a diagnosis.

Factor X deficiency is a rare autosomal recessive disorder and severe cases are more frequent in consanguineous parents. Neonates with severe factor X deficiency can have significant bleeding. Both the PT and APTT may be prolonged compared with age-adjusted normal ranges. Definitive diagnosis is made with measurements of factor X after typically finding a prolongation of the PT and APTT on coagulation assays. Levels are physiologically low in the neonate, making age-related references imperative for proper interpretation. Newborn levels for diagnosing a severe deficiency are reliable.

Factor XI deficiency is autosomally inherited, with the most severe deficiencies being found in homozygotes or compound heterozygotes. Bleeding also occurs in heterozygous deficiency. It is a rare deficiency in the general population but symptomatic disease is more common in Ashkenazi Jews in whom the prevalence of two common mutations is high. Spontaneous bleeding is rare and bleeding typically occurs postoperatively or post-traumatically. On account of its variable bleeding tendency an effort should be made to identify infants at risk of bleeding antenatally. There is also a predilection to bleed in areas of the body where there is high fibrinolytic activity – the mouth, nose, and genitourinary tracts. ICH in factor XI-deficient infants has not been reported. Prenatal diagnosis is usually reserved for cases only where there is a risk of severe deficiency. In factor XI-deficient neonates the APTT may be prolonged compared with age-adjusted normal levels. In babies at risk, factor XI levels should be measured on the cord blood and may prove useful to assess bleeding risk in neonates who may be circumcised. Tranexamic acid may be given to neonates with a more severe deficiency to prevent bleeding during circumcision [14]. Neonatal levels are approximately 50% lower than adult levels and increase with age [7, 15], thus mild factor XI deficiency cannot be diagnosed with certainty in a neonate. Repeat testing at a later time may be required to exclude mild factor XI deficiency.

Severe factor XIII deficiency leads to a severe phenotype with possible ICH as the cause of death in about a third of affected individuals. Severe cases with levels under 1% are at greatest risk of spontaneous and severe bleeding. Routine coagulation studies are normal and clot lysis assays or specific factor XIII enzyme-linked immunosorbent assays (ELISAs) are necessary to diagnose this deficiency, especially since the PT and APTT are typically normal. All coagulation screening should include a factor XIII assay to exclude this life-threatening bleeding disorder.

Bleeding in the newborn

The first symptoms of bleeding in a child with a severe bleeding disorder can appear directly after delivery. Cephalohematoma is a typical but relatively uncommon presentation of hemophilia and other bleeding disorders in the newborn. Umbilical stump bleeding may be diagnostic of hemophilia and FXIII deficiency and disorders of fibrinogen. Serious bleeding may also be encountered following venipuncture, intramuscular injections, after circumcision, and following surgery. Such procedures should be avoided or at least deferred temporarily in neonates suspected of a bleeding disorder until a specific diagnosis can be established.

Spontaneous bleeding, especially from mucous membranes may also be seen and should be controlled with non-specific and specific hemostatic agents. Abnormal bruising is a hallmark sign of hemophilia, with muscular bleeds and hemarthroses being more typical of hemophilic bleeds in older children. Circumcision should be deferred until a bleeding disorder is excluded. Most children do not develop any signs until the age of 8 months, when they become more mobile. ICHs occur more frequently in the postnatal period than in any other period of life.

Intracranial hemorrhage

The mode of delivery is highly associated with the occurrence of ICH. Most ICHs have occurred after invasive procedures. Therefore, the use of vacuum extraction and scalp vein sampling is contraindicated in children with an increased risk of bleeding. Some physicians advocate delivery by cesarean section. Apart from higher morbidity that the mother will have in future pregnancies and deliveries, there is a traumatic risk for the child.

The occurrence of ICH is associated with a high risk of severe neurologic damage. It has been shown that in boys who received adequate clotting factor administration, there was a high risk of long-term sequelae [16]. Therefore it is important that ICH is suspected in every child born after a traumatic delivery. Hemostasis should be corrected for 7–10 days after delivery. Although imaging techniques are helpful in making the diagnosis of ICH, it is not logical to wait for abnormal imaging before treating in the case of a child with impaired hemostasis.

ICH and extracranial hemorrhage (ECH) hemophilia occurred in 3.58% of newborns with hemophilia [17]. ICH is the leading cause of mortality and morbidity in hemophilia. These hemorrhagic complications are particularly dreadful, especially considering that 38% or more lead to late neurologic sequelae [17]. There is a 22.8% mortality rate reported in newborns with and without hemophilia and subgaleal hemorrhages. There is no clear evidence that the mode of delivery affects the outcome in hemophilic babies, although there is still controversy over this issue. Current guide-lines do not clearly address optimal peripartum management of affected or potentially affected fetuses born to mothers with bleeding disorders. All babies with suspected hemorrhagic disorders are managed safely with special attention to avoid instrumentation for vaginal deliveries except in certain situations, such as women who are carriers of hemophilia in whom prophylactic cesarean section is considered.

ICH is defined as any bleed occurring within the cranial cavity. ECH is defined as a hemorrhage occurring outside the cranial cavity, including subgaleal and cephalohematoma. Both may be life-threatening and can present with signs and symptoms of hypovolemia, including hemodynamic instability. In a study from Sweden, the total incidence of ICH and ECH was 14.5% in 117 hemophilic newborns – 12 with ECH, four with ICH and one with a retro-orbital hemorrhage [6]. In a survey from the USA, there were 109 episodes of cranial hemorrhage – 71 or 65% ICH and 38 or 35% ECH – in 102 newborns with hemophilia. Among the 71 episodes of ICH, there were 13 subdermal hematoma bleeds, 10 intracerebellar hemorrhages, three subarachnoid hemorrhages, two intraventricular–periventricular hemorrhages, one epidural hemorrhage, and one retro-orbital bleed. Six newborns had combinations of bleeds [18].

ICH from other factor deficiencies are rare. However, ICH has been reported to occur in 30% of factor XIII-deficient children [19].

Two-thirds of bleeds are ICH and one-third ECH in studies where the site of delivery is reported. It seems that ICH occurs irrespective of the severity of the hemophilia. In most published series the majority of newborns with ICH and ECH were hemophilia A rather than hemophilia B [17]. In part, this is explained by the higher frequency of hemophilia A than B. In this series, of the 35 cases of ICH and ECH in hemophilia A (87.5%), 22 were severe, 10 moderate, and three mild, whereas of the five hemophilia B newborns representing 12.5% of all ICH and ECH bleeds, one was severe, two were moderate, one mild and one unknown.

Practices regarding the use of cranial ultrasound scanning (USS) to detect the presence of early ICH and the administration of routine prophylaxis after delivery remains controversial. Only 16% and <6% of hemophilia treatment centers (HTCs) in the UK and in the USA had written guidelines for the management of neonates [18, 20]. Further controversy exists over the choice of imaging technique between cranial ultrasound and computed tomography scan for screening and diagnosing ICH.

Routine use of cranial ultrasound in all neonates with severe hemophilia was reported in 17 of 42 (41%) responses in a nationwide UK survey. A further 38% (16/42) would scan electively in specific circumstances where the chance of bleeding is high, such as following instrumented delivery or prolonged labor. The remaining individuals representing 21% would perform an ultrasound only in the presence of signs and symptoms of bleeding. A slightly higher percentage of survey respondents (47–61%) would opt for routine use of cranial ultrasound before hospital discharge in neonates with severe factor VII, FX, and FXIIII deficiencies [20]. Similar diversity in practice exists in the USA, where only 48% of respondents would check for ICH in male fetuses at risk for hemophilia and only 10% in those with a negative family history [18].

Forty percent of hematologists preferred routine administration of clotting factor concentrates immediately following birth to offset the trauma of delivery prior to hospital discharge and 60% were opposed to routine prophylaxis, although overall 89% favored early prophylaxis [18]. In the UK 19% (8/42) of physicians would consider the use of short temporary prophylaxis for all cases of severe hemophilia whereas a further 50% (21/42) would consider primary prophylaxis for potentially traumatic or premature deliveries [20].

The mean time of diagnosis of ICH in hemophiliacs is 4.5 days after delivery. Although the cranial ultrasound technique is non-invasive, it may miss some intracranial types, primarily subdural hemorrhages and posterior fossa bleeds, and may not detect earlier bleeds prior to discharge [21].

The incidence of an ICH with clinical symptoms is low but by actively looking for neonates with any sign of ICH, the diagnosis will be established without any symptoms. As a consequence, patients will receive intensive treatment when only a small bleed is diagnosed on the ultrasound. Moreover, a single dose of coagulation factor directly after birth will probably only delay the symptoms of ICH and is inadequate treatment.

Treatment for a suspected ICH requires 10–14 days of complete correction of hemostasis. This intensive therapy at such an early age seems to give a much higher chance of developing a high titer inhibitor against factor VIII [22]. If the ultrasound is performed within the first 24 hours, later hemorrhages will be misdiagnosed. Prospective studies are required to elucidate the benefit of early diagnostic head ultrasound in all children born with severe bleeding disorders.

Choice for mode of delivery

Please refer to Chapter 10.

Instrumented deliveries can greatly increase the risk of bleeding and should generally be avoided in affected newborns or at-risk newborns. Vacuum extraction and high forceps seem to lead to the highest incidence of ICH and ECH, with low forceps and unassisted vaginal delivery being the least problematic. It is unclear whether cesarean section protects against this risk.

Arguments in favor of cesarean section relate to the safety of the baby: ample timing and planning the delivery to coordinate care for mother and baby, convenience for planning, and avoiding cases of protracted labor and or arrest of labor, which may lead to instrumentation and possibly cesarean section, respectively, each increasing significantly to neonatal head trauma and hemorrhage risk.

Treatment

When a correct diagnosis has been made, the most appropriate treatment is correction of the missing coagulation factor. For hemophilia A and B both recombinant and plasma products are available. A high purity plasma product and a recombinant product are available for FVII. Only plasma products are currently available for VWD. Recombinant von Willebrand-containing products are currently in development and should be available shortly. For other factor deficiencies fresh-frozen plasma is the product of choice. The duration of treatment depends on the type of bleeding and the location.

References

1 Lippi G, Franchini M, Mantagnana M, Guidi GC. Coagulation testing in pediatric patients: the young are not just miniature adults. *Semin Thromb Hemost* 2007; 33: 816–820.

2 Andrew M, Paes B, Milner R, *et al.* Development of the human coagulation system in the full-term infant. *Blood* 1987; **70**: 165–172.

3 Andrew M, Vegh P, Johnston M, *et al.* Maturation of the hemostatic system during childhood. *Blood* 1992; **80**: 198–205.

4 Mannucci PM. The hemophilias – from royal genes to gene therapy. *N Eng J Med* 2001; **344**: 1773–1779.

5 Chambost H, Gaboulaud V, Coatmélec B, *et al.* What factors influence the age at diagnosis of hemophilia? Results of the French hemophilia cohort. *J Pediatr* 2002; **141**: 548–552.

6 Ljung R, Lindgren AC, Petrini P, Tengborn L. Normal vaginal delivery is to be recommended for haemophilia carrier gravidae. *Acta Paediatr* 1994; **83**: 609–611.

7 Williams MD, Chalmers EA, Gibson BE. Haemostasis and Thrombosis Task Force, British Committee for Standards in Haematology. The investigation and management of neonatal haemostasis and thrombosis. *Br J Haematol* 2002; **119**: 295–309.

8 Sutor AH, von Kries R, Cornelissen EA, *et al.* Vitamin K deficiency bleeding (VKDB) in infancy. *Thromb Hemost* 1999; **81**: 456–461.

9 Monagle P, Barnes C, Ignjatovic V, *et al.* Developmental haemostasis. Impact for clinical haemostasis laboratories. *Thromb Haemost* 2006; **95**: 362–372.

10 Bolton-Maggs PHB, Chalmers EA, Collins PW, *et al.* A review of inherited platelet disorders with guidelines for their management on behalf of the UKHCDO. *Br J Haematol* 2006; **135**: 603–633.

11 Bolton-Maggs PHB, Perry DJ, Chalmers EA, *et al.* Guidelines. The rare coagulation disorders – review with guidelines for management from the United Kingdom Haemophilia Centre Doctor's Organization. *Haemophilia* 2004; **10**: 593–628.

12 Lee CA, Chi C, Pavord SR, *et al.* Guidelines. The obstetric and gynaecological management of women with inherited bleeding disorders – review with guidelines produced by a taskforce of UK Haemophilia Center Doctors' Organization. *Haemophilia* 2006; **12**: 301–36.

13 Kulkarni R, Lusher J. Perinatal management of newborns with haemophilia. *Br J Haematol* 2001; **112**: 264–274.

14 Salomon O, Steinberg DM, Seligshon U. Variable bleeding manifestations characterise different types of surgery in patients with severe factor XI deficiency enabling parsimonious use of replacement therapy *Haemophilia* 2006; **12**: 490–493.

15 Andrew M, Paes B, Milner R, *et al.* Development of the human coagulation system in the healthy premature infant. *Blood* 1988; **72**: 1651–1657.

16 Revel MP. Effect of intracranial bleeds on the health and quality of life of boys with hemophilia. *J Pediatr* 2004; **144**: 490–495.

17 Kulkarni R, Lusher JM. Intracranial and extracranial hemorrhages in newborns with hemophilia: a review of the literature. *J Pediatr Hematol Oncol* 1999; **21**: 289–295.

18 Kulkarni R, Lusher JM, Henry RC, Kallen DJ. Current practices regarding newborn intracranial haemorrhage and obstetrical care and mode of delivery of pregnant haemophilia carriers: a survey of obstetricians, neonatologists and haematologists in the United States, on behalf of the National Hemophilia Foundation's Medical and Scientific Advisory Council. *Haemophilia* 1999; **5**: 410–415.

19 Anwar R, Miloszewski KJ. Factor XIII deficiency *Br J Haematol* 1999; **107**: 468–484.

20 Chalmers EA, Williams MD, Richards M, *et al.* on behalf of the Paediatric Working Party of UKHCDO. Management of neonates with inherited bleeding disorders: a survey of current UK practice. *Haemophila* **11**: 186–187.

21 Smith AR, Leonard N, Heisel Kurth M. Intracranial haemorrhage in newborns with haemophilia: The role of screening radiologic studies in the first 10 days of life. *J Pediatr Hematol Oncol* 2008; **30**: 81–84.

22 Gouw SC, van der Bom JG, van den Berg M. Treatment related risk factors of inhibitor development: a multicenter cohort study among previously treated patients with severe haemophilia A. *J Thromb Haemost* 2007; **5**: 1383–1390.

13 Advocacy for women with bleeding disorders

Rezan A Kadir, Ann-Marie Nazzaro, Rochelle Winikoff, Jane Mathesan, and Peter A Kouides

Introduction

Previous chapters of this book have shown the impact of bleeding disorders on women. Many women suffer a reduced quality of life [1] due to the symptoms of bleeding disorders as well as adverse medical events such as postpartum hemorrhage or prolonged bleeding after surgery. Many of these women, however, are not aware that their symptoms are abnormal and they do not seek medical advice. Even when they seek help, diagnosis of bleeding disorders is overlooked and appropriate treatment is not provided because of lack of awareness among their caregivers [2].

In a survey, conducted by the Haemophilia Society of the UK [3], among 539 women aged 16–45 years, 18% worry that their period is not normal; 45% believe that doctors say everything is normal when they consult about a period problem; and 12% have had to take at least 1 day off work or school each month because of their periods. Even those women with severe discomfort or prolonged bleeding show acceptance of their situation and see it as "bad luck" rather than a physical cause and they are not sure where to go for additional advice other than the GP. Below are examples of comments made by some of the women.

> sometimes I have sat down on a chair and I think I can't get up now, I have made a mess of myself and it's so embarrassing.

> I haven't found a proper pad where I can go for more than 2 hours.

> It's not like there's something called an organization for women with heavy periods.

> If you have had bad periods for God knows how many years you think: I have had it for the last 6 years, what is the point of going (for help)? What can they do? You just plod on.

Over the last decade, there have been increasing and successful efforts by patient advocacy groups and organizations to raise awareness of inherited bleeding disorders in women among the public as well as the healthcare professionals. A Women's Task Force has been developed within the national Haemophilia Society/Foundation in many countries. Their role has been crucial in the campaign to raise the profile of women's bleeding disorders, lobbying governments, and fund raising to promote research in the field as well as means of providing information and support for these women.

"Women Bleed Too": Haemophilia Society – United kingdom

Women Bleed Too was launched in 2005 by the Haemophilia Society in the UK with the aim to create a society in which bleeding disorders are recognized conditions among women and appropriate treatment and support are offered to all those diagnosed (Fig. 13.1). The work is guided by an active and committed women's board. The board comprises specialist

Inherited Bleeding Disorders in Women, 1st edition. By CA Lee, RA Kadir and PA Kouides. Published 2009 by Blackwell Publishing, ISBN: 978-1-4051-6915-8.

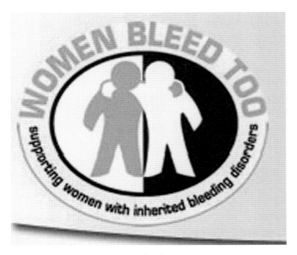

Fig. 13.1 Logo for Women Bleed Too.

healthcare professionals and affected women, who provide advice and guidance for the project.

A 3 year project was set up in 2005 with the objective of promoting appropriate diagnosis and treatment of women with symptoms of bleeding disorders by achieving the following goals:

1 Increase referral of women from primary care and gynecology clinics for appropriate assessment.

2 Increase the number of women members in the Haemophilia Society so that women make up 50% of the Society's overall membership.

3 Increase the average monthly number of helpline enquiries from affected women.

To achieve these goals, media campaigns were undertaken to reach the general public. A public relations company was employed to place stories within the media targeting different age and ethnic groups [3]. The project conducted a research project looking at various menstrual issues among women and young girls. The findings of the research, supported by case studies from women diagnosed with a bleeding disorder, led to a large number of press releases and generated various publications in the media. Following these media campaigns, there was an average of 550 unique visitors to the *Women Bleed Too* website per month and increasing calls to the helpline.

To reach health professionals and raise the awareness of the needs of women with bleeding disorders, the project holds a stand in relevant health professional conferences and organizes workshops and seminars for professionals. The importance of a multidisciplinary approach was soon realized and a first multidisciplinary seminar "Current Thinking in Women's Bleeding Disorders and Haemostasis" was held and attracted hundreds of healthcare professionals from a wide variety of disciplines ranging from GPs, nurses, midwives, women's groups, and health charities. The conference led to links with a number of key groups and professionals.

After the success of the first 3 year project, the future strategy will build on the project's foundations and strengths and incorporate findings from regular needs assessment of women.

Providing information, support, and raising awareness are the pillars for advocacy for these women.

Training tool for health professionals

A training tool was developed to increase awareness among health professionals in the primary care sector (Table 13.1) [4]. Coventry University, UK, was commissioned to pilot the tool locally, and their recommendations were incorporated into the final version of the tool. The tool includes a brief text that provides the health professionals with the following information:

1 The symptoms, diagnosis, and management of bleeding disorders in women.

2 Genetics/inheritance patterns.

Table 13.1 Key messages from the training tool

Women can have a bleeding disorder
• VWD is the most common of these: 1% of the UK population (300 000) is estimated to have this inherited bleeding disorder that affects both males and females
• Carriers of hemophilia A and B can be symptomatic
The indicative symptoms of a bleeding disorder are:
• Heavy and prolonged periods
• Frequent or heavy nosebleeds
• Easy bruising, prolonged bleeding from small cuts
• Heavy or prolonged bleeding after a tooth extraction, surgery or childbirth
• A family member with heavy periods or any of the above symptoms
Bleeding disorders adversely affect quality of life especially if undiagnosed

3 The psychosocial impact of having a bleeding disorder, particularly when it is left undiagnosed.

4 Sources of support and information.

The tool also has 20 multiple-choice questions, offering professionals a chance to test their knowledge in the area. The tool will be used as an online learning resource hosted on the "Women Bleed Too" website.

Publications

A magazine *Female Factors* is produced by the Haemophilia Society twice yearly as a mean of increasing awareness, sharing information, and providing support.

It has been recognized that there is a lack of information leaflets and guides addressing specific issues for girls and women with bleeding disorders. "A guide for women living with von Willebrand disease" was published in 2007. Several thousands of copies have been distributed. A publication targeting girls and young women with bleeding disorders, based on their experiences, is in production. Work is also in progress for providing these leaflets in different community languages.

Website

www.womenbleedtoo.org.uk went live in 2006, providing another opportunity for women to obtain and share information and ideas. A section with information for healthcare professionals is being developed to include the online training tool.

Helpline

The Haemophilia Society runs a free telephone and email helpline. Information and support is offered on a range of issues: carriers with and without symptoms; undiagnosed women with heavy periods; critical times such as contemplating pregnancy; genetic counseling; childbirth; and dental treatment.

A list of women willing to support each other through the telephone network and website discussion forum is being developed.

Guidelines on care and treatment

The Haemophilia Society was a stakeholder in the submission to the National Institute for Health and Clinical Excellence (NICE) [5] for its guidelines on the management of heavy menstrual bleeding. As a result, inherited bleeding disorders, specifically von Willebrand disease (VWD), were accepted as a risk factor and recommendations on testing for these disorders are addressed in the guideline.

Women Bleed Too was also involved in a UK Haemophilia Centre's Doctors Organisation (UKHCDO) commissioned task force to produce guidelines on the management of women with bleeding disorders: "The Obstetric and Gynaecological Management of Women with Inherited Bleeding Disorders" [6]. This guideline is available on the Women Bleed Too website.

Poster and checklist

As part of the awareness-raising campaign, a poster and checklist flyer (Table 13.2) were developed listing the key symptoms of a bleeding disorder. These were piloted in GP surgeries in the South West and Midlands area of England. A recent evaluation suggested that the checklist could have a bigger impact through other venues such as gynecology clinics. The poster has now been distributed to all Haemophilia Centres, community family planning clinics, and gynaecological nurses.

Project Red Flag: United States advocacy efforts for women with bleeding disorders

National Hemophilia Foundation and the Centers for Disease Control

In early 2001, a strategic plan for Project Red Flag (PRF) [7]: *Real talk about women's bleeding disorders* was developed by the National Hemophilia Foundation (NHF) (Fig. 13.2). PRF is a public awareness and education campaign aimed at outreach and educationfor women and education for healthcare providers about the symptoms of bleeding disorders [8–13]. Although concerned about all women's bleeding disorders – rare disorders, platelet disorders, mild to severe hemophilia in women, and other bleeding disorders, PRF strategically focused on the most prevalent bleeding disorder, von Willebrand disease. The PRF has three main goals to:

1 Increase the number of women with VWD who are diagnosed and properly treated.

Table 13.2 Bleeding disorder checklist flyer

Women bleed too

If you have more than one of the symptoms below you may
have a bleeding disorder

Do you . . . ?

Have heavy and prolonged periods

Have frequent or heavy nosebleeds

Bruise easily or have prolonged bleeding from small cuts and
scratches

Have experience of heavy or prolonged bleeding after having
a tooth removed, surgery or giving birth

Have a family member with heavy periods or any of these
symptoms

1% of the population is estimated to have von Willebrand
disease, an inherited bleeding disorder that affects both
males and females

There is currently no cure for von Willebrand disease but in
most cases symptoms can be treated easily

Diagnosis of a bleeding disorder is vital to prevent
complications following surgery, accident or childbirth

What do I do next . . . ?

If you think you might have a bleeding disorder then talk to
your GP and ask him/her to refer you to a hematologist
for investigation.

Contact us for further information, Women Bleed Too
is a project of the Haemophilia Society and can be
contacted on:

Helpline 0800 018 6068 (Mon–Fri 10 am–4 pm)
womenbleedtoo@haemophilia.org.uk
www.womenbleedtoo.org.uk

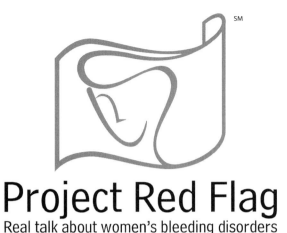

Project Red Flag
Real talk about women's bleeding disorders

Fig. 13.2 Project Red Flag logo.

identify undiagnosed women with VWD and other
bleeding disorders.

4 Develop strategic alliances and information links
with key health, women, minority, academic and gov-
ernment organizations.

5 Help women's healthcare providers identify and
establish a relationship with bleeding disorder specialists at HTCs.

6 Offer meaningful benefits for women with VWD to
encourage them to establish a relationship with NHF
and with its chapters/associations.

To raise awareness in the general population of
women, PRF needed a basic piece of information – it
should signal the leading symptoms that could mean
an underlying bleeding disorder or VWD. This basic
information card, "Heavy Periods – or a Bleeding
Disorder?," designed in a slim-format handout,
known as a "slim jim," was created for use at women's
health fairs, general health fairs, doctors' surgeries and
for distribution through any other relevant channel
for reaching women.

The companion piece to this "slim jim," is "Facts
You Should Know About Bleeding Disorders," a
larger, two-sided card, which again lists the symptoms
and offers such helpful facts as who can best diagnose
a bleeding disorder, how to contact a local chapter,
and the following points:

1 It's a myth that women cannot have a bleeding
disorder! Women can have VWD as well as platelet
disorders, factor deficiencies, and hemophilia.

2 Reduce inappropriate treatment of women with
bleeding disorders.

3 Establish the National Hemophilia Foundation as
the resource for women with bleeding disorders, con-
necting women to the NHF, chapters, independent
associations, and hemophilia treatment centers.

Core strategies to achieve PRF's objectives from the
early plan have evolved over the years. Initial and
evolved strategies are now to:

1 Prepare women and their healthcare providers to
discuss VWD and pursue appropriate treatment.

2 Define basic information needs for women with
possible bleeding symptoms at different decision
stages and tailor information to those stages.

3 Engage NHF chapters, independent associations
and hemophilia treatment centers in local initiatives to

179

2 Although it is estimated that 1 or 2 in 100 people can have VWD, very few are ever properly diagnosed. Most people who have VWD are unaware of it.

3 A good place to find a hematologist who specializes in bleeding disorders is at a HTC, a federally supported health center that focuses on the treatment of bleeding disorders. You can locate your nearest HTC at www.hemophilia.org or by calling 800 42-HANDI.

4 If you suspect you may have a bleeding disorder, discuss your symptoms with your doctor or healthcare professional. If you need more information or further help, please call the National Hemophilia Foundation at (800) 42-HANDI or write to info@projectredflag.org.

PRF also developed a brochure "For You and Your Doctor," to target women with bleeding symptoms such as heavy periods or chronic nosebleeds wanting to discuss these symptoms with their physicians. The brochure contains key information for the patient and for the physician. For those women and girls who had already been diagnosed "Tips for Living with Your Bleeding Disorder" was created. Highlights from this brochure are:

1 It is important to visit your local hemophilia treatment center to manage your bleeding disorder. Your HTC can provide you with the latest information, treatment and care.

2 Make sure your healthcare providers (dentists, obstetricians and primary care physicians) know you have a bleeding disorder to help you receive integrated and appropriate care.

3 You're not alone! The National Hemophilia Foundation can provide information, support and networking opportunities . . . Call (800) 42-HANDI or write NHF at info@projectredflag.org for more information.

Next steps for Project Red Flag

A barrier to raising awareness about women's bleeding disorders has been the lack of medical consensus on diagnosis and treatment of VWD; and even on what to call it – disease, disorder, or risk factor. The National Heart, Lung and Blood Institute (NHLBI) produced guidelines for diagnosis and management of VWD [14]. In the next phase of its work, PRF will be printing and distributing the final version of the guidelines to healthcare providers. The guidelines will also be translated into a reader-friendly, brief-format document for the public, describing VWD, its causes, symptoms, treatment, and tips for living with this bleeding disorder. These guidelines will represent the closest thing to medical consensus for diagnosis and treatment of VWD. The NHF will use the guidelines as a vehicle for overcoming existing barriers in communicating PRF messages.

As part of PRF's strategy to target adolescents, the NHF will provide to all chapters and associations a curriculum on women's bleeding disorders for middle school and high school health educators. This curriculum, POWER, originally developed by the Great Lakes Hemophilia Foundation, is designed for health educators to use with their classes, teaching adolescent boys and girls about bleeding disorders and that *anyone* can be affected. The teachers in a school district are introduced to the curriculum through an in-service training day, conducted by chapter and HTC professionals and consumers.

In a two-pronged approach to reaching adolescents in schools, along with the POWER program, PRF will work with school nurses. The nurses will learn about the American Academy of Pediatrics and ACOG "normal" period definition and they will be provided with a checklist of bleeding disorder symptoms as outlined in Table 13.3.

NHF will use its annual Washington Days, during which patients and families advocate for their needs with federal legislators in Washington, DC, to promote the NHLBI Guidelines and the unmet needs in the area of research, and diagnosis and treatment of women with VWD and other bleeding disorders. Understanding the need for advocacy for women's bleeding disorders and the sharing of best practices on the international level, PRF is working with NFH to help establish and strengthen a world coalition for women's bleeding disorders.

LadyBugs

LadyBugs is an organization dedicated to identifying and providing support for women with bleeding disorders (WWBDs). It provides support though social events, education of staff and patients, networking in part through a toll-free telephone number and web email, and empowerment through inspirational and motivational contacts and positive associations. The LadyBugs logo symbolizes women putting their heads together to help each other. For further information, the contact is Barbara Forss: barbforss@yahoo.com

Table 13.3 School nurses checklist

Heavy periods or a bleeding disorder?

Do you need to change your tampon or pad within an hour because it is saturated or leaks? Yes/No

Do you wake up from sleep to change your tampon or pad because it is saturated or leaks? Yes/No

Do you pass clots larger than one inch in diameter? Yes/No

Do you ever need to use more than one tampon or pad at a time? Yes/No

Have you ever been absent from school because of heavy bleeding during your period? Yes/No

Do you bruise easily or have bruises accompanied by lumps under the skin? Yes/No

Do you have prolonged bleeding after dental procedures or after simple cuts? Yes/No

Do you get frequent nose bleeds? Yes/No

Do your nose bleeds last longer than 10 minutes? Yes/No

Are there other family members who have symptoms similar to these? Yes/No

Have you been told by a medical professional that you are anemic? Yes/No

These symptoms can be signs of a bleeding disorder. If a woman answers yes to two or more of these questions, encourage her to contact her healthcare provider for further screening. For more information contact HANDI, the information resource center of the National Hemophilia Foundation: 800.42.HANDI handi@hemophilia.org Visit: www.hemophilia.org and click on the Project Red Flag section for women.

Canadian Hemophilia Society advocacy initiatives for women with bleeding disorders

The first recognition of women with bleeding disorders was in the early 1990s when HIV support groups organized by the Canadian Hemophilia Society (CHS) included women affected by HIV (Fig. 13.3). It was realized some women were infected through blood transfusions because of a bleeding disorder. Subsequently, lack of recognition, information and support for women with bleeding disorders was recognized by the CHS and the Women's Task Force was formulated in 1995. The task force includes women with various bleeding disorders, two nurse coordinators, a gynecologist, and two hematologists.

Fig. 13.3 Canadian Hemophilia Society Logo.

With the main goals of increasing awareness and providing support for women with bleeding disorders, the following strategies were planned and achieved:

1 The Female Factor column in the CHS newsletter "Hemophilia Today" was created in 1996 and is still ongoing. The column includes various topics, from personal stories to the latest in treatment options and research to specific medical information. A resource binder for women that included articles and information about all types of bleeding disorders as they pertain to women was developed by the CHS. Presentations about women's issues were included in the provincial workshops.

2 During the second national conference on comprehensive care (Winnipeg II) in 1998, women's issues were brought forward as a specific need for the first time, including their access to comprehensive care programs. The first CHS session for women with bleeding disorders was held during the CHS Bi-annual Medical Symposium in 1999.

3 In 2001, the VWD Public Awareness Campaign was developed. A survey to measure awareness about VWD among healthcare providers was conducted. A public relations firm was hired to coordinate development of key messages, identify and train spokespersons, and launch a media campaign. Awareness tools targeted at women are being developed, including posters, brochures, folders, and reference materials in community newspapers and magazines, and a community education kit on VWD developed by lay people for lay

181

people. In 2003, the Bleeding Disorders Initiative was launched. CHS developed a campaign to reach out to all people with bleeding disorders, not just hemophilia A or B or VWD. Pamphlets describing various other rare factor deficiencies were developed. Public displays on bleeding disorders were set up across the country in shopping malls, at women's health fairs, in hospitals. All documents produced by CHS are in French and English.

Resource and publications

1 The CHS website was developed in 1999 with specific information about women's issues (www.hemophilia.ca).
2 CHS also recognized the need to develop a way to make the public aware of the prevalence of VWD and reach out to healthcare providers and to people yet to be diagnosed with VWD. The VWD Advisory Group was established by the CHS and includes hematologists, family physicians, gynecologists, haemophilia clinic nurses and people affected by VWD. "All About von Willebrand Disease," the first ever comprehensive resource on VWD was published. One section dealt specifically with women's issues
3 A resource book for carriers of hemophilia VIII and IX entitled *All About Carriers* was produced. Contributors included carriers, parents of carriers, a hematologist, an obstetrician, a nurse-coordinator, a social worker, a psychologist, a geneticist, and a naturopathic doctor. *All About Carriers* was launched during the CHS bi-annual medical symposium in 2007. A workshop was held for carriers from across the country with medical presentations (heredity and treatment options), a psychosocial session and a workshop model to take back to provincial chapters.
4 Management guidelines: the CHS subcommittee on women with bleeding disorders developed guidelines on the management of women with bleeding disorders, including guidelines for establishing a multidisciplinary clinic for women. In 2005, the Society of Obstetricians and Gynecologists of Canada (SOGC) published *Clinical Practice Guidelines for Gynecological and Obstetric Management of Women with Inherited Bleeding Disorders* [15], based on the women's subcommittee document.
5 All About Teen Carriers: a CHS resource tool for girls 9–16 years of age who are either obligate or possible carriers is being developed for publication in autumn 2008.
6 The CHS organizes a National workshop to train women from across the country to use the VWD Community Education Kit. The workshop includes medical presentations, public speaking tips, hands-on practice for both visual presentations and kiosks and discussion of opportunities to set up kiosks and/or do provincial presentations.

The future

There is no doubt that the women's advocacy programs have been successful and crucial in raising the profile of bleeding disorders in women and improving their quality of care and life. These efforts have led to an increase in the number of women diagnosed with these disorders and the number of women attending the HTCs. In the USA, the number of women seen at HTCs increased by 44% from 1998 to 2004 [16]. Despite this increase, there is no doubt that there are many women for whom a bleeding disorder remains a hidden disease and who are struggling for a diagnosis and appropriate care.

Joint efforts among women's advocacy groups, interested professionals, and organizations as well as the development of a group of "ambassadors" for the women and bleeding disorders are of paramount importance to increase awareness not only among women and professionals but also with the governments. This will ensure continued progress and success of these projects. Collaboration between successful projects in the developed countries, such as Women Bleed Too in the UK, the Red Flag in the USA, CHS in Canada, etc., and sharing strategies across countries and cultures will make the initiative an international priority and extend the benefits to women in the developing countries.

Useful websites

www.womenbleedtoo.org.uk
www.haemophilia.org.uk
www.hemophilia.org
www.projectredflag.org
www.ladybugsupport.com

www.hemophilia.ca
www.haemophilia.org.nz
www.hemophilia.org.au
www.womenshealth.about.com

References

1 Shankar M, Chi C, Kadir RA. Review of quality of life: menorrhagia in women with or without inherited bleeding disorders. *Haemophilia* 2008; **14**: 15–20.

2 Lee CA, Chi C, Kadir RA. Women Bleed Too. *Acta Obstet Gynecol Scand* 2007; **86**: 772–3.

3 Coverage and Key Message Analysis for Female Factors Launch. Female Factors. Prepared by Red Door Communications for the Haemophilia Society. May 2006.

4 Barlow J, Stapley J. Development of a training tool for health professionals in relation to inherited bleeding disorders in women: Pilot Phase. Coventry University commissioned by the Haemophilia Society, UK, 2007.

5 National Collaborating Centre for Women's and Children's Health. *Heavy Menstrual Bleeding.* London: RCOG Press, 2007.

6 Lee CA, Chi C, Pavord SR, *et al.* The obstetric and gynaecological management of women with inherited bleeding disorders – review with guidelines produced by a task-force of UK Haemophilia Centre Doctors' Organization. *Haemophilia* 2006; **12**: 301–36.

7 National Hemophilia Foundation. *Project Red Flag woman-to-woman trainer manual.* New York: NHF, 2005.

8 National Hemophilia Foundation. Reaching out to culturally diverse hemophilia populations. Report on the Chapter Outreach Demonstration Project, NY: 1992.

9 US Office on Women's Health. *Women's health issues: an overview.* May 2000.

10 Helping women understand bleeding disorders. Health Matters for Women. Centers for Disease Control and Prevention. Newsletter, Summer, 2002.

11 Kaiser Family Foundation Issue Brief: Update on Women's Health Policy. Women, Work and Family Health: A Balancing Act. April 2003.

12 American Academy of Pediatrics & American College of Obstetricians and Gynecologists. Menstruation in girls and adolescents: using the menstrual cycle as a vital sign. *Pediatrics* 2006; **118**: 2245–2250.

13 Zuckerman, AM, Markham, CH. Why women's health business development? *Healthcare Financial Management* 2006: **October**: 122.

14 Nichols WL, Hultin MB, James AH, *et al.* von Willebrand disease (VWD): evidence–based diagnosis and management guidelines, the National Heart, Lung, and Blood Institute (NHLBI) Expert Panel report (USA) 1. *Haemophilia* 2008; **14**: 171–232

15 Demers C, Derzko C, David M, Douglas J. Gynaecological and obstetric management of women with inherited bleeding disorders. *Int J Gynaecol Obstet* 2006; **95** (1): 75–87.

16 Report of the Universal Data Collection Program (UDC), Centers for Disease Control and Prevention. 2005; **7** (1): 1–39.

Appendix i
Bleeding score with assigned score for each bleeding symptom

Symptom	Score					
	−1	0	1	2	3	4
Epistaxis	–	No or trivial (less than 5)	>5 or more than 10′	Consultation only	Packing or cauterization or antifibrinolytic	Blood transfusion or replacement therapy or desmopressin
Cutaneous	–	No or trivial (< 1 cm)	> 1 cm and no trauma	Consultation only		
Bleeding from minor wounds	–	No or trivial (less than 5)	> 5 or more than 5′	Consultation only	Surgical hemostasis	Blood transfusion or replacement therapy or desmopressin
Oral cavity	–	No	Referred at least once	Consultation only	Surgical hemostasis or antifibrinolytic	Blood transfusion or replacement therapy or desmopressin
Gastrointestinal bleeding	–	No	Associated with ulcer, portal hypertension, hemorrhoids, angiodysplasia	Spontaneous	Surgical hemostasis, blood transfusion, replacement therapy, desmopressin, antifibrinolytic	
Tooth extraction	No bleeding in at least two extractions	None done or no bleeding in one extraction	Referred in < 25% of all procedures	Referred in > 25% of all procedures, no intervention	Resuturing or packing	Blood transfusion or replacement therapy or desmopressin
Surgery	No bleeding in at least two surgeries	None done or no bleeding in one surgery	Referred in < 25% of all surgeries	Referred in > 25% of all procedures, no intervention	Surgical hemostasis or antifibrinolytic	Blood transfusion or replacement therapy or desmopressin
Menorrhagia	–	No	Consultation only	Antifibrinolytics, pill use	Dilation and curettage, iron therapy	Blood transfusion or replacement therapy or desmopressin or hysterectomy

Symptom	Score					
	−1	0	1	2	3	4
Postpartum hemorrhage	No bleeding in at least two deliveries	No deliveries or no bleeding in one delivery	Consultation only	Dilation and curettage, iron therapy, antifibrinolytics	Blood transfusion or replacement therapy or desmopressin	Hysterectomy
Muscle hematomas	–	Never	Post trauma no therapy	Spontaneous, no therapy	Spontaneous or traumatic, requiring desmopressin or replacement therapy	Spontaneous or traumatic, requiring surgical intervention or blood transfusion
Hemarthrosis	–	Never	Post trauma no therapy	Spontaneous, no therapy	Spontaneous or traumatic, requiring desmopressin or replacement therapy	Spontaneous or traumatic, requiring surgical intervention or blood transfusion
Central nervous system bleeding	–	Never	–	–	Subdural, any intervention	Intracerebral, any intervention

References

Rodeghiero F, Castarman G, Tosetto A, *et al*. The discriminant power of bleeding history for the diagnosis of type 1 von Willebrand disease: an international multicenter stydy. *J Thromb Haemost* 2005; 3: 2619–2626.

Tosetto A, Rodeghiero F, Castaman G, *et al*. A quantitative analysis of bleeding symptoms in type 1 von Willebrand disease: results from a multicentre European study. *J Thromb Haemost* 2006; 4: 766–773.

Appendix ii
Pictorial blood assessment chart

The pictorial blood assessment chart (PBAC) (Fig. Aii.1) consists of a series of diagrams representing lightly, moderately and heavily soiled towels and tampons. The numbers at the top of the chart represent the day of menstruation. The women are instructed to insert a mark in the appropriate box at the time each towel and/or tampon is discarded and if sufficient they are counted in groups of five. Passage of clots (size equated with the size of different coins) and episodes of flooding are also recorded.

The woman is given the chart to complete with her next menstrual period, with clear instructions and explanation of how it should be used. An example of a completed chart is also provided (Fig. Aii.2). After completion, the woman returns the chart by post (stamped addressed envelops are provided) or during her next appointment to the clinic. The chart is scored using the scoring system devised by Higham *et al.* 1990 (Fig. Aii.3). A baseline score is established, subsequent treatment cycles are then assessed and success can be indicated by a decreasing score.

Patient Name:	Date of Birth: DD/MM/YY		Hospital Number:

Date of Start: DD/MM/YY

Towel	1	2	3	4	5	6	7	8
Clots/Flooding								

Tampon	1	2	3	4	5	6	7	8
Clots/Flooding								

Clots: size of a coin = 1p/50p etc.

Fig. Aii.1 Menstrual pictorial chart.

Date of Start: Score:

Towel	1	2	3	4	5	6	7	8
	//	/	/		/	/		
			///	//				
		//	//					
Clots/Flooding		50p × 1	1p × 3					

Tampon	1	2	3	4	5	6	7	8
		/			//	/		
		//	///	//				
		/	////					
Clots/Flooding								

Clots: size of a coin = 1p/50p etc.

Fig. Aii.2 An example of a completed chart.

Towels

1 point	For each lightly stained towel
5 points	For each moderately soiled towel
20 points	If the towel is completely saturated with blood

Tampons

1 point	For each lightly stained tampon
5 points	For each moderately soiled tampon
20 points	If the tampon is completely saturated with blood

Clots

1 point	For small clots (size of 1p coin)
5 points	For large clots (size of 50p coin)

Fig. Aii.3 Scoring system.

Reference

Higham JM. O'Brien PM, Shaw RM. Assessment of menstrual blood loss using a pictorial chart. *Br J Obstet Gynaecol* 1990; 8: 734–739.

Index

Page numbers in **bold** represent tables, those in *italics* represent figures.